Welcome to

Atkins Diet World

Unlock EVERY Secret of Cooking

Through 500 AMAZING

Atkins Diet Recipes

(Unlock Cooking, Book 17)

Annie Kate

Content

Chapter 1: Breakfast Recipes

***

All Purpose Low-Carb Baking Mix

Servings: 9 | *Prep:* 5 mins | *Style:* American

Ingredients

- 1/4 cup Wheat Bran (Crude)
- 1 1/8 cups Whole Grain Soy Flour
- 2/3 cup Vanilla Whey Protein
- 1/4 cup Organic 100% Whole Ground Golden Flaxseed Meal
- 2/3 cup Vital Wheat Gluten Flour

Directions

It is not necessary to use vanilla flavored whey protein powder, unflavored is ideal but the vanilla will not contribute much flavor to the mix so if it is what you have on hand, use it.

1. Combine all ingredients and mix thoroughly.
2. Use immediately or store in an airtight container in the refrigerator for up to 1 month. Each recipe makes 9 servings or 3 cups.
3. Each serving size is 1/3 cup.

Almond and Coconut Muffin in a Minute

Servings: 1 | *Prep:* 3 m | *Style:* American | *Phase:* 2

Ingredients

- 1/8 cup Almond Meal Flour
- 1/3 tbsp Organic High Fiber Coconut Flour
- 1 tsp Sucralose Based Sweetener (Sugar Substitute)
- 1/2 tsp Cinnamon
- 1/4 tsp Baking Powder (Straight Phosphate, Double Acting)
- 1/8 tsp Salt
- 1 large Egg (Whole)

- 1/3 tbsp Extra Virgin Olive Oil

Directions

1. Place all dry ingredients in a coffee mug. Stir to combine.
2. Add the egg and oil. Stir until thoroughly combined.
3. Microwave for 1 minute. Use a knife if necessary to help remove the muffin from the cup, slice, butter, eat.

Note

- Your MIM can be toasted once it's cooked and topped with cream cheese if you like. Replace the cinnamon with other spices, sugar-free syrup or 1/2 tsp unsweetened cocoa (net carb count will be .2g higher). Add a tablespoon of sour cream for a moister MIM. Change the shape by making it in a bowl.

Almond Muffin in a Minute

Servings: 1 | Prep: 3 m | Style: American | Cook time: 1 m

Ingredients

- 1/4 cup Almond Meal Flour
- 1 tsp Sucralose Based Sweetener (Sugar Substitute)
- 1/4 tsp Baking Powder (Straight Phosphate, Double Acting)
- 1/8 tsp Salt
- 1/2 tsp Cinnamon
- 1 large Egg (Whole)
- 1 tsp Canola Vegetable Oil

Directions

1. Place all dry ingredients in a coffee mug. Stir to combine.
2. Add the egg and oil. Stir until thoroughly combined.
3. Microwave for 1 minute. Use a knife if necessary to help remove the muffin from the cup, slice, butter, eat.

Note

- Your MIM can be toasted once it's cooked and topped with cream cheese if you like. Replace the cinnamon with other spices, sugar-free syrup or 1/2 tsp unsweetened cocoa (net carb count will be .2g higher). Add a tablespoon of sour cream for a moister MIM. Change the shape by making it in a bowl.

Almond Protein Pancakes with Blueberries

*Servings: 1 | **Prep:** 5 m | **Style:** American | **Cook: 10** m*

Ingredients

- 1/16 cup Blanched Almond Flour
- 3/4 large Egg (Whole)
- 1/8 cup dry Whole Grain Soy Flour
- 1/4 tsp Baking Powder (Straight Phosphate, Double Acting)
- 1/2 oz Large or Small Curd Creamed Cottage Cheese
- 2 tbsps Vanilla Whey Protein
- 1/4 cup Fresh Blueberries

Directions

1. Combine the almond flour, protein powder, soy flour and baking powder together. Stir in the beaten egg and cottage cheese until blended.
2. Heat a large nonstick skillet or griddle over medium heat. Lightly grease with butter or canola oil.
3. Using about 1/4 cup per pancake, drop batter onto the skillet. When bubbles begin to form in the middle of each pancake, turn over and cook another 2 minutes or until firm.
4. Serve with blueberries Or add blueberries to the pancake batter before cooking.

Almond Protein Pancakes

*Servings: 4 | **Prep:** 5 m | **Style:** American | **Cook**: 10 m*

Ingredients

- 2 oz Vanilla Whey Protein
- 1/4 cup Almond Meal Flour
- 3 tbsps Whole Grain Soy Flour
- 1 tsp Baking Powder (Straight Phosphate, Double Acting)
- 3 large Eggs (Whole)
- 1/3 cup Large or Small Curd Creamed Cottage Cheese

Directions

Serve with almond butter or sugar-free pancake syrup. Garnish with toasted almonds, if desired.

1. Mix the protein powder (1oz is about 4 Tbsp), almond meal, soy flour and baking powder together. Whisk the eggs, then blend together with the cottage cheese (substitute cream cheese if cottage cheese is not on your accepted foods list).
2. Heat a large nonstick skillet or griddle over medium heat. Lightly grease with butter or canola oil.
3. Using about 1/4 cup per pancake, drop batter onto the skillet. When bubbles begin to form in the middle of each pancake, turn over and cook another 2 minutes or until firm.
4. Repeat, keeping pancakes warm in the oven.

Almond-Pineapple Smoothie

Servings: 1 | Prep: 5 m | Style: American

Ingredients

- 1/2 cup (8 fl oz) Plain Yogurt (Whole Milk)
- 2 1/2 oz Pineapple
- 20 whole Blanched & Slivered Almonds
- 1/2 cup Pure Almond Milk - Unsweetened Original

Directions

1. Feel free to substitute other fruits or nuts for the pineapple and/or almonds (about 20 whole almonds, 3 Tbsp slivered). Be sure to use fresh pineapple in this smoothie. Canned pineapple is swimming in sugar.
2. Combine the yogurt, pineapple, almonds and almond milk in a blender and purée until smooth and creamy.

Almond-Pumpkin Pancakes

Servings: 6 | Prep: 5 m | Style: American | Cook: 10 m

Ingredients

- 4 oz Vanilla Whey Protein
- 4 large Eggs (Whole)
- 1/4 cup Blanched Almond Flour
- 1/4 cup dry Whole Grain Soy Flour
- 1 tsp Baking Powder (Sodium Aluminum Sulfate, Double Acting)
- 1/2 tsp Pumpkin Pie Spice
- 1/4 cup Large or Small Curd Creamed Cottage Cheese
- 1/2 cup Pumpkin (Without Salt, Canned)

Directions

Be sure to use canned pumpkin purée, not pumpkin pie mix (which has added sugar), to make these pancakes. Serve with sugar-free pancake syrup or almond butter.

1. Mix the protein powder, almond meal, soy flour, baking powder and pumpkin pie spice mix in a medium mixing bowl. Stir in the beaten eggs, cottage cheese and pumpkin purée until blended.
2. Heat a large nonstick skillet or griddle over medium heat. Lightly grease skillet with butter or canola oil.
3. Using about 1/4 cup per pancake, drop batter onto the skillet. When bubbles begin to form in the middle of the pancakes, turn and cook another 2 minutes or until firm.
4. Repeat, keeping pancakes warm in the oven before serving.

Almond-Raspberry Smoothie

*Servings: 1 | **Prep:** 5 m | **Style:** American*

Ingredients

- 4 oz Greek Yogurt - Plain (Container)
- 1/2 cup Red Raspberries
- 20 whole Blanched & Slivered Almonds
- 1/2 cup Pure Almond Milk - Unsweetened Original

Directions

1. Feel free to come up with your own combination of other berries and nuts for this protein-packed smoothie. If you use frozen raspberries, make sure they contain no added sugar.
2. Combine the yogurt, raspberries, almonds and almond milk in a blender and purée until smooth and creamy.

Ancho Macho Chili

*Servings: 10 | **Prep:** 10 m | **Style:** American | **Cook:** 165 m*

Ingredients

- 5 lbs Beef Top Sirloin (Trimmed to 1/8" Fat)
- 2 tsps Salt
- 1/2 tsp Black Pepper
- 3 tbsps Extra Virgin Olive Oil
- 1 medium (2-1/2" dia) Onions
- 2 tsps Garlic
- 3 tbsps Chili Powder
- 14 1/2 oz Red Tomatoes (with Green Chilies, Canned)
- 6 fl ozs Red Table Wine

Directions

Cooking evaporates alcohol, which is why this recipe is suitable for Induction despite the red wine. But feel free to use chicken broth instead. Jarred roasted garlic cloves can be found in the produce section of most supermarkets or simply mince a whole clove of garlic.

1. Heat oven to 325°F.
2. Season beef with salt and pepper. Heat 1 1/2 teaspoons oil in a Dutch oven over high heat. Add one-third of the beef and brown on all sides, about 1 minutes per side.
3. Transfer to a bowl and repeat two more times with beef and oil.
4. Chop the onion and add to a Dutch oven preheated with the remaining 1 1/2 teaspoons oil. Cook onion and garlic until lightly browned. Stir in chile powder, tomatoes and wine; bring to a simmer. Return beef and accumulated juices to Dutch oven. Cover and bake 2 1/2 hours, stirring once halfway through cooking time, until beef is very tender. One serving is about 3/4-1 cup.

Apple Muffins with Cinnamon-Pecan Streusel

Servings: 8 | Prep: 15 m | Style: American | Cook: 25 m

Ingredients

- 1 2/3 cups Almond Meal Flour
- 1/2 cup half Pecans
- 6 1/2 tsps Cinnamon
- 1/3 tsp Salt
- 24 tsps Erythritol
- 1 pinch Stevia
- 2 tbsps Unsalted Butter Stick
- 2 large Eggs (Whole)
- 1/4 cup Coconut Milk Unsweetened
- 2 tsps Vanilla Extract
- 2 tbsps Organic High Fiber Coconut Flour
- 1 tsp Baking Powder (Straight Phosphate, Double Acting)
- 2/3 cup quartered or chopped Apple

Directions

1. Preheat oven to 350 F. Prepare a muffin tin with 8 cupcake papers.
2. Combine 2/3 cup almond flour, chopped pecans, 2 tablespoons cinnamon, 1/8 teaspoon salt, 2 tablespoons granular sugar substitute (eryhtritol), a pinch of stevia and 2 tablespoons melted butter in a small bowl. Mix with a fork until it begins to crumble. Set aside while making the muffin batter.
3. For the muffins: whisk together the eggs, 1/4 cup coconut milk, 2 teaspoons vanilla, 6 tablespoons granular sugar substitute (erythritol), a pinch of stevia, and 1/2 teaspoon ground cinnamon. Add 1 cup almond flour, 2 tablespoons coconut flour, 1/4 teaspoon salt and 1 teaspoon baking powder; mix to combine then fold in 2/3 cup finely chopped apples.
4. Divide into muffin 8 wells topping each with about 2 tablespoons of the struesal. Bake for 25 minutes, remove from oven and allow to sit for 10-20 minutes to cool before removing. These may be eaten immediately or stored in an airtight container in the refrigerator for up to 1 week.

Asian Beef Salad Single Serving

Servings: *1 |* ***Prep:*** *720 m |* ***Style:*** *American |* ***Cook:*** *5 m*

Ingredients

- 1/2 clove Garlic
- 1/2 tbsp Tamari Soybean Sauce
- 1/4 tbsp Sodium and Sugar Free Rice Vinegar
- 1/4 tsp Sesame Oil
- 1/8 tsp Sucralose Based Sweetener (Sugar Substitute)
- 1/8 tsp Curry Powder
- 1/16 tsp Ginger
- 4 1/4 oz Beef Top Sirloin (Trimmed to 1/8" Fat, Choice Grade)
- 3/4 cup Spring Mix Salad
- 1/2 tbsp Canola Vegetable Oil
- 1/4 large (2-1/4 per lb, approx 3-3/4" long, 3" dia) Sweet Red Peppers
- 2 oz Waterchestnuts
- 1 large Scallions or Spring Onion

Directions

Note: Because only half of the marinade is used in this recipe for the salad dressing and the rest is used as a marinade and discarded, please double the first six ingredients. (The nutritionals shown are correct.) For added flavor, use dark (toasted) sesame oil instead of regular sesame oil.

1. Mix green onions, garlic, soy sauce, rice wine vinegar, sesame oil and sugar substitute in a small bowl. Pour half into a resealable plastic bag; add steak and marinate overnight in the refrigerator.
2. To remaining soy sauce mixture, add curry powder and ginger.Heat canola oil in a large skillet over high heat until very hot.
3. Drain beef and discard marinade; quickly stir-fry beef 2 to 3 minutes in hot oil for medium doneness. Transfer to a large mixing bowl. Add salad greens, bell pepper, water chestnuts and reserved soy dressing. Toss to coat and serve immediately.

Atkins Cinnamon Pie Crust

Servings: 8 | Prep: 10 m | Style: American

Ingredients

- 1/4 tsp Salt
- 1 tsp Sucralose Based Sweetener (Sugar Substitute)
- 1 tsp Cinnamon
- 1/2 cup Unsalted Butter Stick
- 3 3/4 servings All Purpose Low-Carb Baking Mix
- 2 tbsps Tap Water

Directions

1. Use the Atkins recipe to make All Purpose Low-Carb Baking Mix. You will need 1 1/4 cups to make one pie crust.
2. Pulse the baking mix, salt, sugar substitute, and cinnamon in a food processor to incorporate; add butter and pulse until mixture resembles a coarse meal, about 30 seconds. Pulse in water until dough just comes together, about 30 seconds (add up to 1 more tablespoon if necessary).
3. Transfer dough to a sheet of plastic wrap; form into a a disk about 6 inches in diameter. Wrap tightly in plastic; refrigerate until firm, about 30 minutes.
4.   Rol
l and bake as directed in pie recipe. Makes 1 pie crust.

Atkins Cuisine Biscuits

Servings: 18 | Prep: 25 m | Style: American | Cook: 20 m

Ingredients

- 1 1/2 tsps Baking Powder (Straight Phosphate, Double Acting)
- 3/4 tsp Salt
- 1 individual packet Sucralose Based Sweetener (Sugar Substitute)
- 1/2 cup Unsalted Butter Stick
- 6 servings All Purpose Low-Carb Baking Mix
- 1 cup Heavy Cream

Directions

1. Preheat oven to 425°F degrees.
2. Blend together 2 cups low-carb baking mix, baking powder, sugar substitute and salt in a large mixing bowl.
3. Cut butter into small chunks and add to the dry ingredients, using a pastry blender or your fingertips to work until the mixture resembles coarse crumbs. Do not over-mix.
4. Pour in heavy cream and stir lightly.
5. Coat cutting board with olive oil spray. Using a spatula, transfer the dough to a cutting board. Coat hands with oil spray and lightly knead dough a few times until blended. Do not over knead.
6. Pat out dough into a circle 1/2 3/4-inch thick. Using a biscuit cutter with a 2¼-inch diameter, form biscuits. Make an extra biscuit out of scraps instead of re-rolling the dough.
7. Place biscuits on a baking sheet coated with oil spray. Brush tops with melted butter, if desired.
8. Bake 15 -18 minutes or until golden brown.
9. Remove biscuits from oven and place on a wire rack to cool.

Atkins Cuisine Pancakes

Servings: 10 | Prep: 5 m | Style: American | Cook: 15 m

Ingredients

- 1 individual packet Sucralose Based Sweetener (Sugar Substitute)
- 1 large Egg (Whole)
- 2 tsps Baking Powder (Straight Phosphate, Double Acting)
- 1/4 tsp Salt
- 1 cup Cream (Half & Half)
- 3 servings All Purpose Low-Carb Baking Mix

Directions

1. Blend together 1 cup baking mix, sugar substitute, baking powder and salt in a large mixing bowl.
2. Add the half and half and egg. Whisk batter. Let the mixture sit for at least 5 minutes to activate the baking powder.
3. Coat the griddle with olive oil spray. Over medium heat, cook 4 pancakes at a time. When bubbles appear on the top and the edges are firm, flip the pancakes and cook another 2 3 minutes. Keep warm in the oven.
4. Repeat with remaining pancakes.

Atkins Cuisine Pie Crust

Servings: 8 | Prep: 10 m | Style: American

Ingredients

- 1/3 cup 100% Stone Ground Whole Wheat Pastry Flour
- 1/3 cup Whole Grain Soy Flour
- 2 oz Vital Wheat Gluten
- 3 tbsps Plain Wheat Germ
- 1/2 tsp Salt
- 1/2 cup Unsalted Butter Stick
- 1 tbsp Tap Water

Directions

1. In a food processor, pulse flours, wheat gluten, germ, salt and butter until mixture resembles a coarse meal. Slowly add water and continue pulsing until the dough begins to come together. Turn onto a sheet of plastic wrap,

form into a ball and cover with plastic. Flatten to a 7-inch disc and chill in the freezer for 15 minutes.

2. Roll dough out between 2 sheets of plastic wrap to a 12-inch circle (if needed, sprinkle on 1/2 teaspoon wheat gluten flour per side to facilitate rolling). Remove the top sheet of plastic and invert onto a 9-inch pie plate. Center dough and press onto the bottom and sides of plate. Remove plastic, roll under the edges and crimp decoratively. Chill in the freezer for 15 minutes.
3. Use unbaked crust as indicated in recipe of your choice. Or for a prebaked crust, preheat oven to 400° F. Prick the bottom and corners of the pie shell with a fork. Line the pie shell with foil, fill halfway with pie weights or dried beans and turn the foil over to cover the pastry edge. Bake for 16 minutes. Remove the foil and weights, cover loosely with foil and bake an additional 4 to 6 minutes or until golden. Cool on a rack for 20 minutes before using.
4. Makes 8 servings.

Atkins Cuisine Waffles

Servings: 5 | Prep: 10 m | Style: American | Cook: 10 m

Ingredients

- 1 individual packet Sucralose Based Sweetener (Sugar Substitute)
- 1 large Egg (Whole)
- 2 tsps Baking Powder (Straight Phosphate, Double Acting)
- 1/4 tsp Salt
- 1 cup Cream (Half & Half)
- 3 servings All Purpose Low-Carb Baking Mix

Directions

Use the Atkins recipe to make All Purpose Low-Carb Baking Mix for this recipe. This recipe makes 5 waffles. Assuming your waffle iron makes 4 servings, use four-fifths of the batter and then make a single waffle with the remaining batter. Freeze extra waffles and just pop in the toaster before serving.

1. In a large bowl, blend together 1 cup baking mix, baking powder, sugar substitute and salt.
2. In another large bowl, mix the half-and-half and beaten egg.

3. Add dry ingredients to the liquid ingredients and whisk batter until any lumps are removed. Don't overbeat.
4. Let the mixture sit for at least 5 minutes to activate the baking powder.
5. Heat the waffle iron and pour the batter in the center of the waffle iron.
6. Close the top and cook waffles for about 1 1 1/2 minutes or until golden brown.
7. Repeat with last waffle.

Bacon, Avocado and Jack Cheese Omelets with Fresh Salsa

Servings: 2 | Prep: 10 m | Style: American | Cook: 10 m

Ingredients

- 1 medium whole (2-3/5" dia) Red Tomato
- 3 medium (4-1/8" long) Scallions or Spring Onions
- 1/2 Jalapeno Peppers
- 1 oz Cilantro
- 1 tbsp Fresh Lime Juice
- 4 large Eggs (Whole)
- 1 fl oz Tap Water
- 3 medium slice (yield after cooking) Bacon
- 1 tbsp Unsalted Butter Stick
- 1/2 California Avocados
- 1 cup shredded Monterey Jack Cheese

Directions

1. Prepare salsa: Chop the tomatoes; finely chop the green onions and jalapeno (de-seed if you would like less heat). In small bowl, combine tomato, green onions, jalapeño, cilantro and lime juice and mix well. Season to taste with salt and pepper. Set aside.
2. In medium bowl, whisk eggs with water and season with salt and pepper. Prepare bacon, cook thoroughly, crumble and set aside.
3. Melt half the butter in a small nonstick skillet over medium-high heat. When foam subsides, add half the egg mixture. Tilt pan to coat bottom and cook 1 minute, until almost set. Sprinkle half the omelet with half the crumbled bacon, avocado and cheese and cook 1 minute.
4. Fold empty half of omelet over filling and slide omelet onto a plate. Keep warm.

5. Repeat with remaining butter, egg mixture, bacon, avocado and cheese. Serve with salsa.

Baked Eggs and Asparagus

*Servings: 1 | **Prep:** 5 m | **Style:** American | **Cook:** 10 m*

Ingredients

- 8 spear small (5" long or less) Asparagus
- 1/4 cup Heavy Cream
- 2 large Eggs (Whole)
- 2 tbsps Almond Meal Flour
- 1 tbsp Parmesan Cheese (Shredded)
- 1/8 tsp Garlic
- 1/8 tsp Black Pepper

Directions

1. Preheat oven to 400°F. Prepare a small oven safe casserole or 4-inch by 3-inch dish with a little bit of oil. Set aside.
2. Boil the asparagus spears for 2 minutes until tender-crisp. Drain and run under cold water then pat dry. Arrange in the prepared baking dish.
3. Pour cream over the asparagus and then crack two eggs on top.
4. In a small bowl blend together the almond meal, Parmesan cheese, garlic and black pepper. Sprinkle over the eggs and place in the oven. Cook for 5-10 minutes depending upon how you like your eggs cooked. Longer time will result in a firmer yolk. The cream will puff over the edges of the eggs and the topping should be golden brown and fragrant.

Basque Eggs with Ham, Tomatoes and Bell Peppers

*Servings: 6 | **Prep:** 30 m | **Style:** American | **Cook:** 12 mins*

Ingredients

- 3 tbsps Extra Virgin Olive Oil
- 1 medium (2-1/2" dia) Onions
- 8 oz Roasted Bell Peppers
- 2 plums Red Tomatoes
- 5 1/2 tbsps Basil
- 1/4 tsp Red or Cayenne Pepper
- 12 large Eggs (Whole)
- 6 tbsps Unsalted Butter Stick
- 6 oz boneless, cooked Fresh Ham
- 3 tsps Garlic

Directions

1. Heat oil in large heavy skillet over medium heat. Sauté onion 5 minutes, until softened; add garlic and cook 1 minute more.
2. Add roasted peppers, tomatoes, and cayenne. Cover and cook 10 minutes, until vegetables are very soft, stirring occasionally.
3. Uncover and simmer over medium heat until sauce is thick, about 10 minutes, stirring often. Season to taste with salt and pepper. (Mixture can be made up to 2 days ahead and reheated).
4. In large bowl, beat eggs until blended. In large nonstick skillet, melt butter over low heat. Add eggs and basil. Cook, stirring constantly with rubber spatula, 12 minutes, until soft curds form and eggs are barely set.
5. Add pepper mixture and ham; stir just until mixed.

Béchamel Sauce

Servings: 6 | **Prep:** 10 m | **Style:** American | **Cook:** 20 m

Ingredients

- 1 cup Heavy Cream
- 1 cup Tap Water
- 2 tbsps chopped Onions
- 1 tsp Salt
- 1/8 tsp Black Pepper
- 1/8 tsp Nutmeg (Ground)
- 3 tsps Thick-It-Up
- 1 tbsp Unsalted Butter Stick

Directions

Béchamel is a mild sauce that can be used in soufflés or simmered with finely chopped vegetables or meats. Traditionally thickened with a mixture of flour and fat, our version uses heavy cream and a low-carb thickener instead. Each serving is 1/4 cup.

1. Combine cream, water, white onion, salt, pepper and nutmeg in a small saucepan over medium heat; bring to a simmer. Remove from heat; let stand for 15 minutes.
2. Strain cream mixture; return to saucepan over medium heat. Whisk in 1 tablespoon Thick-It-Up thickener; cook until sauce thickens, about 3 minutes.
3. Remove from heat; swirl in butter until melted. Use immediately

Beef Huevos Rancheros on Canadian Bacon

Servings: 4 | **Prep:** 10 m | **Style:** American | **Cook:** 20 m

Ingredients

- 6 oz Ground Beef (80% Lean / 20% Fat)
- 1/2 cup Green Chili Peppers (Canned)
- 1/4 tsp Garlic Powder
- 1 tsp Chili Powder
- 1/4 tsp Cumin
- 1/4 tsp leaf Oregano
- 1/4 tsp Salt
- 1/4 tsp Black Pepper
- 4 slices Canadian Bacon
- 4 large Eggs (Whole)
- 1/2 cup shredded Cheddar Cheese
- 4 sprigs Cilantro

Directions

The directions for this dish call for scrambled eggs, but you can also serve them fried or poached.

1. In a greased medium skillet, brown the beef over medium heat.
2. Stir in chiles, garlic powder, chili powder, cumin, oregano, salt and pepper. Cook 5-10 minutes to blend the flavors.
3. Lay the Canadian bacon slices over the top of the beef mixture to warm. Remove pan from heat and set aside.
4. In another skillet, scramble eggs until firm.
5. Place 1 piece of Canadian bacon on each plate, top with a quarter of the beef mixture and a quarter of the eggs. Sprinkle with cheese and chopped cilantro.

Beef Sautéed with Green Bell Pepper and Onions Topped with Cheese

Servings: 1 | Prep: 5 m | Style: American | Cook: 10 m

Ingredients

- 1/4 cup chopped Onions
- 1 tbsp Extra Virgin Olive Oil
- 1/2 cup chopped Green Sweet Pepper
- 1/2 cup shredded Cheddar Cheese
- 5 oz Ground Beef (80% Lean / 20% Fat)

Directions

1. Sauté ground beef in a skillet over medium-high heat with small amount of cooking oil for 1-2 minutes. Add green bell pepper and white onions.
2. Sauté until beef is browned and the peppers and onions are soft. Add salt and pepper to taste.
3. Drain off any excess fat and put onto a serving plate. Sprinkle cheese on top and allow to melt. Serve immediately.

Bell Pepper Rings Filled with Egg and Mozzarella with Fruit

Servings: 1 | Prep: 10 m | Style: American | Cook: 5 m

Ingredients

- 1/4 cup shredded Whole Milk Mozzarella Cheese
- 1 tsp Extra Virgin Olive Oil
- 1/4 small (6" to 6-7/8" long) Bananas
- 1/4 small (2-1/2" dia) (approx 4 per lb) Apples
- 1/2 fruit Kiwi Fruit
- 2 large Eggs (Whole)
- 1/4 cup Raspberries
- 1/2 medium (approx 2-3/4" long, 2-1/2" dia) Sweet Red Peppers

Directions

1. Cut bell pepper into two 1- inch rounds.
2. Place rounds in a skillet with a small amount of oil over medium high heat.
3. Crack 1 egg into each round, cook for 2 minutes then add 1-2 Tbsp water to pan and steam the egg and pepper for 3-5 additional minutes until the egg is cooked to your liking.
4. Top with cheese. Leave in the pan and cover for about 1 minute to melt cheese.
5. Combine the fruits and serve with the pepper rings.

Blackberry Smoothie

*Servings: 1 | **Prep:** 5 m | **Style:** American*

Ingredients

- 1/4 cup Frozen Blackberries
- 1 cup Coconut Milk Unsweetened
- 1/4 tsp Cinnamon
- 1/2 tsp Vanilla Extract
- 1 scoop Vanilla Whey Protein
- 1/16 tsp Allspice Ground
- 1/16 cup Organic 100% Whole Ground Golden Flaxseed Meal

Directions

1. For this recipe unsweetened coconut, almond or soy milk may be used. Combine the frozen balckberries, milk of choice, protein powder, vanilla and spices in a blender. Blend until smooth.

Blueberry Cloud Muffin

Servings: 1 | Prep: 1 m | Style: American | Cook: 1 m

Ingredients

- 1 oz Cream Cheese
- 1 large Egg
- 2 tbsps Vanilla Whey Protein
- 1/4 tsp Baking Powder (Sodium Aluminum Sulfate, Double Acting)
- 1/8 tsp Nutmeg (Ground)
- 1/4 cup Blueberries

Directions

1. Place cream cheese in a microwave safe mug. Heat for 10-15 seconds (enough to warm the cream cheese but not to fully melt it).
2. Add the egg and whisk it with the cream cheese.
3. Add the whey protein powder (use a protein powder that has 1g NC or less per serving, one serving is about 1 oz), baking powder, and nutmeg; whisk to combine. Add the blueberries mixing to combine. Heat the mug in the microwave for 1 min and 20 seconds (the blueberries need additional time to cook since they contain so much moisture. Microwave times vary so you may need to increase the time by 10-20 seconds if it does not cook through. Remove muffin by turning over onto a plate. Run a knife around the inside of the mug to more easily release it.

Breakfast Burrito

Servings: 2 | Prep: 15 m | Style: American | Cook: 5 m

Ingredients

- 1/2 tsp Salt
- 1/4 tsp Red or Cayenne Pepper
- 1 tbsp Canola Vegetable Oil
- 4 large Eggs (Whole)
- 3 tbsps Sweet Red Peppers
- 2 tbsps chopped Scallions or Spring Onions
- 1 Jalapeno Pepper
- 2 tortillas Low Carb Tortillas
- 1/8 tsp Tabasco Sauce
- 2 oz Salsa

Directions

1. Whisk eggs, salt and cayenne together in a bowl.
2. In a medium skillet over medium heat, toast tortillas 1 minute per side until brown in spots; set aside and cover with foil to keep warm.
3. In the same skillet add oil, red pepper, scallion whites and jalapeno. Cook until vegetables are softened, about 3 minutes.
4. Add eggs and continue to cook, stirring, until eggs are set, about 2 minutes.
5. Place tortillas on plates. Divide eggs between tortillas, season with hot sauce and gently roll up.
6. Serve with salsa and scallion greens.

Note: This can be made with a whole wheat or low-carb tortilla if you are in an acceptable phase. The whole wheat tortillas used here have 20g NC each so be sure to adjust the NC to the tortilla you are using. Low-carb tortillas typically have less NC than the whole wheat.

Breakfast Mexi Peppers

*Servings: 4 | **Prep**: 30 m | **Style**: American | **Cook**: 30 m*

Ingredients

- 4 oz Pork and Beef Chorizo
- 4 oz Ground Beef (80% Lean / 20% Fat)
- 1/2 cup chopped Onions
- 1/4 cup shredded Cheddar Cheese
- 3 large Eggs (Whole)

- 2 medium (approx 2-3/4" long, 2-1/2" dia) Sweet Red Peppers

Directions

1. Preheat oven to 400°F. Line a baking sheet with foil.
2. Cook chorizo, stirring to break up lumps, until browned. Drain excess fat.
3. Place chorizo and ground beef in mixing bowl and combine with the onion, cheese and eggs.
4. Cut peppers in half lengthwise. Scoop out seeds and cut away ribs.
5. Fill each pepper with one-quarter of the meat mixture. Place on the prepared baking sheet. Bake for 25 30 minutes and serve hot.

Breakfast Sausage Sautéed with Red and Green Bell Peppers

Servings: 1 | Prep: 5 m | Style: Other | Cook: 10 m

Ingredients

- 1 tsp Canola Vegetable Oil
- 4 link cookeds Turkey Breakfast Sausage
- 1/4 large (2.25 per pound, approx 3-3/4" long, 3" dia) Red Sweet Pepper
- 1/4 large (2.25 per pound, approx 3-3/4" long, 3" dia) Green Sweet Pepper
- 1 slice (1 oz) Monterey Jack Cheese

Directions

1. Heat a skillet with 1 teaspoon oil over medium-high heat.
2. Crumble the sausage link or leave whole and slice after cooking. Sauté until just beginning to brown. About 3 minutes. Add in red and green bell peppers. Cook until sausage is browned and peppers are softened, about 5 minutes.
3. Sprinkle cheese on top and allow to melt 1-2 minutes. Serve immediately.

Buttermilk Cinnamon Waffles

Servings: 8 | Prep: 10 m | Style: American | Cook: 4 m

Ingredients

- 1 cup Whole Grain Soy Flour
- 2 tbsps Sucralose Based Sweetener (Sugar Substitute)
- 2 tsps Cinnamon
- 3 tsps Baking Powder (Straight Phosphate, Double Acting)
- 1/2 tsp Baking Soda
- 3/4 cup Buttermilk (Reduced Fat, Cultured)
- 6 tbsps Unsalted Butter Stick
- 3 large Eggs (Whole)
- 1 1/2 oz Sugar Free French Vanilla Syrup
- 1/2 cup Tap Water
- 1/3 second spray Original Canola Cooking Spray

Directions

1. Heat waffle iron per manufacturers instructions.
2. Whisk together soy flour, sugar substitute, cinnamon, baking powder and baking soda. Add buttermilk, butter, eggs and syrup and stir until well blended (batter will be stiff).
3. Add cold water 1 tablespoon (8 tbsp in a 1/2 cup) at a time until batter is easily spoonable and spreadable, about the consistency of a thick pancake batter.
4. Spray waffle iron with oil spray. Place approximately 3 tablespoons of batter in center of a waffle iron.
5. Cook according to manufacturer's instructions until crisp and dark golden brown.
6. Repeat with remaining batter. Serve warm. Enjoy!

California Breakfast Burrito

Servings: 4 | Prep: 20 m | Style: Mexican | Cook: 5 m

Ingredients

- 4 tortillas Low Carb Tortillas
- 1 tbsp Canola Vegetable Oil
- 3 large Scallions or Spring Onions
- 4 oz Green Chili Peppers (Canned)

- 1 medium whole (2-3/5" dia) Red Tomato
- 1/2 tsp Salt
- 1/4 tsp Black Pepper
- 8 large Eggs (Whole)
- 1/8 tsp Red or Cayenne Pepper
- 9 sprigs Cilantro (Coriander)
- 1/2 cup shredded Cheddar Cheese
- 1 serving Tomatillo Salsa

Directions

Use 1/4 cup total of the Atkins recipe for Tomatillo Salsa.

1. Heat oven to 325° F.
2. Wrap tortillas in foil and heat in oven 5-10 minutes. Chop tomatoes and dice green onions.
3. In a medium nonstick skillet, heat oil over medium-high heat. Add green onions, chiles, tomato, salt and pepper. Sauté for 3 minutes.
4. Push mixture to side of pan. Add eggs and cayenne to skillet. Cook, 1-2 minutes, stirring occasionally with rubber spatula, until soft, creamy curds form.
5. Stir vegetable mixture into eggs.
6. Divide mixture among warm tortillas, sprinkle with cilantro, one tablespoon of salsa and 2 tablespoons cheese. Roll up tortillas.

Canadian Bacon, Cheddar and Tomato Stacks

Servings: 1 | Prep: 5 m | Style: American | Cook: 5 m

Ingredients

- 2 slices (6 per 6-oz pkg.) Canadian-Style Bacon (Cured)
- 1 large whole (3" dia) Red Tomato
- 1/4 cup shredded Cheddar Cheese

Directions

1. In a skillet over medium-high heat sauté the Canadian bacon until nicely browned and warmed through.

2. Top with a slice of tomato and then cheddar while still in the pan. Cover with a lid and allow to steam with a teaspoon of water for about 1 minute to heat the tomato and melt the cheese.
3. Plate and serve immediately.

Carrot-Zucchini Latkes

*Servings: 8 | **Prep:** 15 m | **Style:** Middle Eastern | **Cook:** 40 m*

Ingredients

- 12 oz Zucchini
- 3/4 tsp Salt
- 5 medium Carrots
- 1 small Onion
- 4 large Eggs (Whole)
- 1/2 tsp Black Pepper
- 1/2 cup Canola Vegetable Oil
- 1 1/2 servings Atkins Cuisine Bread

Directions

Use the Atkins recipe to make Atkins Cuisine Bread for this recipe.

1. Heat oven to 300°F. Set a rack on a baking sheet.
2. Grate zucchini in a food processor fitted with shredding blade or with a box grater, using the side with the largest holes. Transfer to a bowl; sprinkle with 1/4 teaspoon of the salt and toss. Let stand while you prepare the remaining ingredients.
3. Grate carrots and white onion in food processor or with the grater. Transfer to a large bowl.
4. Put bread on a baking sheet and toast in the oven until dried out, 10 to 14 minutes. Leave oven on. Transfer bread to food processor and pulverize to make crumbs. Add crumbs, eggs, remaining 1/2 teaspoon salt and pepper to carrots. Transfer zucchini to a clean dish towel and squeeze out excess liquid. Add zucchini to carrot mixture and stir well to combine.
5. Heat 1/2 cup of canola oil (may need to add more during cooking) in a large skillet over medium heat until very hot. Drop batter by heaping tablespoons into oil and flatten to 3-inch pancakes; do not crowd pan. Cook until golden brown, 3 to 4 minutes per side. Transfer to paper towels to drain; then set on prepared baking sheet and keep latkes warm in oven.

Repeat, adding more oil if necessary, making a total of 24 latkes. Serve with sour cream or a squeeze of lemon (optional).

Cheddar Omelet with Avocado and Salsa

Servings: 1 | Prep: 5 m | Style: American | Cook: 10 m

Ingredients

- 1 tsp Canola Vegetable Oil
- 2 large Eggs (Whole)
- 1 oz Cheddar Cheese
- 1/2 fruit without skin and seed California Avocados
- 1 oz Salsa

Directions

1. Heat oil in a nonstick skillet over medium high heat. Add slightly beaten eggs to skillet. Cook 3 minutes, flip over, cook other side for 2 minutes.
2. Add shredded Cheddar and avocado to half of the omelet. Flip other half over top. Cook an additional 1-2 minutes to melt cheese.
3. Top with salsa and serve immediately.

Cheddar Omelet with Sautéed Onions and Shiitake Mushrooms

Servings: 1 | Prep: 5 m | Style: American | Cook: 8 m

Ingredients

- 1/4 cup shredded Cheddar Cheese
- 1/3 cup chopped Onions
- 1 tsp Canola Vegetable Oil
- 2 large Eggs (Whole)
- 1/4 cup Shiitake Mushrooms

Directions

- Heat oil in a nonstick skillet or omelet pan over medium-high heat. Add onions and mushrooms. Sauté for about 5 minutes until onions are translucent and mushrooms are soft. Remove from pan and set aside.
- Add eggs to the skillet. Cook 3 minutes, lifting the edges of the egg to allow uncooked eggs to flow over and cook. Flip over and cook another 2 minutes.
- Add onions and mushrooms to half of omelet and top with cheese. Fold other half over and cook 1 -2 minutes more to melt cheese. Serve immediately.

Cheddar Omelet with Sautéed Onions

Servings: 1 | Prep: 5 m | Style: American | Cook: 10 m

Ingredients

- 1/3 cup chopped Onions
- 1 tbsp Extra Virgin Olive Oil
- 1/2 cup shredded Cheddar Cheese
- 2 large Eggs (Whole)

Directions

1. Sauté white onions in 1 tablespoon virgin olive oil in a small skillet over medium heat until translucent and tender. Remove from pan and set aside.
2. Lightly beat eggs and add to the same skillet. Allow to form bubbles then carefully flip over. Spread cheese and onions over half the surface. Cook for 1 minute more, fold other side over onions and cheese. Cook 1 more minute.
3. Slide off skillet and on to plate. Season to taste with salt and freshly ground black pepper.

Cheddar Omelet with Sautéed Tomato and Zucchini

Servings: 1 | Prep: 5 m | Style: American | Cook: 10 m

Ingredients

- 1 tsp Olive Oil
- 1/2 cup chopped Zucchini
- 1/2 medium whole (2-3/5" dia) Red Tomatoes
- 2 large Eggs (Whole)
- 1/2 cup shredded Cheddar Cheese

Directions

1. Preheat a skillet with 1 teaspoon oil. Add chopped zucchini to pan and sauté until soft about 2-3 minutes. Add chopped tomatoes and heat through about 1 minute. Remove from skillet and set aside.
2. Pour slightly beaten eggs into the skillet and cook 2-3 minutes until large bubbles begin to form and bottom edge is set. Carefully lift one edge of omelet and flip over. Cook an additional 2 minutes.
3. Layer half of cheese onto half of the omelet then top with tomatoes and zucchini. Layer the second half of cheese over the vegetables then carefully flip over the other half of the omelet to sandwich in the cheese and veggies. Heat through until cheese begins to melt. Remove from heat to a serving plate and top with remaining vegetables.

Cheddar Omelet with Sautéed Watercress

*Servings: 1 | **Prep:** 5 m | **Style:** American | **Cook:** 8 m*

Ingredients

- 1/2 cup chopped Watercress
- 2 large Eggs (Whole)
- 1/2 cup shredded Cheddar Cheese
- 1 tsp Extra Virgin Olive Oil

Directions

1. Heat oil in small nonstick skillet over medium-high heat. Add watercress and sauté for 1 minute until tender. Add salt and freshly ground black pepper to taste. Remove from skillet and set aside.

2. Add eggs to skillet and cook for 2 minutes on medium heat until underside is lightly browned. Flip and cook 1 more minute.
3. Add watercress to half of omelet and top with cheese. Fold over other half and cook for 1 more minute to melt cheese. Serve immediately.

Cheddar Omelet with Swiss Chard and Onions

Servings: 1 | Prep: 5 m | Style: American | Cook: 8 m

Ingredients

- 1 tbsp Light Olive Oil
- 2 cups Swiss Chard
- 1/4 cup shredded Cheddar Cheese
- 2 large Eggs (Whole)
- 1/4 cup chopped Onions

Directions

1. Heat a nonstick skillet with 2 teaspoons oil over medium-high heat. Add white onions and sauté until tender. Quickly add chard and sauté until wilted. Squeeze as much water as possible from the chart by pressing it with the back of a spatula and draining. Remove from pan and set aside.
2. In same pan, add remaining teaspoon of oil and eggs and cook 2 -3 minutes till firm on one side. Flip and cook 1 more minute. To half of the omelet add onions and chard, top with cheese and fold over other half. Cook another 1 -2 minutes to melt cheese. Season to taste with salt and freshly ground black pepper and serve.

Cheese and Spinach Omelet Topped with Avocado and Salsa

Servings: 1 | Prep: 5 m | Style: American | Cook: 10 m

Ingredients

- 1/2 fruit without skin and seed California Avocados
- 2 1/16 cups Baby Spinach

- 1 slice (1 oz) Monterey Jack Cheese
- 1 serving Salsa Cruda
- 2 large Eggs (Whole)
- 1 tbsp Extra Virgin Olive Oil

Directions

Use the Atkins recipe to make Salsa Cruda or use 2 tablespoons of no-sugar-added salsa.

1. Sauté spinach in a nonstick skillet with 1/2 tablespoon oil over medium high heat until wilted. Remove and set aside.
2. Lightly beat the eggs with salt and freshly ground black pepper.
3. Add 1/2 tablespoon oil to the same skillet used for the spinach then add the eggs. Cook for 3 minutes, flip over, and continue to cook on the other side for 2 minutes.
4. Add the cheese and sautéed spinach to half of the omelet. Flip other half over top. Cook an additional 1-2 minutes to melt cheese. Top with avocado and salsa.

Cheese Baked Eggs

Servings: 1 | Prep: 5 m | Style: American | Cook: 10 m

Ingredients

- 1 tsp Unsalted Butter Stick
- 2 large Eggs (Whole)
- 2 tbsps Heavy Cream
- 2 tbsps Parmesan Cheese (Grated)

Directions

1. Melt butter and coat the inside of a small oven safe dish.
2. Combine the eggs and cream in a bowl and lightly beat.
3. Add parmesan cheese and freshly ground black pepper and salt to taste.
4. Bake at 375°F for 10 minutes or until set.

Cheesy Bacon Cloud Muffin

Servings: 1 | Prep: 1 m | Style: American | Cook: 1 m

Ingredients

- 1 oz Cream Cheese
- 1 large Egg
- 2 tbsps Vanilla Whey Protein
- 1/4 tsp Baking Powder (Sodium Aluminum Sulfate, Double Acting)
- 1 slice cooked Bacon (Cured, Pan-Fried, Cooked)
- 1 slice (1 oz) Cheddar Cheese

Directions

1. Place cream cheese in a microwave safe mug. Heat for 10-15 seconds (enough to warm the cream cheese but not to fully melt it).
2. Add the egg and whisk it with the cream cheese.
3. Add the whey protein powder (use a protein powder that has 1g NC or less per serving, one serving is about 1 oz) and baking powder; whisk to combine. Season with a pinch of salt and freshly ground black pepper.
4. Tear the cooked bacon into small pieces and cut the cheese into small pieces. Add them to the mixture, mixing to combine. Heat the mug in the microwave for 1 min (microwave times vary so you may need to increase the time by 10-20 seconds if it does not cook through with 1 minute.) Remove muffin by turning over onto a plate. Run a knife around the inside of the mug to more easily release it.

Chicken Chorizo and Cauliflower Saute with Cheese and Salsa

Servings: 1 | Prep: 5 m | Style: American | Cook: 15 m

Ingredients

- 1 cup Cauliflower
- 1 link Spicy Chorizo Chicken Sausage
- 1 slice (1 oz) Monterey Jack Cheese
- 2 tbsps Chunky Medium Salsa

Directions

1. Cut cauliflower into bite sized pieces and place in a medium non-stick skillet over medium-high heat. Add 2 Tbsp water and cook until water evaporates and cauliflower is crisp-tender (add more water as necessary to prevent burning). Once cauliflower is crisp-tender add the chorizo breaking it up in the pan with a spatula into bite sized pieces. Cook until sausage is cooked through. Remove from heat and place on a serving plate.
2. Top the cauliflower and chorizo with cheese, allowing it to melt. Serve once cheese has melted with 2 Tbsp fresh salsa.

Chicken-Portobello Broilers

Servings: 6 | Prep: 10 m | Style: American | Cook: 20 m

Ingredients

- 2 tbsps Extra Virgin Olive Oil
- 8 oz raw (yield after cooking, bone removed) Chicken Breast
- 3 tbsps chopped Scallions or Spring Onions
- 4 large Eggs (Whole)
- 6 caps Portobello Mushroom Cap
- 1/4 tsp Salt
- 1/4 tsp Black Pepper
- 1/4 tsp Italian Seasoning
- 1/4 cup shredded Mozzarella Cheese (Whole Milk)

Directions

1. Preheat broiler.
2. Cut chicken breast in half lengthwise, then thinly slice crosswise.
3. Heat oil in a large nonstick skillet over medium heat. Add the chicken and green onion and cook 3 4 minutes until chicken is no longer pink. Add the eggs and cook until firm.
4. Meanwhile, place the mushroom caps, ribbed side up, on a foil-lined baking sheet. Sprinkle with salt, pepper and herbs and broil for about 7 minutes, turning once, until slightly soft and dark in color.
5. Remove mushroom caps from oven and spoon egg mixture into them. Optional: add freshly diced tomatoes or red bell pepper to increase your veggies for the day. Top with cheese and broil for 1 minute until melted.

6. Serve immediately.

Chili Spiced "Tortilla" Wraps

*Servings: 4 | **Prep:** 5 m | **Style:** Mexican | **Cook:** 15 m*

Ingredients

- 3 tbsps Organic High Fiber Coconut Flour
- 3/4 tsp Chili Powder
- 1/16 cup Organic 100% Whole Ground Golden Flaxseed Meal
- 1/8 tsp Salt
- 3 large Egg Whites
- 1/2 cup Coconut Milk Unsweetened
- 1 1/3 tbsps Light Olive Oil
- 1/2 tsp Xylitol

Directions

1. Combine the 3 tbsp coconut flour, chili powder, 1 tbsp flax meal, and salt in a small bowl. Set aside.
2. Whisk the egg whites, coconut milk, and sugar substitute. Add the flour mixture, mix to combine, then allow to sit for 5 minutes.
3. Heat a large skillet with 1 teaspoon of oil over medium-high heat. Using a 1/4 cup measure, pour batter into pan and spread out into a 5-inch tortilla shape. Allow to cook for 2-3 minutes, until golden brown underneath and set on the top. Flip over and cook 1 additional minute. Repeat for remaining 3 tortillas.
4. Place cooked tortillas on a paper towel and a paper towel between each. Tortillas may be refrigerated for up to 1 week, store in an airtight container with the paper towels in between or freeze for up to 3 months.

Chocolate and Strawberry Smoothie

*Servings: 1 | **Prep:** 5 m | **Style:** American*

Ingredients

- 1/2 cup Frozen Strawberries
- 1 cup Coconut Milk Unsweetened
- 1 oz or 1 scoop Chocolate Whey Protein
- 2 tsps Cocoa Powder (Unsweetened)
- 1 pinch Stevia

Directions

1. For this recipe unsweetened coconut, almond or soy milk may be used.
2. Combine the frozen strawberries, milk of choice, protein powder, cocoa powder and stevia (to taste) in a blender. Blend until smooth.

Chocolate Cake Donuts

Servings: 6 | Style: American

Ingredients

- 7 tbsps Unsalted Butter Stick
- 3 large Eggs
- 1/8 cup Coconut Milk Unsweetened
- 5 tbsps Sucralose Based Sweetener (Sugar Substitute)
- 1 tsp Vanilla Extract
- 1/2 cup Almond Meal Flour
- 1/4 cup Cocoa Powder (Unsweetened)
- 2 tbsps Organic High Fiber Coconut Flour
- 1/2 tsp Cinnamon
- 1/4 tsp Baking Soda
- 1/4 tsp Baking Powder (Sodium Aluminum Sulfate, Double Acting)
- 1/4 tsp Salt
- 2 tbsps Heavy Cream
- 2 oz Sugar Free Chocolate Chips

Directions

1. Preheat oven to 350°F. Prepare a 6-well donut pan by spraying with oil and set it aside.

2. Melt 5 tbsp butter in a medium microwave safe bowl. Whisk in the eggs, coconut milk, granular sugar substitute, and vanilla until smooth.

3. In a small bowl whisk to combine the almond meal, cocoa power, coconut flour, cinnamon, baking soda, baking powder and salt. Add this mixture to the egg mixture whisking to combine in to a smooth thick batter. Pour into the wells of the donut pan and bake for 16-18 minutes until fragrant and set. Remove from oven to a cooling rack leaving them to sit in the pan for 10 minutes then remove from the pan and continue to cool on a wire rack.

4. Place the remaining 2 tbsp butter, heavy cream and sugar-free chocolate in a small microwave safe bowl that is slightly bigger than the width of the donuts. Melt at 30 second intervals (1 minute total) then whisk until smooth. Dip the tops of the donuts in the glaze and place back on the cooling rack to set the glaze (drizzle any remaining over the tops).. Enjoy immediately or refrigerate for up to 3 days in an airtight container. Serve at room temperature.

Chocolate Cloud Muffin

*Servings: 1 | **Prep**: 1 m | Style: American | **Cook**: 1 m*

Ingredients

- 1 oz Cream Cheese
- 1 large Egg
- 1 tbsp Vegetable Oil
- 2 tbsps Vanilla Whey Protein
- 2 tsps Cocoa Powder (Unsweetened)
- 2 tsps Xylitol
- 1/4 tsp Baking Powder (Sodium Aluminum Sulfate, Double Acting)
- 1/2 tsp Cinnamon
- 1/8 tsp Salt
- 1 packet 100% Natural Stevia Sweetener

Directions

1. Place cream cheese in a microwave safe mug. Heat for 10-15 seconds (enough to warm the cream cheese but not to fully melt it).

2. Add the egg and oil whisking them into the cream cheese.

3. In a small bowl mix to combine the whey protein powder, cocoa powder, xylitol, baking powder, cinnamon, and a pinch of salt and stevia (a whole

packet may be too much or just right for your taste - you may need to experiment).

4. Add the chocolate mixture to the cream cheese mixture in the cup; stir to combine. (Be sure to us a protein powder that has 1g NC or less per serving, one serving is about 1 oz).

5. Heat the mug in the microwave for 1 min (microwave times vary so you may need to increase the time by 10-20 seconds if it does not cook through with 1 minute.) Remove muffin by turning over onto a plate. Run a knife around the inside of the mug to more easily release it.

Chocolate Hazelnut Smoothie

Servings: 2 | Prep: 3 m | Style: American

Ingredients

- 2 scoops Chocolate Whey Protein
- 1 tbsp Heavy Cream
- 12 tsps Sugar Free Hazelnut Syrup

Directions

1. Place protein mix, cream and syrup in a blender with about 1/2 cup of ice; blend until smooth.
2. Pour into 2 glasses. Sprinkle with cinnamon, if desired.

Chocolate Peanut Butter Smoothie

Servings: 1 | Prep: 5 m | Style: American | Cook: 1 m

Ingredients

- 1 cup Coconut Milk Unsweetened
- 2 tbsps Natural Creamy Peanut Butter 1/3 Less Sodium & Sugar
- 1 tbsp Cocoa Powder (Unsweetened)
- 1 scoop Chocolate Whey Protein

- 1/4 tsp Cinnamon
- 1 pinch Stevia
- 1/16 tsp Salt

Directions

1. For this recipe unsweetened coconut, almond or soy milk may be used.
2. Combine the ice, milk of choice, peanut butter, protein powder, cocoa powder, cocoa powder, stevia and salt (to taste) in a blender. Blend until smooth.

Chorizo, Green Chili and Tomato Frittata

Servings: 6 | Prep: 10 m | Style: American | Cook: 15 m

Ingredients

- 6 oz Pork and Beef Chorizo
- 12 large Eggs (Whole)
- 8 oz Green Chili Peppers (Canned)
- 2/3 cup chopped or sliced Red Tomatoes
- 2 oz Cheddar Cheese

Directions

1. Preheat broiler.
2. In a large oven-proof skillet, sauté the chorizo, breaking it up into bite-sized pieces over medium-high heat until cooked through; about 5 minutes. Drain off excess fat and leave in the pan.
3. Add lightly beaten eggs, green chilies, tomatoes and cheese to the chorizo. Cook over medium-high heat for 4-5 minutes then place pan under the broiler for 3-4 minutes until light and slightly puffed. Serve immediately.

Cinnamon Buns

Servings: 12 | Prep: 20 m | Style: American | Cook: 35 m

Ingredients

- 1 1/2 tsps Baking Powder (Straight Phosphate, Double Acting)
- 1/2 tsp Salt
- 1/2 cup Unsalted Butter Stick
- 2 large Egg Yolks
- 1 1/2 cups Tap Water
- 1 tsp Cinnamon
- 6 tbsps Sucralose Based Sweetener (Sugar Substitute)
- 1/2 cup chopped Pecans
- 1 1/2 oz Dried Currants
- 1 tbsp Heavy Cream
- 6 servings All Purpose Low-Carb Baking Mix
- 5 1/4 tbsps Sugar Free Brown Sugar Cinnamon Syrup

Directions

Use the Atkins recipe to make All Purpose Low-Carb Baking Mix for this recipe.

1. In a large bowl mix baking mix (you will need 2 cups of the above recipe), baking powder, salt, water, 4 tablespoons butter, 4 tablespoons sugar substitute and 1 egg yolk until smooth. Cover lightly with plastic wrap and let rise one hour. Stretch dough out to a rectangle measuring 10x15 inches, long side facing towards you.
2. For filling: mix 4 tablespoons butter, 2 tablespoons sugar substitute and cinnamon. Brush mixture over dough, leaving a ½ border at the bottom. Sprinkle dough evenly with nuts and currants. Roll dough up lengthwise from the top, stretching it as you go along. Pinch dough tightly to seal roll and pat to even out shape if necessary. Cut dough roll in half, then halve each half, then cut each quarter into thirds (you will have 12 even slices). Arrange slices on a nonstick baking sheet, lightly cover with plastic wrap and let rise 45 minutes. Heat oven to 375°F.
3. Mix 1 egg yolk and cream. Brush dough slices with mixture. Bake 30 to 35 minutes until lightly browned. Cool buns five minutes then brush with sugar-free cinnamon syrup. Serve warm or at room temperature.

Cinnamon Churritos

Servings: 8 | **Prep:** 10 m | **Style:** American | **Cook:** 10 m

Ingredients

- 1/2 cup Blanched Almond Flour
- 2 tbsps Organic High Fiber Coconut Flour
- 1/4 tsp Baking Powder (Straight Phosphate, Double Acting)
- 2 tsps Cinnamon
- 1/8 tsp Salt
- 1/2 cup Coconut Milk Unsweetened
- 1 tbsp Unsalted Butter Stick
- 3 tbsps Xylitol
- 1 large Egg (Whole)

Directions

These are acceptable only for the fast track of Phase 1 because they contain almonds.

1. Prepare a large skillet or deep fat fryer with 2-3 inches of oil. Heat to 350°F. In a small bowl combine the almond flour, coconut flour, baking powder, 1 teaspoon cinnamon and salt. Mix thoroughly and set aside.
2. In a small sauce pan bring the coconut milk, butter and 1 tablespoon xylitol to a boil. Remove from heat and add the flour mixture stirring until very thick and it forms a ball. Allow to cool for 5 minutes.
3. Once cool add 1 egg and mix until a very thick paste forms, about 1 minute. Drop by tablespoons 4-8 at a time into the fryer and fry until golden brown and crisp on the outside; about 3-4 minutes; rotating halfway through. Repeat until all of batter is used. It should make about 16 balls. Set aside on a paper towel once cooked.
4. In a blender pulse the remaining 2 tablespoons of xylitol with 1 teaspoon of cinnamon 1 -2 times, until xylitol granules are a little smaller. When each batch is finished roll in the xylitol-cinnamon mixture until evenly coated and set on a serving platter. Enjoy immediately or they may be kept at room temperature for 1 day. May also freeze for 3 months or refrigerate for up to 1 week. 2 balls per serving.

Cinnamon Crumb Coffee Cake

*Servings: 12 | **Prep:** 30 m | **Style:** American | **Cook:** 40 m*

Ingredients

- 3/4 cup 100% Stone Ground Whole Wheat Pastry Flour
- 1/2 cup Whole Wheat Flour
- 1 tsp Baking Powder (Straight Phosphate, Double Acting)
- 1 tsp Baking Soda
- 1/2 tsp Salt
- 2 large Eggs (Whole)
- 1 tsp Vanilla Extract
- 1 cup Sour Cream (Cultured)
- 1 1/4 cups Unsalted Butter Stick
- 2 cups Sucralose Based Sweetener (Sugar Substitute)
- 1/2 cup, dry, yield Oatmeal
- 3/4 cup Whole Grain Soy Flour
- 1 1/2 cup halves Pecan Nuts
- 2 tsps Cinnamon

Directions

1. Preheat oven to 350°F. Grease a 9x13 inch baking pan and set aside.
2. For cake: In a medium bowl, whisk together pastry flour, soy flour, whole-wheat flour, baking powder, baking soda and salt. In a large liquid measuring cup whisk eggs, vanilla and sour cream until well combined.
3. In a large bowl, with an electric mixer on medium speed, beat 1/2 cup butter and 1 cup sugar substitute until smooth and fluffy, about 4 minutes. Alternately add the flour mixture and egg mixture to the butter, beginning and ending with the flour mixture.
4. For topping: In a blender, pulse oats, 1 cup sugar substitute, pecans, 3/4 cup butter and cinnamon until texture resembles a coarse meal.
5. To assemble cake: Spread two-thirds of the batter into the prepared pan. Sprinkle half the topping over batter and lightly swirl with a knife to create pockets of topping within the batter.
6. Spoon remaining batter over topping, and sprinkle evenly with remaining topping. Bake until a knife inserted in the center comes out clean, about 40 minutes. Cool cake in pan set over a wire rack. Serve warm or at room temperature. Makes 12 servings.

Cinnamon Mini Muffins

Servings: 24 | Prep: 15 m | Style: American | Cook: 20 m

Ingredients

- 1/2 cup Blanched & Slivered Almonds
- 1/2 cup dry Whole Grain Soy Flour
- 1 tbsp Cinnamon
- 1/4 tsp Salt
- 1/2 tsp Baking Powder (Straight Phosphate, Double Acting)
- 1/2 cup Unsalted Butter Stick
- 3 large Eggs (Whole)
- 2 tsps Vanilla Extract
- 3/4 cup Sucralose Based Sweetener (Sugar Substitute)

Directions

1. Heat oven to 350°F. Spray mini-muffin tins with cooking spray.
2. Pulse almonds in bowl of food processor and 1 tablespoon soy flour until almonds are finely ground (the soy flour will prevent over processing of almonds). Add remaining soy flour, cinnamon, salt and baking powder; pulse to combine.
3. With an electric mixer on medium speed, beat butter and sugar substitute in until fluffy, 3 to 4 minutes. Beat in vanilla extract. Add eggs, one at a time, beating well after each addition. Fold in almond mixture with a spatula.
4. Fill muffin tins 2/3 full with batter. Bake 20 minutes or until set in middle. Transfer to wire rack for 5 minutes to cool. Turn out muffins on to rack to cool completely.

Coconut-Vanilla Shake

Servings: 4 | Prep: 5 m | Style: American

Ingredients

- 1 14 oz can Coconut Cream
- 2 scoops Vanilla Whey Protein
- 1/2 tsp Vanilla Extract

Directions

1. Place coconut cream, protein powder, vanilla and 2 cups of ice cubes in a blender and pulse until smooth and creamy.

Corned Beef Hash

Servings: 4 | Prep: 5 m | Style: Other | Cook: 20 m

Ingredients

- 16 oz Corned Beef Brisket (Cured)
- 2 cups Turnips (with Salt, Frozen, Drained, Cooked, Boiled)
- 1/2 cup chopped Onions
- 1/2 cup Heavy Cream
- 3 tbsps Canola Vegetable Oil

Directions

For this recipe canned or frozen turnips may be substituted for freshly cooked cubed turnips.

1. Toss cubed beef and turnips together in a bowl. Add onion and heavy cream and stir to combine.
2. Heat oil in a heavy nonstick skillet over medium-low heat 1 minute. Add beef-turnip mixture and cook until a crust forms, about 10 minutes.
3. Turn hash and brown other side, about 10 minutes more. Serve with a poached egg, if desired (adds .4g NC to each serving).

Creamy Scrambled Eggs with Dill and Smoked Salmon

Servings: 4 | Prep: 10 m | Style: American | Cook: 15 m

Ingredients

- 4 medium (4-1/8" long) Scallions or Spring Onions
- 3 tbsps Heavy Cream

- 1/2 tsp Salt
- 8 large Eggs (Whole)
- 4 tbsps Unsalted Butter Stick
- 6 oz Smoked Chinook Salmon (Lox)
- 1 tbsp Dill (Dried)

Directions

1. In a large bowl, beat eggs, cream, dill and salt.
2. Melt butter in a large skillet over medium heat. Add scallions; cook 8 minutes until softened. Pour in egg mixture; cook 3 4 minutes, stirring occasionally, until almost set.
3. Mix in salmon, cook 1 minute more or until eggs reach desired doneness.
4. Transfer to warmed plates.

Crunchy Tropical Berry and Almond Breakfast Parfait

Servings: 4 | Prep: 20 m | Style: American | Cook: 15 m

Ingredients

- 1/2 cup Heavy Cream
- 1 1/2 tsps Sucralose Based Sweetener (Sugar Substitute)
- 1/4 tsp Coconut Extract
- 1/2 cup 2% Plain Greek Yogurt
- 1 cup Red Raspberries
- 1 cup Blueberries
- 1/2 cup Dried Coconut
- 4 servings Sweet and Salty Almonds

Directions

Use the Atkins recipe to make Sweet and Salty Almonds for this recipe. You will need 1/2 cup.

1. Combine cream, 1/2 teaspoon sugar substitute, and coconut (or vanilla) extract in a medium bowl; whip with an electric mixer on medium speed until stiff peaks form. Fold in the yogurt.
2. Puree raspberries and remaining sugar substitute in a blender until smooth.

3. Using 4 parfait glasses, alternate layers of whipped cream, raspberry puree, blueberries, nuts, and coconut, making two layers of each. Serve right away.

Crustless Broccoli Quiche

*Servings: 6 | **Prep:** 15 m | **Style:** American | **Cook:** 60 m*

Ingredients

- 1 tsp Extra Virgin Olive Oil
- 1 cup Half and Half Cream
- 1 cup shredded Cheddar Cheese
- 1/2 cup Tap Water
- 1/4 tsp Thyme
- 1/4 tsp leaf Oregano
- 1/2 tsp Salt
- 4 large Eggs (Whole)
- 1/4 tsp Black Pepper
- 1/4 tsp Rosemary (Dried)
- 1 lb Broccoli Flower Clusters
- 1/2 small Onion

Directions

1. Preheat oven to 375°F.
2. Brush a 9- or 10-inch pie plate with virgin olive oil.
3. Heat oil in a small skillet over medium-high heat. Add white onion and cook until softened, about 3 minutes. Transfer to a medium bowl; let cool.
4. Add eggs to onion and lightly beat. Whisk in dairy beverage, 1/2 cup cheese, water, thyme, oregano, salt, pepper and rosemary to blend.
5. Cover bottom of pie plate with broccoli. Pour egg mixture over it and sprinkle with remaining 1/2 cup cheese.
6. Bake until a knife inserted in middle comes out clean and quiche is golden brown, 50 to 60 minutes. Alternatively, these may be baked in a greased muffin tin for 15-20 minutes until fully set. They make an easy on-the-go meal or snack.

Crustless Pumpkin and Ham Quiche

Servings: 8 | Prep: 10 m | Style: American | Cook: 30 m

Ingredients

- 1 medium (2-1/2" dia) Onions
- 2 tbsps Unsalted Butter Stick
- 4 large Eggs
- 1/2 cup Heavy Cream
- 1 cup mashed Cooked Pumpkin
- 1/2 cup Ham (Whole, Cured, Roasted)
- 1 tbsp Parsley
- 1 cup shredded Gruyere Cheese
- 1/8 tsp Red or Cayenne Pepper

Directions

1. Preheat oven to 350°F. Prepare a pie plate with oil. Set aside.
2. In a small skillet saute the dice onion in the butter until soft; about 6 minutes.
3. In a large bowl whisk together the eggs and cream. Add the pumpkin, diced ham, sauteed onion, chopped parsley and cheese. Season with salt and freshly ground black pepper (about 1/4 tsp each) and the cayenne pepper (optional).
4. Pour into prepared pie plate and bake for 30-35 minutes until puffed and set in the center. Transfer to a wire rack to cool. Enjoy warm or cold.

Crustless Spinach Quiche

Servings: 4 | Prep: 20 m | Style: American | Cook: 30 m

Ingredients

- 2 tsps Canola Vegetable Oil
- 6 1/2 oz Frozen Chopped Spinach
- 1/2 cup chopped Scallions or Spring Onions
- 1 cup Heavy Cream

- 1 cup shredded Muenster Cheese
- 1/4 tsp Salt
- 4 large Eggs (Whole)
- 1/8 tsp Nutmeg (Ground)
- 1/4 tsp Black Pepper

Directions

1. Preheat oven to 350°F (175°C). Lightly grease a 9 inch pie pan.
2. Heat oil in a large skillet over medium-high heat. Add onions and cook, stirring occasionally, until onions are soft. Stir in spinach and continue cooking until excess moisture has evaporated.
3. In a large bowl, combine eggs, cream, cheese, salt, 1/8 tsp nutmeg and pepper. Add spinach mixture and stir to blend. Pour into prepared pie pan.
4. Bake in preheated oven until eggs have set, about 30 minutes. Let cool for 10 minutes before serving.

Double-Chocolate Express Smoothie

Servings: 1 | Prep: 5 m | Style: American | Cook: 30 m

Ingredients

- 1/2 cup Tap Water
- 3 tbsps Half and Half Cream
- 1 1/2 oz or 1 scoops Chocolate Whey Protein
- 1 tbsp Cocoa Powder (Unsweetened)
- 3/4 tsp rounded Coffee (Instant Powder, Decaffeinated)

Directions

1. Combine the water, half-and-half, protein powder, cocoa and espresso powders in a blender; blend until smooth. With the machine running, add 3-4 ice cubes, one at a time, and blend until smooth.
2. Pour into a tall glass, and garnish with a dusting of cocoa powder or drizzle with sugar-free chocolate syrup, if desired. Serve immediately.

Dutch Baby Baked Pancake

*Servings: 6 | **Prep:** 15 m | **Style:** American | **Cook:** 15 m*

Ingredients

- 3 tbsps Unsalted Butter Stick
- 1/2 tsp Cinnamon
- 1/4 cup dry Whole Grain Soy Flour
- 1/4 tsp Salt
- 1/2 cup Heavy Cream
- 3 large Eggs (Whole)
- 5 tbsps Sucralose Based Sweetener (Sugar Substitute)
- 1/2 cup 100% Stone Ground Whole Wheat Pastry Flour
- 2 medium (2-3/4" dia) (approx 3 per lb) Apples

Directions

1. Heat oven to 425°F. Place 2 tablespoons of the butter in a 12-inch nonstick ovenproof skillet; set aside.
2. Whisk eggs, pastry flour, soy flour, salt, cream, 3 tablespoons of the sugar substitute and ¼ cup water together until smooth. Place skillet in oven until butter melts. Pour batter into skillet. Bake 15 minutes.
3. While pancake is baking, melt remaining tablespoon of butter in a medium skillet over medium heat. Add remaining 2 tablespoons sugar substitute, cinnamon and ¼ cup water. Bring to a boil; add apples. Cook 15 minutes over a low heat, stirring occasionally, until apples are tender and most of the liquid has evaporated.
4. After removing pancake from the oven, spoon apples into the center. Serve immediately.

Eggs and Spinach

*Servings: 1 | **Prep:** 5 m | **Style:** American | **Cook:** 5 m*

Ingredients

- 1 tbsp Extra Virgin Olive Oil

- 2 1/16 cups Baby Spinach
- 2 large Eggs (Whole)

Directions

1. Add oil to a small skillet over medium heat. Add spinach and sauté until wilted.
2. Add eggs to skillet and scramble together until eggs are set.
3. Season to taste with salt and freshly ground black pepper before serving.

Eggs Scrambled with Asparagus, Bacon and Swiss Cheese

Servings: 1 | Prep: 5 m | Style: American | Cook: 10 m

Ingredients

- 2 medium slice (yield after cooking) Bacon
- 1 large Egg (Whole)
- 1 oz Swiss Cheese
- 2 spear medium (5-1/4" to 7" long) Asparagus

Directions

1. Cook bacon in a small skillet over medium high heat. Reserve some of the bacon fat in the skillet and discard the rest or save for another use. Chop bacon into small pieces and set aside.
2. Cook asparagus in skillet with reserved bacon grease until tender, about 3 minutes. Remove and cut into bite-size pieces.
3. Add eggs, bacon, cheese and asparagus back to pan and scramble together until egg is cooked and cheese is melted, about 3 minutes. Or omit the cheese and instead sprinkle over the eggs after they are cooked.
4. Season to taste with salt and freshly ground black pepper.

Eggs Scrambled with Avocado, Onions and Tomato

Servings: 1 | Prep: 5 m | Style: American | Cook: 10 m

Ingredients

- 1/2 fruit without skin and seed California Avocados
- 2 large Eggs (Whole)
- 1 small whole (2-2/5" dia) Red Tomato
- 2 tbsps chopped Onions
- 1 tsp Extra Virgin Olive Oil

Directions

1. Heat oil in a nonstick skillet over medium-high heat.
2. Sauté white onions in skillet until translucent.
3. Add eggs, avocado and tomatoes and scramble together until eggs are set.
4. Season to taste with salt and freshly ground black pepper and serve immediately.

Eggs Scrambled with Cheddar and Swiss Chard

Servings: 1 | Prep: 5 m | Style: American | Cook: 8 m

Ingredients

- 2 cups Swiss Chard
- 2 large Eggs (Whole)
- 1/4 cup shredded Cheddar Cheese
- 1 tsp Extra Virgin Olive Oil

Directions

1. In a small skillet or sauté pan with 1 teaspoon of canola oil over medium heat, sauté Swiss chard just until decreased in volume and tender, 2 3 minutes.
2. Add eggs to skillet with chard. Using a spatula, mix to combine and scramble until eggs are set.
3. Top with cheese (or add it with the eggs and cook together) and serve immediately.

Eggs Scrambled with Cheddar, Swiss Chard and Canadian Bacon

Servings: 1 | *Prep:* 5 m | *Style:* American | *Cook:* 8 m

Ingredients

- 2 large Eggs (Whole)
- 2 cups Swiss Chard
- 1/4 cup shredded Cheddar Cheese
- 1 tbsp Extra Virgin Olive Oil
- 2 oz Canadian-Style Bacon (Cured)

Directions

1. Sauté Swiss chard in 1 tsp oil until decreased in volume and tender.
2. Beat eggs slightly and add to pan with Swiss chard. Using a spatula mix to combine and cook till eggs are set.
3. Add shredded Cheddar cheese and Canadian bacon to top or it may be added in with the eggs and cooked all together.

Eggs Scrambled with Feta and Spinach

Servings: 1 | *Prep:* 5 m | *Style:* American | *Cook:* 5 m

Ingredients

- 1 tbsp Canola Vegetable Oil
- 2 1/16 cups Baby Spinach
- 2 large Eggs (Whole)
- 1/2 oz Feta Cheese

Directions

1. In a small non-stick skillet, wilt spinach with 1 tablespoon of water over medium heat.
2. Add lightly beaten eggs and cheese and cook until set.
3. Season with salt and freshly ground black pepper and serve immediately.

Eggs Scrambled with Sautéed Mushrooms and Zucchini

Servings: 1 | *Prep:* 5 m | *Style:* American | *Cook:* 10 m

Ingredients

- 1/2 cup Mushroom Pieces and Stems
- 1/2 cup chopped Zucchini
- 1 tbsp Extra Virgin Olive Oil
- 2 large Eggs (Whole)

Directions

1. Dice zucchini.
2. In a small non-stick skillet, saute the zucchini and mushrooms in the olive oil until softened, about 5 minutes. Season with salt and freshly ground black pepper.
3. Pour in slightly beaten eggs and scramble togther with the vegetables until eggs are set.

Eggs Scrambled with Sautéed Onions and Cheddar Cheese

Servings: 1 | *Prep:* 5 m | *Style:* American | *Cook:* 10 m

Ingredients

- 1 tsp Canola Vegetable Oil
- 1/4 cup shredded Cheddar Cheese
- 1/4 cup chopped Onions
- 2 large Eggs (Whole)

Directions

1. Heat oil in a skillet over medium-high heat. Add white onions and sauté for 3 minutes until tender.

2. Add eggs and cheese and scramble together, cooking until eggs are set.
3. Season with salt and freshly ground pepper. Serve immediately.

Eggs Scrambled with Zucchini, Cheddar and Sour Cream

Servings: 1 | Prep: 10 m | Style: American | Cook: 10 m

Ingredients

- 2 tbsps Sour Cream (Cultured)
- 1/2 cup chopped Zucchini
- 2 large Eggs (Whole)
- 1 tsp Extra Virgin Olive Oil
- 1/4 cup shredded Cheddar Cheese

Directions

1. Lightly beat together eggs and sour cream. Set aside.
2. Heat a skillet over medium-high heat. Lightly sauté zucchini in oil for 2 minutes.
3. Add egg-sour cream mixture and cheese to the skillet and scramble together until thoroughly cooked.

Eggs with Avocado and Salsa with Cantaloupe and Sausage

Servings: 1 | Prep: 5 m | Style: American | Cook: 10 m

Ingredients

- 2 large Eggs (Whole)
- 1 oz Salsa
- 1 wedge large (1/8 large melon) Cantaloupe Melons
- 4 oz Turkey Sausage
- 1/2 fruit without skin and seed California Avocados

Directions

1. Fry eggs (scramble or poach if desired instead).
2. Layer avocado then eggs then top with salsa.
3. Heat sausage in a medium skillet over high heat for about 5 minutes, until cooked through and nicely browned on all sides.
4. Cut cantaloupe and serve with turkey sausage and eggs.

Eggs with Avocado and Salsa

Servings: 1 | Prep: 5 m | Style: American | Cook: 5 m

Ingredients

- 1/2 fruit without skin and seed California Avocados
- 1 oz Salsa
- 2 large Eggs (Whole)

Directions

1. Fry eggs in 1 teaspoon of virgin olive oil in a small skillet over medium high heat until desired doneness. Flip, if desired.
2. Season with salt and freshly ground black pepper.
3. Spread the avocado slices on a plate, top with eggs and then salsa.

Eggs with Avocado and Tomato

Servings: 1 | Prep: 5 m | Style: American | Cook: 10 m

Ingredients

- 2 large Eggs (Whole)
- 1/2 medium whole (2-3/5" dia) Red Tomatoes
- 1/2 fruit without skin and seed California Avocados

Directions

1. Cook egg any way desired.
2. Slice tomato and avocado.
3. Layer tomato, avocado, and eggs. Sprinkle with paprika if desired

Eggs with Avocado, Salsa and Turkey Bacon

*Servings: 1 | **Prep:** 5 m | **Style:** American | **Cook:** 15 m*

Ingredients

- 1 oz Salsa
- 2 oz cooked Turkey Bacon
- 1/2 fruit without skin and seed California Avocados
- 2 large Eggs (Whole)

Directions

1. Slice avocado.
2. Fry eggs (scramble or poach if desired instead).
3. Cook turkey bacon slices on frying pan until crispy.
4. Layer avocado, eggs then bacon and top with salsa.

Eggs with Avocado, Tomato and Sausage

*Servings: 1 | **Prep:** 5 m | **Style:** American | **Cook:** 8 m*

Ingredients

- 1/2 avocado, ns as to florida or californium Avocados
- 1/2 medium whole (2-3/5" dia) Red Tomatoes
- 2 large Eggs (Whole)
- 3 oz raw (yield after cooking) Pork Sausage Patty or Link

Directions

1. Prepare eggs as desired by poaching, frying, scrambling or as an omelet.
2. Form non-link sausage into a patty and cook over medium-high heat in a skillet, or if linked cook until no longer pink in the center; about 5 minutes. Cook alone or with the eggs.
3. Top eggs with avocado and tomato (or fill omelet).
4. Serve with sausage.

Eggs with Cheddar, Asparagus, Salsa and Sour Cream

*Servings: 1 | **Prep:** 5 m | **Style:** American | **Cook:** 10 m*

Ingredients

- 4 spear medium (5-1/4" to 7" long) Asparagus
- 2 large Eggs (Whole)
- 1/4 cup shredded Cheddar Cheese
- 1/2 oz Salsa
- 1 tbsp Sour Cream (Cultured)

Directions

1. Steam asparagus in skillet for 3 minutes with 2 Tbsp water. Drain and chop.
2. Beat eggs and add to skillet with 1 tsp oil over medium heat. Add asparagus and cheddar and scramble with eggs till set.
3. Top with salsa and sour cream.

Farmers Breakfast Soup

*Servings: 4 | **Prep:** 10 m | **Style:** American | **Cook:** 45 m*

Ingredients

- 1/2 cup chopped Onions
- 2 medium slice (yield after cooking) Bacon

- 8 oz Turkey Sausage
- 4 oz Ground Beef (80% Lean / 20% Fat)
- 2/3 cup High Protein TVP (Textured Vegetable Protein)
- 1/2 cup chopped Celery
- 1/2 cup chopped Carrots
- 4 cups Chicken Broth, Bouillon or Consomme
- 1/4 tsp Black Pepper

Directions

1. In a large nonstick skillet, over medium heat, cook the bacon until it begins to brown. Add the sausage and beef to brown, breaking up the meat into small bits with a spatula or spoon (about 7 minutes).
2. Stir in the TVP and vegetables. Cook 5 minutes until vegetables begin to soften.
3. Add remaining ingredients and simmer for 20 minutes, skimming off excess fat from the surface of the liquid.
4. Season with salt and pepper to taste.

Fennel, Carrot Hash and Turkey Hash

Servings: 6 | *Prep:* 10 m | *Style:* American | *Cook:* 20 m

Ingredients

- 2 tbsps Canola Vegetable Oil
- 6 oz Fennel Bulk
- 1/2 cup chopped Carrots
- 1/4 cup Freshly Squeezed Orange Juice
- 1 tbsp Orange Peel
- 1/4 tsp Fennel Seed
- 1 tbsp Tamari Soybean Sauce
- 1/2 cup chopped Scallions or Spring Onions
- 12 oz Turkey Breast Meat (Fryer-Roasters, Cooked, Roasted)

Directions

Top each serving with a poached egg, if desired

1. In a large skillet over medium heat, heat oil; add the fennel and carrot and sauté for about 3 minutes.
2. Add orange juice and zest. Simmer until liquid is almost absorbed, about 4 minutes.
3. Stir in fennel seeds, tamari, scallions and turkey. Cook for another 6 minutes until the turkey is heated through.

Feta and Red Bell Pepper Omelet

Servings: 1 | Prep: 5 m | Style: American | Cook: 10 m

Ingredients

- 1 tsp Extra Virgin Olive Oil
- 1/2 cup chopped Sweet Red Peppers
- 2 large Eggs (Whole)
- 2 oz Feta Cheese

Directions

1. Heat oil in a nonstick skillet over medium-high heat. Add bell pepper and sauté until tender. Remove from pan and set aside.
2. Add eggs to pan and cook 2 minutes till underside is golden. Using a spatular and tilting the skillet, flip over. Place the sautéed bell pepper topped with cheese on half the eggs.
3. Gently flip the other half over the mixture and cook an additional 1 2 minutes to melt the crumbled feta cheese.
4. Slide from the skillet to a plate. Season with salt and freshly ground black pepper.

Fluffy Flax Waffles with Turkey Sausage

Servings: 2 | Prep: 10 m | Style: American | Cook: 15 m

Ingredients

- 1 oz raw (yield after cooking) Turkey Breakfast Sausage
- 1 large Egg (Whole)
- 1/16 cup Coconut Milk Unsweetened
- 1/2 tsp Vanilla Extract
- 1/2 tbsp Canola Vegetable Oil
- 1/4 cup Organic 100% Whole Ground Golden Flaxseed Meal
- 1/2 oz Vanilla Whey Protein
- 1 1/2 tsps Sucralose Based Sweetener (Sugar Substitute)
- 1/4 tsp Baking Powder (Straight Phosphate, Double Acting)
- 1/16 tsp Nutmeg (Ground)
- 1/16 tsp Salt
- 1/4 cup Sugar Free Maple Flavored Syrup

Directions

- Brown sausage in a skillet over medium-high heat until cooked through. Remove excess fat by placing on a paper towel and set aside.
- While the sausage is cooking, preheat a non-stick waffle maker. Spray wells with non-stick spray just before pouring in the batter.
- Combine the egg, 1 Tbsp coconut milk, vanilla and oil in a small bowl. Mix thoroughly with a fork for about 1 minute. Add the flax meal, protein powder, granular sugar substitute, baking powder, nutmeg and salt. Mix thoroughly for 1-2 minutes.
- Pour the batter into the waffle maker (it should fill 4 regular 1/2 -inch waffle slots). Otherwise, simply fill with batter according to your waffle maker instructions. For Belgium waffles this recipe makes 2 1/2 squares.
- Cook for 3-5 minutes until golden brown and set. Or follow your waffle maker instructions. Serve with sugar-free pancake syrup and sausage. These waffles freeze well. Reheat in a toaster for 1-2 minutes.

Fluffy Flax Waffles

Servings: 2 | **Prep:** 5 m | **Style:** American | **Cook:** 10 m

Ingredients

- 1/8 cup Coconut Milk Unsweetened
- 2 large Eggs (Whole)
- 1 tbsp Canola Vegetable Oil

- 1 tsp Vanilla Extract
- 1/2 cup Organic 100% Whole Ground Golden Flaxseed Meal
- 1 oz Vanilla Whey Protein
- 1/2 tsp Baking Powder (Straight Phosphate, Double Acting)
- 1 tbsp Sucralose Based Sweetener (Sugar Substitute)
- 1/8 tsp Nutmeg (Ground)
- 1/8 tsp Salt

Directions

1. Preheat a non-stick waffle maker. Spray wells with non-stick spray just before pouring in the batter.
2. Combine 2 Tbsp coconut milk, eggs, oil and vanilla in a small bowl. Mix thoroughly with a fork for about 1 minute.
3. Add the flax meal, protein powder, baking powder, granular sugar substitute, nutmeg and salt. Mix thoroughly for 1-2 minutes.
4. Pour 1/2 of batter into the waffle maker (it should fill 4 waffle slots). Otherwise, simply fill with batter according to your waffle maker then equally divide the cooked waffles into two servings once cooked.
5. Cook for 3-5 minutes until golden brown and set. Or follow your waffle maker instructions.
6. Serve with a pad of butter and sugar-free pancake syrup. If you are in Phase 2 or higher add fresh berries!

French Quesadillas

***Servings:** 4 | **Prep:** 10 m | **Style:** American | **Cook:** 5 m*

Ingredients

- 3 oz boneless, cooked Fresh Ham
- 1 medium (approx 2-1/2 per lb) Pears
- 4 tortillas Low Carb Tortillas
- 4 oz Brie Cheese
- 1/4 cup sliced Almonds

Directions

1. Preheat oven to 350°F.

2. Lay tortillas flat onto a sheet pan. Layer onto half of each tortilla the pear, ham, Brie cheese and almonds (in that order).
3. Fold the tortilla over and bake for 5 minutes; cut in half and enjoy immediately.

French Toast Casserole

Servings: 4 | Prep: 45 m | Style: American | Cook: 80 m

Ingredients

- 14 large Eggs (Whole)
- 10 tbsps Unsalted Butter Stick
- 3 tbsps Xylitol
- 1 cup Organic High Fiber Coconut Flour
- 1 1/2 tsps Baking Powder (Straight Phosphate, Double Acting)
- 3/4 tsp Salt
- 1 cup Heavy Cream
- 1 cup Coconut Milk Unsweetened
- 1 tsp Cinnamon
- 1/4 tsp Nutmeg (Ground)
- 1/2 cup Sugar Free Maple Flavored Syrup

Directions

It is best but not necessary to make the bread portion of this recipe a day or more ahead (a week in advance works great).

1. Preheat oven to 350°F. Grease a small bread pan (8x4-inches). Set aside.
2. Whisk together 8 eggs, 1 tablespoon xylitol and melted butter in a medium bowl.
3. Sift together the coconut flour, baking powder and 3/4 teaspoon salt. Add to the egg mixture and blend until thickened. Bake for 35-40 minutes until the sides pull away from the pan and are golden brown. Allow to cool in the pan for 10 minutes then transfer to a wire rack to finish cooling; about 30 minutes. If baking in advance, once cool, place in an airtight container or zip top bag and refrigerate for up to 2 weeks. If using immediately, once cool, break into 1-inch pieces and place in the same pan used to bake the bread or a small casserole dish.
4. In a medium bowl, whisk together 6 eggs, heavy cream, coconut milk (soy milk or water can replace the coconut milk), 2 tablespoons xylitol,

cinnamon, nutmeg and a pinch of salt. Pour over bread and bake for 50 minutes at 350°F until it is set in the center. Serve immediately by dividing into 8 servings and drizzle each serving with 2 teaspoons sugar-free pancake syrup (or about 1/3 cup over the whole casserole).

French Toast Loaf

Servings: 10 | Prep: 15 m | Style: American | Cook: 50 m

Ingredients

- Soy Flour
- 3/4 cup Whole Grain Wheat Flour
- 1 1/4 cups Sucralose Based Sweetener (Sugar Substitute)
- 1 1/2 tbsps Cinnamon
- 1 tsp Salt
- 1 tsp Baking Soda
- 1 cup Buttermilk (Reduced Fat, Cultured)
- 1 tbsp Vanilla Extract
- 1/4 tsp Cream Of Tartar
- 6 large Eggs (Whole)

Directions

1. Preheat oven to 350°F. Grease an 8x4 loaf pan; set aside.
2. In a large bowl, whisk soy flour, whole wheat flour, sugar substitute, cinnamon, salt and baking soda.
3. In another bowl, combine buttermilk, yolks and vanilla. Pour into dry ingredients and using an electric mixer on low speed, beat until smooth.
4. In another bowl, beat whites and cream of tartar with an electric mixer on high speed until medium peaks form, about 4 minutes. Using a rubber spatula, fold whites into batter in three additions. Pour batter into prepared pan and smooth top.
5. Bake 45-50 minutes until golden and a toothpick inserted in center comes out clean. Cool on wire rack for 5 minutes.
6. Invert pan, remove loaf and cut into 10 slices. Serve with warm sugar free maple syrup or fruit preserves.

Frittata Lorraine

Servings: 6 | *Prep*: 20 m | *Style:* American | *Cook:* 10 m

Ingredients

- 8 large Eggs (Whole)
- 1/4 cup Tap Water
- 1/4 tsp Salt
- 1/4 tsp Black Pepper
- 1 small Onion
- 1 cup shredded Gruyere Cheese
- 4 medium slice (yield after cooking) Bacon

Directions

1. Heat a 10-inch nonstick ovenproof skillet over medium-high heat. Add bacon and sauté until it begins to crisp, 3 to 5 minutes. Add white onion and sauté until soft, about 5 minutes.
2. Whisk eggs, water, salt, and pepper in a medium bowl. Add egg mixture and cheese to skillet; cook until eggs are set on bottom but top remains slightly runny, about 5 minutes.
3. Heat broiler to high. Transfer skillet to oven and broil until eggs are set and golden, about 2 minutes. Cut into wedges and serve.

Garden Frittata

Servings: 4 | *Prep*: 15 m | *Style:* American | *Cook:* 20 m

Ingredients

- 5 whole Mushroom Pieces and Stems
- 2 leeks Leeks
- 1/4 head large (6-7" dia) Cauliflower
- 2 tbsps Basil
- 1/2 tsp Rosemary (Dried)
- 3 tbsps Parmesan Cheese (Grated)
- 8 large Eggs (Whole)

- 3 tbsps Extra Virgin Olive Oil

Directions

1. Preheat broiler.
2. Heat oil in a medium ovenproof skillet over medium heat. Add leeks and cauliflower; sauté until crisp-tender, about 10 minutes. Add mushrooms, cook 5 minutes, until mushrooms begin to give off liquid.
3. Reduce heat to low. Pour eggs into skillet, stirring slightly. Add basil and rosemary, along with salt and pepper to taste. Cook, stirring frequently, until eggs begin to form small curds and set. Add cheese and lightly press into egg mixture with a spatula.
4. Place skillet under broiler; cook until top is set but not brown, about 1 minute. Cool slightly.
5. To remove frittata whole, tip skillet to one side and use a spatula to loosen edges. Slide onto a serving platter; cut into quarters and serve.

Giant Zucchini Pancake

*Servings: 4 | **Prep**: 15 m | **Style**: American | **Cook**: 20 m*

Ingredients

- 1 lb Baby Zucchini
- 4 slice (1 oz) Havarti Cheese
- 1/3 cup Whole Grain Soy Flour
- 1/3 cup Parsley
- 2 large Eggs (Whole)
- 1/2 tsp Salt
- 1/4 tsp Black Pepper
- 2 tbsps Extra Virgin Olive Oil

Directions

1. Preheat oven to 350°F.
2. Place grated zucchini in a colander and press to drain any excess liquid. Pat zucchini dry with a paper towel.
3. Beat eggs in a large bowl. Stir in cheese, soy flour, parsley, salt and pepper. Add zucchini to cheese mixture. Stir to combine well.

4. In a 10-inch ovenproof skillet, heat oil over medium heat until it shimmers. Add pancake mixture and press down to spread, forming an even layer. Cook 4 minutes or until bottom is set.
5. Transfer skillet to oven; bake 12 15 minutes until middle is just set.
6. Remove from oven and let cool slightly. Cut into wedges and serve crispy side up.

Green Bell Pepper Filled with Creamy Eggs and Spinach

Servings: 1 | Prep: 5 m | Style: American | Cook: 5 m

Ingredients

- 1/2 medium (approx 2-3/4" long, 2-1/2" dia) Green Peppers
- 1 tbsp Extra Virgin Olive Oil
- 1 cup Baby Spinach
- 2 large Eggs (Whole)
- 1 oz Pepper Jack Cheese

Directions

1. Cut bell pepper in half. Slice small slice off the bottom so it will stand up right. Place in a pan with a small amount of water and steam over medium heat until the pepper is tender. Set aside on a serving plate.
2. Sauté 1 cup spinach in a small amount of oil until wilted, add eggs and cheese. Cook until eggs are barely set with a creamy texture (do not over cook) and season with salt and freshly ground black pepper.
3. Spoon the egg mixture into the pepper and serve immediately.

Ham and Cheese Roll-Ups

Servings: 6 | Prep: 15 m | Style: American

Ingredients

- 6 thin slice (approx 4-1/2" x 2-1/2" x 1/8") Fresh Ham

- 6 slice (1 oz) Swiss Cheese
- 6 spears Pickles
- 2 tbsps Real Mayonnaise
- 2 tbsps Dijon Mustard

Directions

1. Trim ham, cheese and pickles to equal lengths. Lay out ham slices, top with cheese slices.
2. Combine mayo and mustard; spread onto cheese. Lay pickle in center and roll up tightly. Cut into bite-sized pieces.

Ham and Swiss Cheese Frittata

Servings: 6 | Prep: 15 m | Style: Italian | Cook: 25 m

Ingredients

- 1 tbsp Unsalted Butter Stick
- 2 tbsps chopped Onions
- 1/2 medium (approx 2-3/4" long, 2-1/2" dia) Sweet Red Peppers
- 8 oz boneless, cooked Fresh Ham
- 3 tbsps Parsley
- 9 large Eggs (Whole)
- 1/4 cup Heavy Cream
- 1/4 cup Tap Water
- 1/2 tsp Salt
- 1/2 tsp Italian Seasoning
- 1 cup shredded Swiss Cheese

Directions

1. Heat broiler.
2. Melt butter in a large nonstick skillet over medium-high heat; add white onion, pepper, ham and half the parsley. Cook 5 minutes, until onion is softened.
3. Combine eggs, cream, water, salt, Italian seasoning and half the cheese.
4. Add egg mixture to pan. Cook, stirring constantly, until the eggs form soft, creamy small curds, about 5 minutes. Remove from heat; sprinkle remaining cheese over top of eggs.

5. Place skillet under broiler; cook until cheese is bubbly and golden, about 3 minutes. Cool slightly.
6. To remove frittata whole, tip skillet to one side and use a spatula to loosen edges. Slide onto a serving platter; top with remaining parsley.
7. Cut into wedges.

Ham, Cream Cheese and Dill Pickle Roll-Ups

Servings: 1 | *Prep:* 5 m | *Style:* American

Ingredients

- 2 oz boneless, cooked Fresh Ham
- 2 tbsps Cream Cheese
- 2 spears Pickles

Directions

1. Spread 1 tablespoon cream cheese on each slice of ham.
2. Place a pickle spear at one end of each ham slice and roll up. Secure with a tooth pick if desired.

Ham, Monterey Jack and Jicama Roll-Ups with Aioli

Servings: 1 | *Prep:* 5 m | *Style:* American

Ingredients

- 2 oz Yambean (Jicama)
- 2 oz boneless, cooked Fresh Ham
- 1 slice (1 oz) Monterey Jack Cheese
- 1 serving Aioli

Directions

1. Roll ham and cheese around the jicama sticks. Serve with Aioli or spread between ham and cheese before rolling.

Ham, Muenster and Asparagus Roll-Ups

*Servings: 1 | **Prep:** 5 m | **Style:** American*

Ingredients

- 4 spear medium (5-1/4" to 7" long) Asparagus
- 2 slice (1 oz) Muenster Cheese
- 4 oz boneless, cooked Fresh Ham
- 2 tbsps Real Mayonnaise

Directions

1. Slice the ham and Muenster into 4 thin slices.
2. Layer ham with mayonnaise and cheese. Roll around the asparagus. Or roll asparagus with ham and cheese and dip into mayonnaise. Pin roll-ups with tooth picks if desired.

Ham, Swiss Cheese and Avocado Roll-ups

*Servings: 1 | **Prep**: 5 m | **Style:** American*

Ingredients

- 1/2 California Avocados
- 1 oz Swiss Cheese
- 4 oz boneless, cooked Fresh Ham

Directions

1. Place a piece of cheese on each piece of ham. Top with a slice of avocado.

2. Roll up and secure with a toothpick, if desired.

Hatch Green Chile, Cheese and Egg Bake

Servings: 4 | Style: American

Ingredients

- 4 oz Green Chili Peppers (Canned)
- 8 large Egg Whites
- 2 tbsps Heavy Cream
- 1/2 tsp Garlic Powder
- 1/4 tsp Salt
- 1/8 tsp Black Pepper
- 1 1/2 cups shredded Cheddar Cheese

Directions

1. Preheat oven to 350°F. Prepare a square pan with aluminum foil and spray it with oil oil spray.
2. In a blender, blend together the chiles, eggs, half & half, garlic powder, salt, pepper, and 1 cup cheese until smooth. Poor in prepared pan and bake covered for 45 minutes or until eggs are set.
3. Remove from oven and sprinkle remaining 1/2 cup cheese on top, allow to melt and cool slightly then serve.

Hazelnut-Chocolate Spread 1

Servings: 1 | Prep: 10 m | Style: Italian | Cook: 5 m

Ingredients

- 1/2 cup whole Hazelnuts or Filberts
- 2 tbsps Xylitol
- 1 tbsp Cocoa Powder (Unsweetened)
- 1/4 tsp Salt

- 1 tbsp Virgin Coconut Oil
- 5 oz Sugar Free Chocolate Chips

Directions

This recipe is suitable for all phases except the first two weeks of Induction because of the hazelnuts.

1. Toast hazelnuts in a 350°F oven on a sheet pan for 5 minutes. Remove from oven and allow to cool slightly. Put hazelnuts on a clean cloth and rub to remove the outer dark skins. It is not necessary to remove all dark skin but as much as possible is best. Place in a food processor.
2. Powder the 2 tablespoons of granular sugar substitute in a blender to a fine powder. Add to the nuts in the food processor along with the cocoa powder and salt. Pulse until the nuts are finely chopped. Add the coconut oil and continue to pulse to a fairly smooth paste.
3. Melt chocolate in a microwave in a small bowl at 30 second intervals. Do not overheat. Stir between intervals to be sure all chocolate is completely melted. Add melted chocolate to food processor and pulse to combine and make a smooth paste. Use immediately or place in an airtight container in the refrigerator for up to two weeks or freeze for several months. Reheat gently in a microwave for 10-15 seconds or leave at room temperature to soften when serving. Makes 3/4 cup or 6 servings of 2 tablespoons each.

Herb-Butter Blend

Servings: 32 | *Prep: 7 m* | *Style: American*

Ingredients

- 1/2 tsp Salt
- 1 tsp Black Pepper
- 1/2 cup Extra Virgin Olive Oil
- 1 tsp Garlic
- 3 tsps leaves Oregano
- 2 tbsps Basil
- 1 cup Unsalted Butter Stick
- 1/2 cup Canola Vegetable Oil

Directions

This savory butter is delicious on vegetables, fish and meats. Each serving is 1 Tbsp.

1. Place salt, pepper, olive oil, garlic, oregano and basil in a food processor. Pulse until herbs are finely ground and there are no visible specks of pepper (30-60 seconds total).
2. Add butter and canola oil, blending until smooth.
3. Scrape into a container with a snap top and refrigerate up to 1 month.

Herbed Scrambled Eggs

*Servings: 2 | **Prep:** 10 m | **Style:** Other | **Cook:** 10 m*

Ingredients

- 6 large Eggs (Whole)
- 2 tbsps Heavy Cream
- 1/4 tsp Salt
- 1/8 tsp Black Pepper
- 1 tsp Tarragon
- 1 tbsp Unsalted Butter Stick

Directions

1. Using a fork, whisk eggs, cream, salt, pepper and fresh tarragon (use 1/2 as much if using dried) in a bowl.
2. Melt butter in a medium nonstick skillet over medium heat. Pour in the eggs. Cook 1 minute without stirring.With a wooden spoon or heat-resistant rubber spatula, gently turn the eggs from bottom to top, scraping around all edges. Eggs should not brown.
3. When eggs form soft and creamy small curds, turn onto warm plates and serve immediately.

Individual Cloud Muffin

*Servings: 1 | **Prep:** 1 m | **Style:** American | **Cook:** 1 m*

Ingredients

- 1 oz Cream Cheese
- 1 large Egg
- 2 tbsps Vanilla Whey Protein
- 1/4 tsp Baking Powder (Sodium Aluminum Sulfate, Double Acting)

Directions

1. Place cream cheese in a microwave safe mug. Heat for 10-15 seconds (enough to warm the cream cheese but not to fully melt it).
2. Add the egg and whisk it with the cream cheese.
3. Add the whey protein powder (use a protein powder that has 1g NC or less per serving, one serving is about 1 oz) and baking powder; whisk to combine. Season as desired with either savory or sweet spices (for sweet - add a pinch of stevia or other sugar substitute - up to 1/2 tsp).
4. Heat the mug in the microwave for 1 min (microwave times vary so you may need to increase the time by 10-20 seconds if it does not cook through with 1 minute.) Remove muffin by turning over onto a plate. Run a knife around the inside of the mug to more easily release it.

Italian Frittata

Servings: *4 |* **Prep:** *20 m |* **Style:** *Italian |* **Cook:** *20 m*

Ingredients

- 1/2 cup chopped Onions
- 1 tbsp Light Olive Oil
- 1 tbsp Unsalted Butter Stick
- 1 tsp Garlic
- 1 large Zucchini
- 1 tsp leaf Basil (Dried)
- 8 oz raw (yield after cooking) Italian Sausage
- 2 tbsps Tap Water
- 8 large Eggs (Whole)
- 1/4 tsp Salt
- 1/4 tsp Black Pepper
- 1/3 cup Parmesan Cheese (Grated)

Directions

1. Preheat broiler.
2. Heat the oil and butter in a large, ovenproof skillet over medium heat. Add the garlic and white onion and sauté for 2 to 3 minutes, or until softened. Add the zucchini and basil and cook for 5 6 minutes, stirring occasionally, until soft but not limp. Add the sausage and cook for 2 to 3 minutes, stirring occasionally.
3. Meanwhile, in a large bowl, whisk together the eggs, water, salt and pepper. Pour the egg mixture into the hot pan over the meat and vegetable mixture. Let cook for a few seconds, undisturbed, then use a spatula to move the eggs toward the center while tilting the pan to let the uncooked eggs run to the sides. Continue cooking and moving the egg mixture for 4 5 minutes, or until the eggs are almost set (they will still be moist on the top).
4. Sprinkle with cheese and place under the broiler until the eggs are cooked on top and the cheese is melted and bubbly, about 2 3 minutes.
5. Cut in quarters and serve immediately.

Italian Sausage Morning Soup

Servings: 4 | Prep: 10 m | Style: Italian | Cook: 40 m

Ingredients

- 1 tbsp Extra Virgin Olive Oil
- 1/2 cup chopped Onions
- 1 stalk medium (7-1/2" - 8" long) Celery
- 1/2 cup chopped Carrots
- 4 cups Chicken Broth, Bouillon or Consomme
- 1/4 cup Spaghetti/Marinara Pasta Sauce
- 1/4 tsp Italian Seasoning
- 8 oz cooked Italian Sausage
- 4 oz Ground Beef (80% Lean / 20% Fat)
- 1 large Egg (Whole)

Directions

1. Heat olive oil In a large saucepan over medium heat. Add the white onion, celery and carrots and cook until they begin to soften, about 5 minutes.

2. Add the broth, marinara sauce and Italian seasoning. Simmer for 20 minutes.
3. Meanwhile, mix the sausage, ground beef and egg together in a mixing bowl. Using a tablespoon, form meat mixture into balls and drop into the simmering soup. Alternatively, bake the meatballs in a 350°F oven on a jelly roll pan until brown on the outside before adding to the soup.
4. Cook for an additional 20 minutes until the meatballs are cooked through.
5. Season to taste with salt and freshly ground pepper and serve immediately.

Leek Quiche

Servings: 6 | *Prep:* 15 m | *Style:* Other | *Cook:* 45 m

Ingredients

- 1 tbsp Unsalted Butter Stick
- 1 1/2 lbs Leeks
- 1/2 cup Heavy Cream
- 3 large Eggs (Whole)
- 1/2 tsp Salt
- 1/4 tsp Black Pepper
- 1 cup shredded Gruyere Cheese
- 8 servings Atkins Cuisine Pie Crust

Directions

Use 1 Atkins Cuisine Pie Crust recipe (see recipe). Follow instructions to prebake the pie crust. Prebake the shell and pour filling (directions follow) into hot shell.

1. Keep oven on at 350°F. In a medium skillet over medium heat, melt butter. Add leeks and sauté, stirring occasionally, 5 to 6 minutes, until softened. Remove from heat and stir in cream. Let stand 5 minutes.
2. Meanwhile, in a medium bowl, whisk eggs with salt and pepper. Stir egg mixture into the leeks and cream. Sprinkle ¾ cup of cheese on bottom of pie shell.
3. Pour egg mixture into prebaked pie shell; sprinkle remaining cheese on top. Bake 45 minutes, or until just set in middle and browned on top. If necessary, turn on broiler; broil 6 from element 2 minutes, just until top browns.

Lemon Poppy Seed Cloud Muffin

Servings: 1 | *Prep:* 1 m | *Style:* American | *Cook:* 1 m

Ingredients

- 1 oz Cream Cheese
- 1 large Egg
- 1/4 fl oz Lemon Juice
- 1/2 tsp Lemon Peel
- 2 tbsps Vanilla Whey Protein
- 1/4 tsp Baking Powder (Sodium Aluminum Sulfate, Double Acting)
- 1/2 tsp Poppy Seed
- 1 tsp Vanilla Extract
- 1/2 packet 100% Natural Stevia Sweetener

Directions

For Atkins 20 Phase 1, omit the poppy seeds in this recipe.

1. Place cream cheese in a microwave safe mug. Heat for 10-15 seconds (enough to warm the cream cheese but not to fully melt it).
2. Add the egg, lemon zest and lemon juice (1-2 tsp) and whisk it with the cream cheese.
3. Add the whey protein powder (use a protein powder that has 1g NC or less per serving, one serving is about 1 oz), baking powder and poppy seeds; whisk to combine. Season with a pinch of salt,vanilla, and stevia (or up to 1/2 tsp other sugar substitute).
4. Heat the mug in the microwave for 1 min (microwave times vary so you may need to increase the time by 10-20 seconds if it does not cook through with 1 minute.) Remove muffin by turning over onto a plate. Run a knife around the inside of the mug to more easily release it.

Low Carb Coconut Bread

Servings: 16 | *Prep:* 10 m | *Style:* American | *Cook:* 37 m

Ingredients

- 6 large Eggs (Whole)
- 1/2 cup Unsalted Butter Stick
- 1 tsp Xylitol
- 3/4 cup Organic High Fiber Coconut Flour
- 1 tsp Baking Powder (Straight Phosphate, Double Acting)
- 1/2 tsp Salt

Directions

1. Preheat oven to 350°F. Grease a small bread pan (8x4-inches or smaller).
2. Combine the eggs, xylitol and melted butter. Whisk for 1 minute. Sift together the coconut flour, baking powder and salt.
3. Add the flour mixture to the eggs and blend until thickened. Bake for 35-40 minutes until the sides pull away from the pan and are golden brown. Allow to cool in the pan for 10 minutes then transfer to a wire rack to finish cooling; about 30 minutes. Store in an air-tight container in the refrigerator for up to 2 weeks. Makes 16 x 1/2-inch slices. Nutritionals reflect 1 slice per serving.

Low-Carb French Toast

Servings: 3 | Style: American

Ingredients

- 2 large Eggs
- 2 tbsps Heavy Cream
- 1/4 tsp Cinnamon
- 1/8 tsp Nutmeg (Ground)
- 3 servings Low-Carb Bread

Directions

Use the Atkins recipe to make Atkins Cloud Bread for this recipe.

1. Slice 3 thick pieces of Protein Cloud Bread into 2 thinner slices. Set aside. Preheat a non-stick skillet with a small amount of oil over medium-high heat.
2. Whisk together the eggs, heavy cream, cinnamon and nutmeg in a shallow bowl.
3. Dip each slice of bread into the egg mixture, turning to coat both sides. Once coated evenly, place in the hot skillet and repeat with 1 or two more slices of bread to fill the pan; be sure it is not over crowded. Cook 3-4 minutes per side until golden. Place on a serving plate and repeat with the remaining bread and egg mixture. Top with butter and serve with sugar-free maple syrup.

Low-Carb Granola

Servings: 5 | Style: American

Ingredients

- 1/3 cup Coconut Oil
- 1 cup whole Flaxseed Seeds
- 1 cup Raw Sunflower Seeds
- 1 cup half Pecan Nuts
- 9 tbsp raws Unsweetened Shredded Coconut
- 2 tbsps Sucralose Based Sweetener (Sugar Substitute)
- 2 tsps Cinnamon
- 1 tsp Vanilla Extract

Directions

1. Preheat oven to 350°F.
2. In a large skillet over medium heat melt the coconut oil completely, and then stir in the rest of the ingredients. Stir continuously for 10 minutes. Remove from heat, spread mixture on large cookie sheet lined with parchment paper.
3. Bake for 20 minutes. Let cool, and store in an airtight container in the refrigerator. Makes about 2 1/2 cups each serving is 1/2 cup. Tastes great with unsweetened almond or coconut milk!!!

Mexican Stuffed Breakfast Portobello Mushrooms

Servings: 2 | Prep: 15 m | Style: Mexican | Cook: 25 m

Ingredients

- 1 tsp Extra Virgin Olive Oil
- 10 oz Smoked Turkey Italian Sausage
- 1 cup Baby Spinach
- 4 oz Salsa
- 2 large Eggs (Whole)
- 1/2 California Avocados
- 1/2 cup shredded Cheddar Cheese
- 1 sprig Cilantro
- 2 caps Portobello Mushroom Cap

Directions

Use the Atkins recipe to make Diane's Quick Tomato Salsa for this recipe. You will need 1 full recipe to serve two people; or about 1/2 cup of prepared salsa of choice.

1. Preheat oven to 400 degrees.
2. Place mushrooms smooth side up on baking sheet lined with parchment paper. Bake 10 minutes. Remove from oven and place mushroom caps smooth side up on a platter lined with paper towels to drain some of the water.
3. Heat oil in a medium frying pan over medium heat. Brown sausage and break into small pieces with the back of a wooden spoon while cooking. Stir in chopped spinach and salsa. Transfer mixture to a mixing bowl to cool slightly.
4. Carefully separate egg yolks and place whites in one bowl and yolks in 2 separate small bowls. Beat egg whites with a fork.
5. Place mushrooms smooth side down on a baking sheet lined with parchment paper. Slice the avocado and divide them onto the bottom of the mushrooms.
6. Add egg whites and cheddar cheese to sausage mixture and combine well. Divide mixture in half and stuff into portobello caps on top of the avocado.
7. For each mushroom make a well in the center of the sausage mixture that is large enough for the egg yolk. Bake 10 minutes then and carefully pour yolk in each well.
8. Bake until the yolks are set, about 5 more minutes, then sprinkle tops with chopped cilantro.

Mini Breakfast Sausage, Bell Pepper and Scallion Casseroles

Servings: 4 | *Prep:* 5 m | *Style:* American | *Cook:* 20 m

Ingredients

- 8 oz Turkey Sausage
- 4 large Eggs (Whole)
- 2 medium (4-1/8" long) Scallions or Spring Onions
- 1/4 cup shredded Cheddar Cheese
- 1/2 large (3-3/4" long, 3" dia) Yellow Sweet Peppers

Directions

1. Preheat oven to 400°F. Arrange rack in the middle of the oven.
2. In a medium skillet over medium heat, cook the sausage, about 3 minutes. Add the peppers and scallions and cook until soft, about 3 minutes.
3. Divide sausage mixture in 4 individual souffle dishes; top with cheese. Add 1 beaten egg to each dish.
4. Bake for 15 -17 minutes until eggs are firm.

Mini Chocolate Chip Muffins

Servings: 24 | *Prep:* 10 m | *Style:* American | *Cook:* 15 m

Ingredients

- 1 cup Whole Grain Soy Flour
- 1 tsp Baking Powder (Straight Phosphate, Double Acting)
- 1/2 cup Sucralose Based Sweetener (Sugar Substitute)
- 1/4 tsp Salt
- 1/2 cup Sour Cream (Cultured)
- 2 tbsps Unsalted Butter Stick
- 2 tbsps Heavy Cream
- 1 fl oz Tap Water
- 2 tsps Vanilla Extract

- 4 oz Sugar Free Chocolate Chips

Directions

1. Heat oven to 350°F. Grease two 12-compartment mini muffin pans.
2. In a bowl, combine soy flour, baking powder, sugar substitute, and salt.
3. In another bowl, whisk sour cream, butter, heavy cream, water and vanilla to combine.
4. Add the sour cream mixture to the soy mixture. Stir until well combined. Fold in chocolate chips.
5. Divide batter (it will be somewhat thick) in pan compartments, using about 1 rounded tablespoon per muffin. Bake 15-20 minutes, or until lightly browned on top and toothpick inserted in center comes out clean.
6. Cool muffins in pans for 2 minutes, then turn out onto wire racks to cool completely.

Mixed Berry Shortcakes

Servings: 6 | Prep: 35 m | Style: Other | Cook: 15 m

Ingredients

- 1 cup Whole Grain Soy Flour
- 1 tsp Baking Powder (Straight Phosphate, Double Acting)
- 2 2/3 tbsps Sucralose Based Sweetener (Sugar Substitute)
- 1 tsp Salt
- 6 tbsps Unsalted Butter Stick
- 1 2/3 cups Heavy Cream
- 1/4 cup Sour Cream (Cultured)
- 1 cup whole Strawberries
- 1 large Egg (Whole)
- 1 cup Blueberries
- 1 cup Raspberries
- 1/2 cup half Pecans

Directions

1. In a food processor, pulse flour, baking powder, pecans, 3 tablespoons of the sugar substitute and salt until nuts are finely ground. (If you don't have a food processor, grind the nuts in a nut or coffee grinder.)

2. Add the butter and pulse until its the texture of cornmeal. In a liquid measuring cup or bowl, whisk 2/3 cup of the heavy cream, sour cream and egg. Pour evenly over the dry mixture and pulse just until combined.

3. Chill dough for 30 minutes. Separate dough into 12 equal-sized pieces (you'll need about 3 1/2 tablespoons of dough for each piece). Put each piece into a disk measuring 2 1/2 to 3-inches across. Space disks evenly on baking sheet, leaving 1 inch between biscuits to allow for spreading during the baking process.

4. Bake shortcakes about 20 minutes, until bottoms are golden brown. Cool on baking sheet set on a wire rack.

5. With an electric mixer on medium speed, beat remaining cup of heavy cream with remaining 2 teaspoons sugar substitute until soft peaks form.

6. To assemble: Dollop 1/4 cup whipped cream on 6 six shortcakes, top with 1/2 cup berries and cover with remaining shortcakes.

Muffin in a Minute

Servings: 1 | Prep: 3 m | Style: American | Cook: 1 m

Ingredients

- 4 tbsps Organic 100% Whole Ground Golden Flaxseed Meal
- 1/2 tsp Baking Powder (Straight Phosphate, Double Acting)
- 1/2 individual packet Sucralose Based Sweetener (Sugar Substitute)
- 1 tsp Cinnamon
- 1 large Egg (Whole)
- 1 tsp Unsalted Butter Stick

Directions

1. For this recipe 1 packet of sucralose equals 2 teaspoons; use 1 teaspoon per muffin.
2. Mix the flax meal, baking powder, sugar substitute and cinnamon in a coffee mug or single-serving soufflé dish.
3. Add the egg and butter (or oil). Mix with dry ingredients.
4. Microwave 1 minute or more, until firm
5. Turn out and serve with butter or cream cheese. Or toast before applying spread. Makes 1 serving.

Chapter 2: Desserts Recipes

***

Black Velvet Cupcakes

Servings: 6 | Prep: 5 m | Style: American | Cook: 17 m

Ingredients

- 3 large Eggs (Whole)
- 1/4 cup Coconut Milk Unsweetened
- 1/4 cup Xylitol
- 2 tsps Vanilla Extract
- 7 tbsps Unsalted Butter Stick
- 1/4 cup Organic High Fiber Coconut Flour
- 1/4 tsp Baking Powder (Straight Phosphate, Double Acting)
- 2 tbsps Cocoa Powder (Unsweetened)
- 1/4 tsp Baking Soda
- 1/4 tsp Salt
- 4 oz Cream Cheese
- 6 tsps Erythritol

Directions

For this recipe you will need black food coloring (either liquid or gel; for liquid you will need 1/2 tsp and for gel just a small amount is needed). You will also need orange or other color for the frosting; amount will depend upon desire for color depth. The cupcakes may be sprinkled with edible glitter which is made of food coloring and guar gum (no sugar). The glitter and food colorings can be found at some hobby stores or online.

1. Preheat oven to 375°F. Prepare a muffin tin with 6 paper cups. Set aside.
2. In a medium bowl whisk the eggs with the coconut milk, granular sugar substitute, vanilla, black food coloring and 3 tablespoons melted butter. Set aside.
3. In a small bowl whisk together the coconut flour, baking powder, cocoa powder, baking soda and salt. Add to egg mixture whisking to incorporate all ingredients for about a minute. Divide batter into the 6 paper cups, place in the oven and bake until fully set in the center; about 15-18 minutes. When done, set on a wire rack to cool.
4. Make Frosting: In a small bowl, beat the cream cheese with an electric mixer until smooth. Add 4 tbsp (1/4 cup) softened butter and continue to beat another minute. Add the erythritol; beat another minute then add

vanilla and food coloring as desired. Adjust for sweetness by adding a pinch of stevia if desired. Frost cupcakes using a piping bag or by hand.

Caramelized Pear Custard

Servings: 8 | *Prep*: *5 m* | *Style*: *American* | *Cook*: *20 m*

Ingredients

- 2 tbsps Butter
- 2 tbsps Xylitol
- 1/4 tsp ground Cardamom
- 2 medium (approx 2-1/2 per lb) Pears
- 3 large Eggs (Whole)
- 2 large Egg Yolks
- 2 cups Heavy Cream
- 1/8 cup Sugar Free Low Calorie Maple Flavor Syrup
- 1/2 fl oz (no ice) Rum
- 1 tsp Vanilla Extract

Directions

1. Preheat oven to 375°F.
2. Heat the butter, xylitol and cardamom in a large sauce pan over medium-high heat. Slice the pears into 1/2-inch wedges. Once the butter has melted add the pears and allow to caramelized for 4 minutes on each side. Remove from heat and arrange in a pie plate or 3-4 cup casserole dish. Reserve about 2 Tbsp syrup and pour the remaining over the pears (keep remaining in the sauce pan and set aside).
3. In a small bowl, whisk the eggs, egg yolks, heavy cream, sugar free syrup, rum and vanilla until combined. Pour mixture over the pears and bake for 15-20 minutes until golden brown and custard has set. Remove from oven and allow to cool slightly.
4. Using a pastry brush, brush the top with reserved caramel syrup. If the syrup has hardened, reheat in the sauce pan until liquid.

Cardamom Butter Cookies

*Servings: 12 | **Prep:** 10 m | **Style:** American | **Cook:** 23 m*

Ingredients

- 1/2 cup Blanched Almond Flour
- 1/4 tsp Baking Powder (Straight Phosphate, Double Acting)
- 1/2 tsp Salt
- 10 tbsps Unsalted Butter Stick
- 1/2 cup Sucralose Based Sweetener (Sugar Substitute)
- 1 large Egg (Whole)
- 1 tbsp Tap Water
- 2 tsps Vanilla Extract
- 4 2/3 servings All Purpose Low-Carb Baking Mix
- 3/4 tsp ground Cardamom

Directions

Please use the Atkins recipe for All Purpose Low-Carb Baking Mix (or the Gluten Free version) for this recipe. To make 12 servings you will need 1 1/2 cups of the mix. If you change the serving size for the recipe to up or downsize it you will need to adjust accordingly. Each serving of bake mix is 1/3 cup.

1. Heat oven to 350°F. Line 2 baking sheets with parchment paper; set aside.
2. Combine 1 1/2 cups baking mix, 1/2 cup almond flourl, baking powder, and salt in a medium bowl. Combine butter and sugar substitute in a large bowl; cream with an electric mixer on high speed until light and fluffy. Add egg, water, vanilla, and cardamom; beat on medium speed until combined, scraping down sides of bowl as necessary (mixture may look watery). Add flour mixture; mix on low speed until dough comes together.
3. Divide dough in half, and then in half again. Make 6 equal balls from each quarter portion of dough. Place 12 balls on each baking sheet. Press each gently with the tines of a fork in a crisscross pattern (optional); bake until lightly browned on the edges, about 10 minutes. Alternatively, place in the refrigerator for 30 minutes and then roll out between parchment; cut out shapes and bake. Transfer cookies to a wire rack to cool completely. Store in an airtight container for up to 1 week. Makes 2 cookies per serving.

Cherry Cobbler

*Servings: 8 | **Prep:** 30 m | **Style:** American | **Cook:** 40 m*

Ingredients

- 1/4 cup half Pecans
- 1/2 cup Sucralose Based Sweetener (Sugar Substitute)
- 3/4 tsp Cinnamon
- 1/4 tsp Salt
- 3 tbsps Unsalted Butter Stick
- 1/3 cup Heavy Cream
- 2 tbsps Sour Cream (Cultured)
- 1 large Egg (Whole)
- 3 cup, without pits Sweet Cherries
- 1/4 tsp Pure Almond Extract
- 2 1/4 servings All Purpose Low-Carb Baking Mix

Directions

Use the Atkins recipe to make All Purpose Low-Carb Baking Mix for this recipe. You will need 3/4 cup.

1. For biscuit: In a food processor, pulse baking mix, pecans, 2 tablespoons sugar substitute, 1/2 teaspoon cinnamon and salt until medium ground. Add butter and pulse until mixture resembles a coarse meal.
2. In a liquid measuring cup or bowl, whisk heavy cream, sour cream and an egg. Pour into food processor and pulse just until combined. Remove dough and pat into a flat disk. Cover with plastic wrap and chill 1 to 2 hours.
3. For filling and cobbler: Preheat oven to 400°F. In a medium bowl, toss cherries with 1/3 cup sugar substitute, almond extract and 1/4 teaspoon cinnamon. Pour filling into an 8-inch square or round baking dish. Divide dough into 8 pieces and pat into disks about 3 across.
4. Stagger biscuits over filling and bake cobbler 35 to 40 minutes, until biscuits are browned and cooked through and fruits are bubbly and tender. Serve with freshly whipped cream (optional).

Cherry Hazelnut Biscotti

Servings: 8 | Prep: 90 m | Style: Italian | Cook: 51 m

Ingredients

- 1 1/2 cups chopped Hazelnuts or Filberts
- 1 cup Whole Grain Soy Flour
- 3/4 cup Sucralose Based Sweetener (Sugar Substitute)
- 1 tsp Cinnamon
- 1/4 cup Sour Cream (Cultured)
- 4 large Eggs (Whole)
- 12 tbsps Unsalted Butter Stick
- 1/3 cup Bake-Dried Cherries
- 1/4 tsp Salt

Directions

1. Heat oven to 350°F.
2. Whisk together finely chopped hazelnuts, soy flour, ground cinnamon and salt. In a medium bowl mix sour cream, and eggs.
3. In a large bowl, with an electric mixer on medium speed, beat butter with sugar substitute for 3 minutes until creamy.
4. Add half the egg mixture, beat 30 seconds and scrape down the sides of the bowl with spatula. Repeat with remaining egg mixture. Turn mixer on low and add dry ingredients, mixing until just combined. Fold in cherries and coarsely chopped hazelnuts. Chill dough for 1 hour.
5. Divide dough in half. On ungreased baking sheets, form each dough half into a log measuring 12 x 2½ inches (moisten hands if necessary to keep dough from sticking). Bake logs 30 minutes, until almost firm. Transfer sheets to wire rack to cool 10 minutes.
6. Reduce oven temperature to 325°F. Carefully cut logs crosswise, with a serrated knife, into ½ wide slices. Arrange slices on baking sheets. Bake 17-20 minutes until firm and crisp. Cool slices on baking sheets before storing.

Chocolate and Flan Layered Mini Cakes

Servings: 8 | Prep: 20 m | Style: American | Cook: 50 m

Ingredients

- 2 1/2 tbsps Organic 100% Whole Ground Golden Flaxseed Meal
- 2 tsps Cocoa Powder (Unsweetened)
- 1/8 tsp Baking Soda

- 1/16 tsp Salt
- 2 large Eggs (Whole)
- 2 oz Sugar Free Chocolate Chips
- 1 1/2 tbsps Unsalted Butter Stick
- 1 tbsp Tap Water
- 2 tbsps Sour Cream (Cultured)
- 1 tsp Vanilla Extract
- 3 tbsps Cream Cheese
- 3/4 cup Heavy Cream
- 2/3 cup Coconut Cream
- 1 large Egg Yolk
- 2 tbsps Sucralose Based Sweetener (Sugar Substitute)
- 6 tbsps Sugar Free Caramel Syrup

Directions

Note: For best results, this recipe requires 6 hours of refrigeration before serving.

For the Cake:

1. Preheat oven to 350°F and adjust rack to the middle position. Grease six wells of a muffin tin.
2. Combine the flax meal, cocoa, baking soda and salt in a small bowl; set aside.
3. In a medium microwave safe bowl, combine the chocolate and butter. Microwave at 30 second intervals, stirring at each interval until melted; about 3 minutes total.
4. Whisk together the water, sour cream, 1/2 egg and 1/2 tsp vanilla. Add to the melted chocolate and stir until fully incorporated.
5. Stir in flax mixture until just combined. Divide the batter equally among the six muffin wells.

For the Flan:

1. Combine the cream cheese, heavy cream, coconut milk, 1 1/2 eggs, egg yolk, granular sugar substitute and 1/2 tsp vanilla in a blender and blend until smooth.
2. Pour the flan mixture over the cake batter until almost filled to the top. Place muffin tin in a large roasting pan and fill roasting pan with hot water until it reaches halfway up the sides of the muffin wells.
3. Bake until a toothpick inserted in the cake comes out clean and the flan reaches 180°F. As it cooks the cake will rise to the top of the muffin tin and the flan will remain below, if the cake is done on top and it has cooked for at least 50 minutes the flan should be the correct temperature.

4. Transfer the muffin tin to a wire rack and allow it to cool to room temperature, about 1 hour, cover with plastic wrap and refrigerate until fully set, about 6 hours or overnight.
5. To release the cakes, place bottom of muffin tin in the same roasting pan used for cooking and fill with 1-inch of hot tap water; allow to sit for 1 minute. Gently turn muffin tin upside down to release the flan and carefully transfer each to serving plates.
6. Drizzle 2 tablespoons sugar-free caramel or maple syrup over the cakes before serving.

Chocolate Donut Delight

Servings: *6 |* ***Prep:*** *5 m |* ***Style:*** *American |* ***Cook:*** *13 m*

Ingredients

- 1 large Egg (Whole)
- 4 oz Almond Butter
- 2 tbsps Cocoa Powder (Unsweetened)
- 6 tsps Erythritol
- 1/4 tsp Baking Powder (Straight Phosphate, Double Acting)
- 1/4 tsp Baking Soda
- 1/4 tsp Salt
- 1/2 14 oz can Coconut Cream
- 2 tsps Vanilla Extract

Directions

Note: For best results, this recipe requires 6 hours of refrigeration before serving.

For the Cake:

1. Preheat oven to 350°F and adjust rack to the middle position. Grease six wells of a muffin tin.
2. Combine the flax meal, cocoa, baking soda and salt in a small bowl; set aside.
3. In a medThis recipe is suitable for all phases except for the first two weeks of Induction due to the almond butter.
4. Preheat oven to 350°F. Prepare a 6-well donut pan with non-stick spray.
5. Place all ingredients in a blender or food processor, pulse a few times, scraping the container between pulses.

6. Pour into donut pan and bake for 13 minutes. Cool in pan for 10 minutes then turn out on a wire rack to cool completely.

Chocolate Ice Cream

Servings: 8 | Prep: 240 m | Style: American | Cook: 10 m

Ingredients

- 2 cups Heavy Cream
- 4 large Egg Yolks
- 10 packets Sucralose Based Sweetener (Sugar Substitute)
- 1/4 cup Cocoa Powder (Unsweetened)
- 2 tbsps Sugar Free Chocolate Syrup
- 1 tsp Vanilla Extract

Directions

1. Heat cream in a heavy saucepan over low heat. Whisk in egg yolks, one at a time. Cook over low heat, stirring constantly, until mixture coats the back of a spoon. Do not let boil.
2. Remove from heat. Whisk in sugar substitute, cocoa powder, chocolate syrup, and vanilla extract.
3. Cool to room temperature. Pour custard into an ice cream maker and freeze according to manufacturers instructions.

Chocolate Mint Cheesecake Bars

Servings: 24 | Prep: 270 m | Style: American | Cook: 20 m

Ingredients

- 2 oz Unsweetened Baking Chocolate Squares
- 2 1/4 cups Heavy Cream
- 1/4 cup Unsalted Butter Stick
- 1/2 cup Erythritol Powder

- 2 tsps Vanilla Extract
- 2 large Eggs (Whole)
- 1 1/3 cups Tap Water
- 1 3/4 cups Sucralose Based Sweetener (Sugar Substitute)
- 1/4 cup Cocoa Powder (Unsweetened)
- 1 cup Blanched Almond Flour
- 1 1/2 tsps Baking Powder (Straight Phosphate, Double Acting)
- 1/2 tsp Salt
- 1 package (1 oz) Gelatin Powder (Unsweetened)
- 16 oz Cream Cheese
- 1 tsp extract of Peppermint (Mint)
- 8 tbsps Sugar Free Chocolate Syrup

Directions

Be sure to use powdered erythritol (you will need about 1/2 cup granulated to make 1 cup powdered). It can be easily powdered in a blender. Measure it after it is powdered.

Bottom layer:

1. Preheat an oven to 350°F and grease a 9x13x2-inch non-stick pan; set aside. Melt the chocolate and 1/4 cup heavy cream in a small bowl in the microwave at 20 second intervals. Once melted mix to combine and set aside to cool.
2. Cream the butter and 1 cup powdered erythritol in a mixer for 5 minutes until light and fluffy. Add the vanilla and the eggs one at a time blending for 30 seconds between each egg. Add the cooled chocolate mixture, beating until thoroughly combined. Add 1/3 cup water and 1/2 cup sucralose, beat for 1 minute.
3. In a small bowl whisk together the cocoa powder, almond flour, baking powder and salt. Add to the batter and mix for another minute until fully blended. Pour batter into prepared pan and bake for 20 minutes or until a toothpick inserted in the center comes out clean. Allow to cool. While cooling prepare the top layer.

Top layer:

1. Add the packet of gelatin to 1 cup boiling water. Mix until all the gelatin dissolves then place in the refrigerator about 10 minutes (do not allow it to fully set-up, cool to room temperature only.)
2. In a medium bowl beat the softened cream cheese with 1 cup sucralose until fully blended and smooth. Add the peppermint extract and enough green food coloring to achieve desired color depth (about 1/4 teaspoon). When the gelatin has fully cooled, blend it into the cheese mixture.

3. Whip the remaining 2 cups cream with the remaining 1/4 cup sucralose until semi-stiff peaks form. Gently fold the cream into the cheese mixture until fully incorporated. Pour this over the cooled brownie layer in the pan and refrigerate for 4 hours or overnight.
4. When ready to serve, cut into 24 squares and top with 1 teaspoon of sugar-free chocolate syrup (Smucker's Sugar Free Sundae Syrup works great as it is a little thicker than regular syrup.) To make spider web: starting in the middle of the square make a spiral. Take a toothpick and from the center pull out in a straight line to the outer edge. Repeat 5-6 times spacing them equally.

Chocolate Mousse Mini Cheesecakes

Servings: 8 | *Prep:* 270 m | *Style:* American | *Cook:* 20 m

Ingredients

- 3 oz Unsweetened Baking Chocolate Squares
- 16 oz Cream Cheese
- 1/2 cup Sucralose Based Sweetener (Sugar Substitute)
- 3 large Eggs (Whole)
- 3/4 cup Heavy Cream
- 3/4 tsp Pure Almond Extract
- 1/2 tsp Vanilla Extract

Directions

Prep time includes 4 hours to chill. You'll need to bake the cheesecakes in a water bath. If you don't have instant boiling water, begin to boil a pot of water after Step 4. This recipe can be prepared ahead of time; wrap each custard cup tightly in plastic, place in an airtight container and freeze for up to 1 month.

1. Heat oven to 325°F.
2. Place eight 6-ounce ramekins in a roasting pan; set aside.
3. Heat chocolate in the microwave in 30-second increments until fully melted, about 1-2 minutes; set aside to cool slightly.
4. In the large bowl of an electric mixer, beat cream cheese on medium speed until lightened, scraping down sides of bowl as needed. Add chocolate and beat until combined. Add sugar substitute, beating until combined.
5. Add eggs, one at a time, beating well after each addition. Add cream and almond and vanilla extracts, beating until completely smooth.

6. Pour mixture into prepared custard cups. Carefully pour enough boiling water into roasting pan to come halfway up sides of ramekins.
7. Bake until the cheesecakes are puffed and the centers are just set, about 20 minutes. Remove from oven and let sit in the water bath for 10 minutes.
8. Transfer custard cups to a wire rack; cool to room temperature. Refrigerate until well chilled, 4 hours or overnight.
9. Garnish with mint sprigs, chocolate shavings and raspberries, if desired.

Chocolate Mudslide

Servings: 4 | Prep: 120 m | Style: American | Cook: 10 m

Ingredients

- 1 cup Heavy Cream
- 1/2 cup Tap Water
- 8 tbsps Sugar Free Chocolate Syrup
- 3 tbsps Cocoa Powder (Unsweetened)
- 1 tsp Vanilla Extract

Directions

1. In a medium saucepan combine cream, 1/2 cup syrup, water and cocoa powder.
2. Bring to a boil over medium heat.
3. Reduce heat to low; cook, stirring occasionally, 5 minutes. Remove from heat and stir in vanilla.
4. Pour mixture into two ice cube trays. Freeze 2 hours.
5. Before serving transfer cubes into a food processor and process until mixture is finely chopped and slushy. Serve immediately.

Chocolate Peanut Butter Haystacks

Servings: 18 | Prep: 10 m | Style: American | Cook: 5 m

Ingredients

- 1/4 cup Heavy Cream
- 2 tbsps Unsalted Butter Stick
- 3 tbsps Cocoa Powder (Unsweetened)
- 2 tbsps Xylitol
- 1 pinch Stevia
- 1/16 tsp Salt
- 1/4 cup Natural Creamy Peanut Butter 1/3 Less Sodium & Sugar
- 2 cups Unsweetened Flaked Coconut

Directions

1. Toast the coconut flakes on a sheet pan for 5 minutes at 350°F. Once toasted, fold into the chocolate mixture until coated.
2. Drop by tablespoons onto wax paper or a silicon mat on a sheet pan forming 18 mounds. Allow to cool and harden or place in refrigerator to harden quickly. May be stored in the refrigerator in an air tight container for up to two weeks or frozen for up to 3 months. Serve cold or at room temperature. One haystack = 1 serving.

Chocolate Peppermint Cupcakes

*Servings: 6 | **Prep:** 15 m | **Style:** American | **Cook:** 17 m*

Ingredients

- 1 large Eggs (Whole)
- 1/4 cup Coconut Milk Unsweetened
- 1/4 cup Xylitol
- 1 tsp Vanilla Extract
- 7 tbsps Unsalted Butter Stick
- 4 tbsps Organic High Fiber Coconut Flour
- 2 tbsps Cocoa Powder (Unsweetened)
- 1/4 tsp Baking Powder (Straight Phosphate, Double Acting)
- 1/4 tsp Salt
- 4 oz Cream Cheese
- 6 tsps Erythritol
- 1 serving Bob's Starlight Mints Peppermint Sugar Free Candy

Directions

1. Please powder the erythritol before making the frosting for this recipe. Place 2 tablespoons in a blender and pulse 3-4 times until powdered. To crush peppermint candies place them in a zip top bag and hit with a hammer.
2. Preheat oven to 375°F. Prepare a muffin tin with 6 paper cups. Set aside.
3. In a medium bowl whisk the eggs with the coconut milk, granular sugar substitute, vanilla, peppermint extract and 3 tablespoons melted butter. Set aside.
4. In a small bowl whisk together the coconut flour, cocoa powder, baking powder and salt. Add to egg mixture whisking to incorporate all ingredients for about a minute. Pour into the 6 paper cups, place in the oven and bake until fully set in the center; about 15-18 minutes. When done, set on a wire rack to cool.
5. Make Frosting: In a small bowl, beat the cream cheese with an electric mixer until smooth. Add 1/4 cup softened butter and continue to beat another minute. Add the powdered erythritol; beat another minute then add peppermint extract and food coloring as desired (optional; red is pretty as pictured and green is festive with the red and white candies). Adjust for sweetness by adding a pinch of stevia if desired. Frost cupcakes using a piping bag or by hand. Sprinkle with crushed peppermint candies.

Chocolate Walnut Cookies

Servings: *32 |* ***Prep:*** *20 m |* ***Style:*** *American |* ***Cook:*** *6 m*

Ingredients

- 1/8 cup 100% Stone Ground Whole Wheat Pastry Flour
- 2 tbsps Whole Grain Soy Flour
- 1/8 tsp Baking Soda
- 3/4 cup Sucralose Based Sweetener (Sugar Substitute)
- 1 1/2 oz Unsweetened Baking Chocolate Squares
- 5 tbsps Heavy Cream
- 2 large Eggs (Whole)
- 2 tbsps Unsalted Butter Stick
- 1 tsp Vanilla Extract
- 1/4 cup chopped English Walnuts

Directions

1. Preheat over to 350°F. Lightly toast walnuts in an even layer on a cookie sheet for 6 to 8 minutes. Cool, coarsely chop the walnuts and set aside.
2. Put oven up to 375°F. Line two baking sheets with parchment paper or aluminum foil; set aside.
3. Whisk 2 tbsp whole-wheat flour 2 tbsp soy flour and baking soda together in a bowl; set aside.
4. In the large bowl of an electric mixer, beat eggs and sugar substitute together on medium until light and slightly thickened. Place chocolate, cream and butter in a microwavable bowl; microwave on medium until butter has melted and chocolate has softened (it need not be completely melted), 1½ to 2 minutes. Let stand 5 minutes; stir until smooth.
5. Gradually beat the slightly warm chocolate mixture and vanilla extract into the egg mixture. Reduce speed to low, and beat in flour mixture, just until combined. Cover, and chill until thickened, 30 minutes.
6. Drop slightly rounded teaspoonfuls of dough, 1 inch apart, onto prepared sheet. Sprinkle tops of cookies with walnuts, lightly pressing into dough. Bake until cookies are just set but soft on top, 5½ to 6 minutes. Cool cookies on baking sheet 1 minute before transferring to wire racks to cool completely. Store in an airtight container.

Chocolate Yule Log

Servings: 10 | Prep: 20 m | Style: American | Cook: 12 m

Ingredients

- 1/3 second spray Original Canola Cooking Spray
- 1 1/3 cups Sucralose Based Sweetener (Sugar Substitute)
- 5 tbsps Cocoa Powder (Unsweetened)
- 9 large Eggs (Whole)
- 2 tbsps Whole Grain Soy Flour
- 1/4 tsp Salt
- 1 1/3 cups Heavy Cream
- 2 oz Unsweetened Baking Chocolate Squares
- 8 tbsps Unsalted Butter Stick
- 1/4 tsp Vanilla Extract

Directions

1. Preheat oven to 375°F. Spray a jellyroll pan with oil spray; line with parchment, leaving a 2-inch border, spray again. Set aside.
2. In a large bowl, whisk together 1 cup sugar substitute, 4 tablespoons cocoa powder and soy flour.
3. In another large bowl, beat egg yolks with an electric mixer on high speed until pale yellow and fluffy, about 3 minutes. Turn speed down to low and slowly mix in cocoa mixture until just combined.
4. In another bowl, beat egg whites and salt with an electric mixer on high speed until stiff peaks form, about 3 minutes. Fold 1/3 of the whites into yolk mixture until just combined. Fold in remaining egg whites. Spread batter evenly in prepared pan. Bake 15 minutes, until cake springs back when lightly touched and pulls away from sides of the pan. Cool cake in pan on wire rack for 30 minutes to 1 hour.
5. While cake is cooling, prepare filling and frosting. For the filling, whip 1 cup cream and 1 1/2 tablespoon sugar substitute in a medium bowl until stiff peaks form (do not overbeat).
6. For the frosting, gradually combine 1/3 cup cream and melted chocolate in a large bowl. With an electric mixer on medium speed, beat in butter, 5 tablespoons sugar substitute, 1 tablespoon cocoa powder and vanilla. Beat until smooth and fluffy, about 4 minutes. Chill in refrigerator until ready to use.
7. When cake is cool, slide cake from pan with parchment underneath. Place on counter top. Spread filling over cake, leaving a ½ inch border. Roll up cake from narrow end, using parchment to help. Cut 1-inch diagonal pieces from each end. Transfer roll to a serving platter; place cut diagonal pieces on either side to form log stumps. Set aside.
8. To assemble: Use a generous dab of frosting to attach stumps to main log. Frost entire log, and run fork tines through frosting to create a bark-like texture.

Chocolate-Cappuccino Mini Cupcakes

Servings: 18 | Prep: 15 m | Style: Other | Cook: 20 m

Ingredients

- 1 cup sliced Almonds
- 1 cup Whole Grain Soy Flour
- 1 tsp Baking Powder (Straight Phosphate, Double Acting)
- 1/2 cup Unsalted Butter Stick
- 1/2 cup Sucralose Based Sweetener (Sugar Substitute)

- 1 tbsp Cocoa Powder (Unsweetened)
- 1 tsp dry Coffee (Instant Powder)
- 2 oz or 1 scoops Chocolate Whey Protein
- 3 large Eggs (Whole)

Directions

1. Heat oven to 350°F. Spray mini muffin tins with cooking spray.
2. Process almonds in a food processor in pulses until finely ground. Add soy flour and baking powder; pulse to combine.
3. In a large bowl, beat butter and sugar substitute with an electric mixer until fluffy, about 2 minutes. Beat in cocoa powder, coffee powder, and 2 oz protein powder. Add eggs one at a time. Mix in almond mixture with a spatula. Divide batter in muffin tins, filling each 2/3 full. Bake 20 minutes, until set.

Chocolate-Coconut Haystacks

Servings: 32 | Prep: 15 m | Style: American | Cook: 12 m

Ingredients

- 2 large Egg Whites
- 1 cup Sucralose Based Sweetener (Sugar Substitute)
- 2 tbsps Cocoa Powder (Unsweetened)
- 16 oz Dried Coconut
- 2 tbsps Sugar Free Chocolate Syrup

Directions

1. Heat oven to 325°F. Line baking sheets with aluminum foil.
2. Whip egg whites on low until medium peaks form; gradually beat in sugar substitute and cocoa powder; continue beating until stiff peaks form. Fold in coconut and syrup.
3. Drop mixture by rounded teaspoonfuls onto prepared baking sheets. Shape into little pyramids with wet fingertips. Bake 12 minutes. Cool on sheets 1 minute before transferring to wire racks to cool completely.

Chocolate-Cream Frosty

Servings: *32* | **Prep:** *15 m* | **Style:** *American* | **Cook:** *12 m*

Ingredients

- 1/2 cup Tap Water
- 2 tbsps Heavy Cream
- 2 tbsps Sugar Free Chocolate Syrup

Directions

1. Place water, cream and syrup in a blender along with 3 ice cubes and blend until frothy.

Chocolate-Ginger Cake

Servings: *16* | **Prep:** *20 m* | **Style:** *Other* | **Cook:** *45 m*

Ingredients

- 1/3 second spray Original Canola Cooking Spray
- 3/4 cup half Pecans
- 4 oz Unsweetened Baking Chocolate Squares
- 1/3 cup Tap Water
- 1/3 cup Canola Vegetable Oil
- 1/4 cup Cocoa Powder (Unsweetened)
- 1/4 cup dry Whole Grain Soy Flour
- 2 1/4 cups Sucralose Based Sweetener (Sugar Substitute)
- 12 large Eggs (Whole)
- 2 tsps Ginger (Ground)
- 1/4 tsp Cream Of Tartar

Directions

1. Preheat over to 350°F. Toast pecans in an even layer on a cookie sheet for 8 minutes. Cool, coarsely chop the pecans and set aside.

2. Lower oven to 325°F. Grease the bottom of a 10-inch tube pan, and line with parchment or waxed paper.
3. Place chocolate and the water in a microwavable bowl; microwave on high 1 to 2 minutes, until chocolate is melted, checking at 1-minute intervals. Stir until smooth, cool to lukewarm, then stir in oil; set aside.
4. In a food processor, pulse pecans, cocoa powder and soy flour until pecans are finely ground. In a large bowl, beat egg yolks with cup sugar substitute on high speed with an electric mixer, until light and fluffy, about 5 minutes. Stir in melted chocolate, pecan mixture and ginger.
5. In another large bowl, beat egg whites and cream of tartar on medium-high speed with an electric mixer, until frothy. Gradually add remaining sugar substitute, beating until stiff peaks form. With a rubber spatula, fold one-third of the meringue into the yolk mixture to lighten; fold in the remaining meringue until just combined.
6. Pour batter evenly in prepared pan and bake until a toothpick inserted in center of cake comes out clean, about 45 minutes. Allow cake to cool for 30 minutes before removing from pan.
7. To remove: Run a knife around the inner and outer rim of cake, place a wire rack or plate over pan, and invert. Remove pan, and peel off paper. Cool completely before cutting into 16 servings.

Chocolate-Mint Mousse Layer Cake

Servings: 8 | Prep: 180 m | Style: Other | Cook: 25 m

Ingredients

- 1/3 second spray Original Canola Cooking Spray
- 1 cup Heavy Cream
- 2 tsps Vanilla Extract
- 1/2 oz Coffee (Instant Powder)
- 1 1/4 cup dries Whole Grain Soy Flour
- 1/2 cup Cocoa Powder (Unsweetened)
- 1/2 cup half Pecans
- 1/2 tsp Baking Powder (Straight Phosphate, Double Acting)
- 1/2 tsp Salt
- 1 cup Unsalted Butter Stick
- 1 cup Sucralose Based Sweetener (Sugar Substitute)
- 8 servings Chocolate Mint Mousse
- 4 large Eggs (Whole)

Directions

Use the Atkins recipe for Chocolate-Mint Mousse (See recipe).

1. Preheat oven to 325°F. Grease two 8 round cake pans with oil spray.
2. In a small bowl, mix cream, vanilla and coffee. Set aside. In a medium bowl, whisk together soy flour, cocoa, pecans, baking powder and salt. Set aside. In a large bowl, with an electric mixer on medium speed, beat butter with half of the sugar substitute until light and fluffy, about 5 minutes. Separate the eggs into yolks and whites. Add egg yolks, one at a time, beating well and scraping down the sides of the bowl after each addition. Add heavy cream mixture and beat until well-blended. Turn mixer speed down to low, and slowly add dry ingredients, one third at a time, beating until just-combined. Set aside.
3. In another large bowl, beat egg whites until soft peaks form, about 3 minutes. Add remaining sugar substitute and beat until stiff peaks, about 1 more minute. Using a rubber spatula, fold whites into chocolate batter in three parts, combining thoroughly after each addition.
4. Divide batter in prepared pans; smooth tops. Bake 20 minutes, or until cake springs back when touched in the middle. Cool in pans on racks 5 minutes; invert onto racks to cool completely, about 2 hours.
5. To assemble cake: Cut off rounded tops of each cake. Place one cake layer on a serving plate, cut side down. Spread top with half of mousse filling, leaving a 1/2 border. Place cut side of the other cake layer down on top of the mousse, pressing gently, being careful not to let mousse squirt out. Top this with remaining mousse and swirl decoratively. Garnish with raspberries and mint leaves. Makes 8 servings.

Chocolate-Peanut Whip

Servings: 1 | Prep: 5 m | Style: American

Ingredients

- 1 tbsp Cocoa Powder (Unsweetened)
- 1 tbsp Natural Creamy Peanut Butter 1/3 Less Sodium & Sugar
- 2 tsps Sucralose Based Sweetener (Sugar Substitute)
- 2 tbsps Heavy Cream

Directions

1. Using a spatula, blend together 1 Tbsp unsweetened cocoa powder, 1 Tbsp smooth peanut butter and 1 packet of sweetener.
2. Whip 2 Tbsp heavy cream until soft peaks form.
3. Gently fold into the peanut butter mix. This is also delicious with almond butter instead of peanut butter.

Chunky Mocha Ice Cream

Servings: 8 | Prep: 240 m | Style: American | Cook: 5 m

Ingredients

- 1 tsp Gelatin Powder (Unsweetened)
- 1 cup Tap Water
- 6 large Egg Yolks
- 1 cup Sucralose Based Sweetener (Sugar Substitute)
- 2 1/2 cups Heavy Cream
- 1/2 cup Cocoa Powder (Unsweetened)
- 4 tsp roundeds Coffee (Instant Powder, Decaffeinated)
- 1 tsp Vanilla Extract
- 1/2 tsp Salt
- 3 bars Snack Caramel Double Chocolate Crunch Bar

Directions

1. Sprinkle gelatin over water and let soften, about 5 minutes.
2. In a medium bowl, whisk yolks and sugar substitute to combine.
3. In a medium pot, mix cream, gelatin mixture, cocoa powder and coffee. Cook over medium-low heat, stirring occasionally, until cocoa and coffee granules have dissolved and mixture has begun to simmer.
4. Slowly pour 1 cup of hot cocoa mixture over egg yolk mixture, whisking constantly. Pour mixture back into pot. Cook, stirring constantly, until mixture is thick enough to coat the back of a spoon. Remove from heat. Stir in vanilla and salt. Chill mixture 4 hours.
5. Pour mixture into ice cream maker. Process according to manufacturer's directions. About 5 minutes before ice cream is finished, add the chopped bars.

Cinnamon Custard

Servings: 6 | Prep: 20 m | Style: Mexican | Cook: 30 m

Ingredients

- 2 cups Heavy Cream
- 1/2 tsp Cinnamon
- 2 large Eggs (Whole)
- 1/2 cup Sucralose Based Sweetener (Sugar Substitute)
- 1/8 tsp Salt
- 1/2 tsp Vanilla Extract
- 6 tbsps Caramel Sugar Free Syrup
- 2 large Egg Yolks

Directions

This delectable Mexican dessert can be prepared a day ahead, covered with plastic wrap and refrigerated.

1. In a medium-size heavy saucepan, combine cream and cinnamon. Heat over medium heat, whisking constantly to thoroughly blend cinnamon into cream, just until cream begins to steam. Do not boil. Remove from heat.
2. Heat oven to 300°F.
3. In a medium bowl, whisk eggs, egg yolks, sugar substitute and salt together until pale yellow and slightly thickened.
4. Using a soup ladle and whisking constantly, very gradually pour in the hot cream. When all the cream has been added, whisk in the vanilla extract.
5. Pour about 1/2 cup of the cream mixture into each of six 4-ounce custard cups (or pour entire mixture into a 2-quart round baking dish).
6. Place the cups or baking dish in a roasting pan. Carefully pour enough boiling water(about 4 cups) in the roasting pan to come halfway up the sides of the cups or baking dish.
7. Bake until custard is still slightly loose in center, about 30 minutes. (Bake the baking dish about 5 minutes more).
8. Using an oven mitt, carefully remove cups from water bath.
9. Serve warm, at room temperature or cold, toping each serving with 1 tablespoon of caramel syrup.

Cinnamon-Almond Meringues

Servings: 8 | *Prep*: 120 m | *Style*: French | *Cook*: 90 m

Ingredients

- 1/2 cup whole Almonds
- 10 individual packets Sucralose Based Sweetener (Sugar Substitute)
- 3 large Egg Whites
- 1/2 tsp Pure Almond Extract
- 1/2 tsp Cinnamon
- 1/8 tsp Cream Of Tartar

Directions

This recipe is suitable for all phases except the first two weeks of Induction due to the almonds.

1. Heat oven to 200°F. Line a baking sheet with aluminum foil.
2. In a food processor, chop nuts with sugar substitute until nuts are finely ground.
3. In a large bowl, with electric mixer at high speed, beat egg whites until soft peaks form. Add the cream of tartar, almond extract and cinnamon beating until stiff peaks form. Gently fold in nut mixture.
4. With a spoon, drop 8 evenly spaced mounds onto prepared baking sheet. Make a depression in center of each with the back of the spoon. Bake meringues on center oven rack 1½ hours, until golden and very dry. Turn off oven and let meringues dry in oven until cool. Carefully peel meringues off foil.

Classic Apple Tart

Servings: 8 | *Prep*: 30 m | *Style*: American | *Cook*: 45 m

Ingredients

- 5 medium (2-3/4" dia) (approx 3 per lb) Apples (Without Skin)
- 1/4 cup Sucralose Based Sweetener (Sugar Substitute)

- 3/4 tsp Cinnamon
- 1/8 tsp Nutmeg (Ground)
- 1 serving Atkins Cuisine Pie Crust
- 1 tbsp Unsalted Butter Stick

Directions

1. Prepare Atkins Cuisine Pie Crust (see recipe) and press evenly into a 10-inch tart pan with removable bottom. Freeze 15 minutes.
2. Heat oven to 350°F. In a large bowl, combine apples, sugar substitute, cinnamon and nutmeg. Toss until apples are evenly coated. Spoon into crust; dot top with butter.
3. Bake tart 30 minutes. Cover loosely with foil and bake 10 to 20 minutes more, until apples are tender when pierced with the tip of a knife. Cool tart on wire rack.
4. Serve warm or at room temperature, with ice cream and praline sauce, if desired.

Classic Chocolate Cupcakes

Servings: 12 | **Prep:** 10 m | **Style:** American | **Cook:** 22 m

Ingredients

- 1 cup Unsalted Butter Stick
- 9 tbsps Xylitol
- 3 large Eggs (Whole)
- 4 tsps Vanilla Extract
- 5 fl ozs Heavy Cream
- 3 tbsps Tap Water
- 2 tbsps Organic High Fiber Coconut Flour
- 1 cup Blanched Almond Flour
- 1/3 cup Cocoa Powder (Unsweetened)
- 1/2 tsp Baking Powder (Straight Phosphate, Double Acting)
- 1/4 tsp Baking Soda
- 1/4 tsp Salt
- 2 oz Unsweetened Baking Chocolate Squares
- 1 tsp dry Coffee (Instant Powder)

Directions

Cupcakes:

1. Preheat oven to 325°F. Line a muffin tin with 12 paper or foil liners.
2. Beat 1/2 cup softened butter with 5 tablespoons xylitol until light and fluffy; about 3 minutes. Add the eggs one at a time until fully incorporated, then add 3 tsp vanilla, 2oz (about 1/4 cup) heavy cream, water and coconut flour. Blend thoroughly.
3. In a sepatate bowl whisk to combine the almond flour, cocoa powder, baking powder, baking soda and salt. Add to the wet ingredients and beat until smooth and thick. Divide into the muffin liners and bake for 20-25 minutes or until fully cooked, be careful not to over bake or they will be bitter. Allow to cool in the muffin tin for 5 minutes then transfer to a baking rack to cool.

Frosting:

1. Melt the chocolate with 3oz (about 1/3 cup) heavy cream in the microwave at 20 second intervals. Stir and allow to cool completely. Once cooled whisk in 4 tablespoons xylitol. Set aside.
2. In a very small bowl stir to combine the 1 tsp vanilla, 1 tsp cocoa powder (optional) and 1 tsp instant coffee. Set aside.
3. Transfer cooled chocolate to a medium bowl and beat with the remaining 1/2 cup butter on medium speed until lighter in color and fluffy. Add the reserved vanilla mixture and beat to combine.
4. Using a piping bag and fancy tip or simply a quart-sized plastic bag with a corner cut off, pipe the frosting onto the cupcakes. Garnish with an Atkins Endulge Chocolate Peanut Candy if desired.

Coconut Cookies

Servings: 12 | Prep: 8 m | Style: American | Cook: 27 m

Ingredients

- 1/3 second spray Original Canola Cooking Spray
- 1/2 cup Whole Grain Soy Flour
- 1/3 cup Dried Coconut
- 1/4 cup whole Hazelnuts or Filberts
- 2 large Egg Whites
- 1/8 can Seltzer Water
- 1 1/2 tsps Coconut Extract

- 1/2 tsp Vanilla Extract
- 1/2 tsp Salt
- 8 tbsps Unsalted Butter Stick
- 7 tbsps Sucralose Based Sweetener (Sugar Substitute)

Directions

1. Preheat oven to 350°F. Toast hazelnuts in an even layer on a cookie sheet for 8 minutes. Cool, coarsely chop and set aside.
2. Increase oven temperature to 375°F. Grease baking sheet with cooking spray.
3. In large bowl, combine soy flour, unsweetened coconut, hazelnuts, egg whites, 2 Tbsp seltzer, 1 1/2 tsp coconut and 1/2 tsp vanilla extract., salt, butter and sugar substitute. Mix well.
4. Drop by rounded 1 tablespoonful (12 cookies) onto prepared baking sheet. Bake 20 minutes, or until light golden brown. Cool cookies on baking sheet 1 minute before transferring to wire racks to cool completely.

Coconut Lemon Ice Cream with Blackberry-Peach Compote

Servings: 8 | Prep: 480 m | Style: American | Cook: 10 m

Ingredients

- 1 pinch Stevia
- 1/2 cup Xylitol
- 3 cups Coconut Cream
- 1/16 tsp Salt
- 4 large Egg Yolks
- 1/2 cup Lemon Juice
- 4 servings Blackberry-Peach Compote

Directions

1. Use the Atkins recipe to make Blackberry-Peach Compote. The recipe suggests 4 servings of the compote, 1 serving is 1/4 cup. Based on the serving size recommended for the ice cream, it is suggested to use only 2 tablespoons of the compote for each serving. If you would like to add more please add 2.1g NC for each additional 2 tablespoons of compote to the NC value listed for this recipe.

2. Combine 2 cups coconut cream and a pinch of salt in a medium sauce pan. Heat until almost boiling. While the coconut cream is heating, combine the egg yolks, granular sugar substitutes and lemon zest. Whisk to combine.
3. Slowly pour the coconut cream into the egg yolk mixture while whisking continuously. Once incorporated transfer mixture back to the sauce pan over medium-high heat. Cook while stirring continuously until it reaches 170°F and begins to coat the back of a wooden spoon, do not allow the mixture to boil.
4. Set mixture over an ice water bath and stir in the remaining 1 cup coconut cream and 1/2 cup lemon juice. Cool to room temperature then transfer to the refrigerator. Keep in the refrigerator overnight or at least 4 hours to intensify flavors and chill properly.
5. Once chilled, place into ice cream maker and follow manufacturers instructions to make ice cream. Enjoy immediately or put into a freezer-safe container and freeze for at least 4 hours or up to one month. Makes about 1 quart of ice cream, 1 serving is about 1/2 cup. Before serving place in the refrigerator 20-30 minutes. To serve, dip ice cream scoop into hot water and dish up ice cream. Top with 2 tablespoons Blackberry-Peach Compote.

Coconut Macaroons

Servings: 30 | Prep: 20 m | Style: American | Cook: 12 m

Ingredients

- 1/3 second spray Original Canola Cooking Spray
- 4 large Egg Whites
- 2/3 cup Sucralose Based Sweetener (Sugar Substitute)
- 1/2 tsp Vanilla Extract
- 1/4 tsp Salt
- 2 cups Dried Coconut

Directions

1. Heat oven to 325°F. Spray two baking sheets with oil spray.
2. With an electric mixer on medium speed, beat egg whites until medium peaks form. Gradually beat in sugar substitute, vanilla extract and salt. Turn speed up to high and continue beating until stiff (but not dry) peaks form.
3. Using a rubber spatula, fold in coconut.

4. Drop tablespoon-sized mounds of mixture onto prepared baking sheets. Bake 15 minutes. Cool on sheets 1 minute before carefully transferring to wire racks to cool completely.

Coconut Panna Skullotta

Servings: 12 | Prep: 240 m | Style: American

Ingredients

- 1 14 oz can Coconut Cream
- 2 oz Gelatin Powder (Unsweetened)
- 2 cups Heavy Cream
- 1/2 cup Sucralose Based Sweetener (Sugar Substitute)
- 1 tsp Vanilla Extract
- 2 tsps Coconut Extract

Directions

1. Plastic skull molds can be found at hobby stores in the baking section and during seasonal promotions. Cake pans also work nicely, just be sure your mold will hold 4 fluid cups.
2. Pour 1 cup of the coconut milk into a medium bowl. Sprinkle with the gelatin and let stand until softened, about 1 minute
3. In a small saucepan, combine the remaining coconut milk with the cream. Heat over medium heat, stirring, until small bubbles begin to form along the sides of the pan. Pour over the gelatin mixture. Stir in sucralose and mix well. Allow to cool to room temperature.
4. Once the mixture has cooled, stir in the vanilla and 2 tsp coconut extract. Spray a 4-cup mold with cooking spray, pour in the gelatin mixture, cover with plastic wrap and refrigerate overnight or until set; at least 4 hours. To serve, pull the panna cotta away from the mold at the edges then carefully invert onto a plate. Garnish with unsweetened shredded coconut if desired.

Coconut Shortcakes with Berries and Cream

Servings: 6 | Prep: 20 m | Style: American | Cook: 12 m

Ingredients

- 1/4 cup Whole Grain Soy Flour
- 1 tsp Baking Powder (Straight Phosphate, Double Acting)
- 6 tbsp raws Unsweetened Shredded Coconut
- 4 tbsps Sucralose Based Sweetener (Sugar Substitute)
- 3 tbsps Unsalted Butter Stick
- 1 large Egg (Whole)
- 1 tsp Coconut Extract
- 1 2/3 cups Heavy Cream
- 1 tsp Vanilla Extract
- 1 1/4 cups Red Raspberries
- 1 1/4 cups Strawberries
- 1/2 cup Blueberries

Directions

1. Heat oven to 375°F. In a large mixer bowl, combine soy flour, baking powder, ¼ cup coconut, 3 tablespoons sugar substitute and the melted butter. Make a well in center and add egg, coconut extract and 2/3 cup heavy cream. Whisk the liquid ingredients together until blended, then combine with the dry mixture, mixing just until blended.
2. Drop the mixture by slightly rounded ¼ cupfuls onto a baking sheet to make 6 mounds. Using fingertips, shape each into 2½ rounds; divide and sprinkle remaining coconut over tops. Cover with plastic wrap and refrigerate 20 minutes. Bake 12 minutes, until lightly golden around edges and firm to the touch. Transfer to a wire rack and cool completely.
3. Meanwhile, with an electric mixer on medium-high, beat together remaining 1 cup heavy cream, 1 tablespoon sugar substitute and the vanilla extract to soft peaks. Whisk 1 tbsp sugar-free jam (if using) in a medium bowl until smooth; add raspberries, sliced strawberries and blueberries, tossing gently until coated.
4. To serve, split the shortcakes in half horizontally. Spread 1/3 cup whipped cream on the bottom of each shortcake. Spoon ½ cup of the berries over whipped cream and cover with shortcake top. Top with a dollop of whipped cream, if desired.

Coconut-Cashew Chocolate Truffles

Servings: 32 | Prep: 10 m | Style: French

Ingredients

- 3/4 cup Heavy Cream
- 2 tbsps Sucralose Based Sweetener (Sugar Substitute)
- 2 tbsps Unsalted Butter Stick
- 14 oz Sugar Free Chocolate Chips
- 3 oz Unsweetened Baking Chocolate Squares
- 3/4 tsp Vanilla Extract
- 8 oz Dried Coconut
- 1/2 cup Organic Raw Cashews

Directions

1. Combine cream, sugar substitute and butter in a small saucepan. Bring to a simmer. Place chopped chocolate in a medium bowl; pour hot cream mixture over chocolate. Let stand 5 minutes.
2. Stir chocolate mixture gently until chocolate is completely melted. Stir in extract and 1/2 cup of the coconut. Refrigerate until firm, about 1 hour 45 minutes, stirring occasionally (Truffles will be easier to form if the mixture is not too stiff).
3. Toast the remaining 1/2 cup coconut in a dry skillet over medium heat, shaking often, until lightly browned; transfer to a bowl and cool.
4. Roll the chocolate mixture into 32 balls about the size of large marbles. Roll half of the balls in cashews and half in toasted coconut. Place in an airtight container between layers of wax paper. Can refrigerate up to one week.

Coconut-Lime Mousse

Servings: 4 | *Prep:* 10 m | *Style:* American

Ingredients

- 2 oz Cream Cheese
- 4 individual packets Sucralose Based Sweetener (Sugar Substitute)
- 1/4 cup Fresh Lime Juice
- 1 tsp Vanilla Extract
- 1 cup Heavy Cream

Directions

1. Using an electric mixer, beat together 2 oz soft cream cheese and 4 packets of granular sugar substitute (equivalent to 8 teaspoons) until smooth.
2. Slowly add 1/4 cup lime juice, beating until creamy.
3. Beat in 1 teaspoon coconut extract (vanilla may be used if coconut is unavailable) and 1 cup heavy cream until fluffy.
4. Place in four bowls, sprinkle with 1 Tbsp unsweetened coconut flakes each (optional, don't forget to add in .4g NC carbs) and refrigerate until serving.

Coeur a la Creme

Servings: 6 | Prep: 720 m | Style: French

Ingredients

- 4 oz Cream Cheese
- 1/4 cup, small curd (not packed) Cottage Cheese
- 1/4 cup Sour Cream (Cultured)
- 1/2 cup Heavy Cream
- 4 tsps Sucralose Based Sweetener (Sugar Substitute)
- 1 tsp Vanilla Extract
- 1/8 tsp Salt

Directions

1. To prepare molds: Poke several holes in bottoms of disposable muffin tins. Wet cheesecloth, wring out and fold in half. Drape cheesecloth over tin and press into molds, leaving a 2-inch overhang along border of tin. Set aside.
2. To prepare Coeur: In a food processor, pulse cream cheese, cottage cheese and sour cream until smooth, scraping sides occasionally as needed. Transfer to large bowl and set aside.
3. In another medium bowl, with an electric mixer on medium-high speed, whip cream, sugar substitute, vanilla and salt until stiff peaks form, about 4 minutes. In three additions, fold whipped cream into cheese mixture.
4. Divide among tins, cover with overhanging cheesecloth. Place tin on rack over baking sheet. Refrigerate for 12 to 24 hours or until solid. If desired, serve with a berry purée, sweetened with sugar substitute.

Coffee Eggnog

*Servings: 4 | **Prep:** 5 m | **Style:** Other*

Ingredients

- 1 tsp Sucralose Based Sweetener (Sugar Substitute)
- 1/2 tsp Vanilla Extract
- 1 cup (8 fl oz) Coffee (Brewed From Grounds, Decaffeinated)
- 1 cup Heavy Cream
- 4 fl oz (no ice) Rum
- 2 large Eggs (Whole)
- 1/8 tsp Cinnamon

Directions

1. In a small bowl, beat eggs and sugar substitute. Add vanilla, coffee, cream and rum (if using); mix thoroughly.
2. Sprinkle top with cinnamon. Enjoy!

Cranberry Parfait

*Servings: 8 | **Prep:** 180 m | **Style:** French*

Ingredients

- 1 cup whole Cranberries
- 8 oz Sugar Free French Vanilla Syrup
- 2 scoops Vanilla Whey Protein
- 3 cups Tap Water
- 2 1/2 package (1 oz) Gelatin Powder (Unsweetened)
- 4 individual packets Sucralose Based Sweetener (Sugar Substitute)

Directions

1. In a blender, combine cranberries, vanilla syrup and shake mix. Purée until smooth.

2. In a mixing bowl, pour 1 cup cold water; sprinkle gelatin into water and let stand 1 minute.
3. Combine remaining 2 cups water with sugar substitute and bring to a boil (either in a microwave or on the stovetop). Add hot water mixture to gelatin mixture; stir until gelatin dissolves.
4. Add berry mixture and stir until smooth. Pour into eight custard cups. Chill at least 3 hours to set.

Cranberry-Raspberry Gelatin Dessert

Servings: 6 | Prep: 180 m | Style: American

Ingredients

- 2 package (1 oz) Gelatin Powder (Unsweetened)
- 1/2 cup Tap Water
- 2 cup (8 fl oz) Low Calorie Cranberry Juice Drink with Vitamin C Added
- 8 tbsps Raspberry Sugar Free Syrup
- 2 tsps Fresh Lemon Juice

Directions

1. Place gelatin in a large bowl. Bring water to a boil. Pour water over gelatin; stir until dissolved.
2. Add cranberry juice, raspberry syrup, and lemon juice. Mix well.
3. Divide mixture in 6 dessert glasses. Chill until gelled, about 3 hours.

Dark Mocha Pudding

Servings: 8 | Prep: 10 m | Style: American | Cook: 10 m

Ingredients

- 2 cups Organic Coconut Milk
- 1/2 cup Heavy Cream
- 1/8 tsp Salt

- 1/3 cup Erythritol Powder
- 3 tsps Sucralose Based Sweetener (Sugar Substitute)
- 2 large Egg Yolks
- 1 tsp dry Coffee (Instant Powder)
- 1 tbsp Cocoa Powder (Unsweetened)
- 1/2 tsp Thick-It-Up
- 1 tsp Vanilla Extract
- 2 oz Sugar Free Chocolate Chips
- 1 tbsp Unsalted Butter Stick

Directions

1. Place 1 3/4 cups of the coconut milk in a sauce pan with the heavy cream, salt and granular sugar substitutes. Bring to a simmer over medium heat.
2. While the milk is heating, whisk the egg yolks with the remaining 1/4 cup coconut milk and instant coffee. Once the milk mixture is hot pour a steady stream in the egg yolks while whisking to temper them. Once all the milk has been incorporated pour the mixture back into the sauce pan over medium heat. While it is heating back up, quickly whisk together the cocoa powder and Thick-It-Up in a small bowl then whisk it into the milk and egg mixture. Cook and stir pudding continuously to be sure the egg does not curdle. Cook until it begins to thicken (mixture will still be slightly runny); about 2-3 minutes. Do not allow pudding to boil. Take off the heat once thickened; about 3-5 minutes.
3. Melt the chocolate with the butter in small bowl in a microwave at 30 second intervals. Do not overheat. Stir to blend and then scrape into the hot pudding stirring to blend completely. Remove from heat.
4. Cool quickly over an ice water bath; place plastic wrap on the surface to prevent a skin from forming. Once cooled place in the refrigerator to continue cooling or immediately dish into serving bowls, top with whipped cream if desired and serve. Makes 2 2/3 cups. Each serving is 1/3 cup. This pudding is very rich, consider serving it in a small glass dish layered with whipped cream.

Decadent Chocolate Cake

Servings: 12 | Prep: 15 m | Style: American | Cook: 45 m

Ingredients

- 4 oz Unsweetened Baking Chocolate Squares

- 1/2 cup Unsalted Butter Stick
- 1 tbsp Tap Water
- 3/4 cup Sucralose Based Sweetener (Sugar Substitute)
- 2 tbsps Cocoa Powder (Unsweetened)
- 1 tsp Vanilla Extract
- 6 large Eggs (Whole)

Directions

1. Heat oven to 325°F. Grease an 8-inch spring form pan and line the bottom with parchment paper; grease paper and set aside.
2. Melt chocolate, butter and water in the top of a double boiler set over simmering water, stirring to combine. Remove from heat and transfer to a large bowl; cool to room temperature. Add ¼ cup of the sugar substitute, the cocoa powder and vanilla extract to chocolate mixture, stirring until combined.
3. In a medium bowl, with an electric mixer on medium-high, beat eggs until mixture forms thick ribbons when beater is lifted, about 6 minutes. Reduce speed to medium; gradually add remaining ½ cup sugar substitute and beat until combined, 1 minute. Stir one-third of the egg mixture into the chocolate mixture to lighten. In two additions, fold in remaining egg mixture until well combined.
4. Pour batter into prepared pan, smoothing top. Bake until evenly risen and almost set, 40-45 minutes (it will look like a brownie). Cool completely on a wire rack. To serve, run a knife around edge of pan and remove rim. Cut into 12 pieces and serve with whipped cream (optional).

Decadent Chocolate Ice Cream

Servings: 8 | **Prep:** 240 m | **Style:** American | **Cook:** 20 m

Ingredients

- 2 large Egg Yolks
- 3 cups Heavy Cream
- 4 large Eggs (Whole)
- 3/4 cup Cocoa Powder (Unsweetened)
- 3/4 cup Sucralose Based Sweetener (Sugar Substitute)
- 1/4 tsp Salt
- 2 tsps Vanilla Extract
- 1/2 tsp Pure Almond Extract

Directions

1. Pour heavy cream into a heavy-bottomed 3-quart saucepan and place over medium heat. Allow to simmer but do not boil. Remove from heat and set aside.
2. In a large mixing bowl, combine the eggs, yolks, cocoa powder, sugar substitute and salt. With an electric mixer on medium, beat until thickened and smooth, 2 to 3 minutes, scraping sides of bowl with a rubber spatula. Using a ladle, remove about a cup of the hot cream from the pan, and gradually whisk into egg mixture (this tempers the eggs so they won't curdle). While whisking, pour tempered egg mixture into remaining cream in saucepan.
3. Place over medium heat and whisk until slightly thickened and coats the back of a wooden spoon; temperature should not go over 170°F.
4. Pour into a clean bowl, whisk in extracts and let stand until custard is cooled to room temperature, about 1 1/2 hours or place in a clean bowl set in a larger bowl filled with an ice water bath to chill quickly to room temperature. Refrigerate 2 hours, until well chilled, or cover with plastic wrap and refrigerate overnight to develop more flavor.
5. Freeze in ice cream maker according to manufacturers directions. When freezing process is complete, serve immediately for soft serve ice cream, or for firm ice cream, place in an airtight container and freeze 2 to 4 hours or overnight. (Can be stored in the freezer up to 1 month.) Makes about 1 quart; each serving = 1/2 cup. This recipe is acceptable in Phase 1; however the serving size would need to be decreased to 1/4 cup = 3.6g NC.

Double Chocolate Cookies

Servings: 18 | *Prep*: 10 m | *Style*: American | *Cook*: 20 m

Ingredients

- 1/4 cup Unsalted Butter Stick
- 1/4 cup Xylitol
- 1 tsp Vanilla Extract
- 1 large Egg (Whole)
- 1 1/2 cups Blanched Almond Flour
- 2 tbsps Cocoa Powder (Unsweetened)
- 1/4 tsp Baking Soda
- 1/4 tsp Salt
- 3 packs Endulge Chocolate Candies

Directions

This recipe is suitable for all phases except for the first two weeks of Induction due to the nuts. Xylitol usually comes granulated but does not melt into the wet ingredients as well as regular sugar. For this reason be sure to measure the xylitol first and then powder it in a blender for 3-4 pulses. 1 cookie = 1 serving.

1. Preheat an oven to 350°F. Use a silpat mat or parchment paper on the cookie sheet.
2. Beat the softened butter with the powdered xylitol until light and fluffy; about 3 minues. Add the vanilla and egg and beat until combined.
3. Combine all the remaining dry ingredients except the candies, stir to blend and then add to the wet ingredients. Blend until fully incorporated then add the candies.
4. Form into 18 x 1-inch balls, spacing 1-inch apart and flatten slightly on the prepared cookie sheet. Bake for 10 minutes, remove from oven and allow to sit for 5 minutes then move to a cooling rack. Cookies may be stored in an airtight container at room temperature for up to 2 days.

Earl Grey Tea and Chocolate Pots de Crème

*Servings: 4 | **Prep:** 75 m | **Style:** French | **Cook:** 40 m*

Ingredients

- 1 1/2 oz Unsweetened Baking Chocolate Squares
- 1 cup Heavy Cream
- 2/3 cup Tap Water
- 3 tea bags Tea Bags
- 4 large Egg Yolks
- 5 tbsps Sucralose Based Sweetener (Sugar Substitute)

Directions

1. Heat oven to 325°F. Place chocolate in a small bowl.
2. In a small saucepan over medium heat, bring cream and water to a simmer. Remove from heat.
3. Pour just enough cream mixture over chocolate to cover (about ½ cup). Add tea bags to remaining cream mixture in saucepan and let steep 10 minutes. Squeeze tea bags over mixture and remove.

4. Whisk chocolate mixture until smooth. Whisk egg yolks and sugar substitute into the warm cream mixture in saucepan until well mixed, then whisk in the chocolate until smooth. Pour mixture through a strainer into four 4-ounce ramekins or custard cups.
5. Place cups in a large roasting pan. Place roasting pan in oven and carefully pour boiling water into pan until water comes halfway up sides of cups. Cover entire pan with foil and bake 33-35 minutes, until custards are set but slightly jiggly in center.
6. Let stand in pan at room temperature 15 minutes. Remove cups, cover with plastic wrap (stretch wrap over edges of cup so wrap does not touch custard) and refrigerate until cold. Serve topped with a dollop of whipped cream, if desired.

Endulge Chocolate Cups

Servings: 1 | Prep: 20 m | Style: American

Ingredients

- 1 1/2 oz Sugar Free Chocolate Chips

Directions

1. Line a muffin tin compartment with a paper cupcake liner. Place chocolate pieces in a Pyrex measuring cup. Microwave on 20 percent power for 30 seconds. Stir, and repeat process until pieces are melted but haven't completely lost their shape. Stir until smooth.
2. With a pastry brush, coat inside of cupcake liner with a layer of chocolate. Refrigerate 4 to 5 minutes, until chocolate sets. Repeat process until all the chocolate is used up. When chocolate is hardened, carefully peel off liner.
3. Cups may be made ahead, covered in plastic and stored in a cool place for up to 5 days.

Endulgent Chocolate-Covered Strawberries

Servings: 24 | Prep: 25 m | Style: American

Ingredients

- 8 oz Sugar Free Chocolate Chips
- 24 large (1-3/8" dia) Strawberries

Directions

1. Line a baking sheet with aluminum foil or waxed paper. Break chocolate bars into pieces; place in the top part of a double boiler or a metal bowl set over (but not touching) a pot of simmering water. Stir one to two minutes, until chocolate is melted. Remove from heat.
2. Holding each strawberry by the stem, dip in chocolate, leaving a 1/4inch border at the top. Gently shake off excess chocolate; place berry on foil. Repeat with remaining berries. Reheat chocolate if necessary.
3. Chill berries 40 minutes, until chocolate is set. May be prepared up to a day ahead.

Extra-Creamy Strawberry Shake

Servings: 2 | Prep: 5 m | Style: American

Ingredients

- 6 medium (1-1/4" dia) Strawberries
- 2 scoops Strawberry Whey Protein
- 1/2 cup Heavy Cream
- 1 tsp Vanilla Extract
- 2 cups Tap Water
- 2 individual packets Sucralose Based Sweetener (Sugar Substitute)

Directions

1. Place strawberries, protein mix, cream, vanilla, water, and sugar substitute in a blender and blend at high speed until very smooth.

Firecracker Popsicles

*Servings: 6 | **Prep:** 240 m | **Style:** American*

Ingredients

- 1 cup Blueberries
- 1 cup Raspberries
- 1 cup Coconut Milk
- 6 tsps Xylitol
- 1/2 packet Stevia
- 1/2 tsp Coconut Extract

Directions

1. Puree the blueberries with 2 teaspoons xylitol and a pinch of stevia, set aside in a small bowl.
2. Puree the raspberries with 2 teaspoons xylitol and a pinch of stevia, set aside in a small bowl. If the raspberries are not very sweet add additional stevia to taste.
3. In a small bowl combine the coconut milk with 2 teaspoons xylitol, a pinch of stevia and 1/2 teaspoon of either coconut or vanilla extract.
4. Layer the popsicle mold: Start with the coconut milk, add 2-3 tablespoons then add a couple of tablespoons of each of the raspberry and blueberry purees, layering as you go. Once the popsicle is filled to about 1/2-inch from the top, take a knife, stick it in the center and gently swirl the knife to get the firecracker effect.
5. Freeze for at least 3 hours. May be kept frozen for up to 1 month. To release from the molds, run hot water over the molds until they slip off easily; about 5-10 seconds.

Fresh Berry Tarts with Cream

*Servings: 4 | **Prep:** 15 m | **Style:** American | **Cook:** 10 m*

Ingredients

- 2/3 cup, slivered Almonds
- 1/2 cup Fresh Blueberries
- 1/4 cup Heavy Cream
- 1/2 cup Red Raspberries
- 2 tbsps Sucralose Based Sweetener (Sugar Substitute)

Directions

1. Heat broiler. Chop almonds and divide among 4 small ramekins. Sprinkle 1 tablespoon sugar substitute over the almonds. Place ramekins on a cookie sheet and broil until the tops of the nuts are golden and the sugar substitute has melted. Remove and cool until at room temperature.
2. Whip the heavy cream and remaining tablespoon of sugar substitute until doubled in volume. Place one-quarter of blueberries and one-quarter of raspberries in each ramekin and top with a dollop of whipped cream. Serve immediately.

Frozen Chocolate Fudge Tart

Servings: 12 | Prep: 210 m | Style: American | Cook: 20 m

Ingredients

- 5 tbsps Cocoa Powder (Unsweetened)
- 1/2 tsp Cinnamon
- 7 tbsps Sucralose Based Sweetener (Sugar Substitute)
- 4 tbsps Unsalted Butter Stick
- 3 oz Cream Cheese
- 4 oz Sugar Free Chocolate Chips
- 2 tsps Vanilla Extract
- 2 1/2 cups Heavy Cream
- 1 2/3 servings All Purpose Low-Carb Baking Mix
- 1 tsp dry Coffee (Instant Powder)

Directions

1. Preheat oven to 425°F.
2. For the crust: In a food processor, pulse the 1/2 cup baking mix, 4 tablespoons cocoa powder, cinnamon and 3 tablespoons granular sugar substitute to combine, about 10 seconds. Add cold chopped butter and pulse until mixture resembles a coarse meal, about 30 seconds. Add cream cheese and pulse until mixture begins to come together, about 30 more seconds.
3. Transfer dough to a 9-inch pie plate and pat into an even layer on bottom and sides. Prick the dough about 15 times with a fork and crimp edges decoratively. Cover lightly with aluminum foil and bake 10 minutes, until

set. Uncover and bake 10 more minutes until light golden brown. Cool crust before filling.

4. For the filling: Place chocolate and 1 teaspoon vanilla extract in a medium bowl. Heat one cup cream and instant coffee over medium-high heat until just about to boil, about 4 minutes. Pour over chocolate, let stand 3 minutes, then stir until chocolate is melted. Pour into pie shell, smooth top and chill 30 minutes.

5. In a medium bowl with an electric mixer on high speed, beat remaining cream, 4 tablespoons sugar substitute, 1 teaspoon vanilla extract and 1 tablespoon cocoa powder until medium peaks form, about 4 minutes. Spread over chocolate layer and freeze at least 2.5 hours or until firm. Remove from freezer 10 minutes before serving.

Frozen Peanut Butter Chocolate Cheesecake Bombs

Servings: 12 | *Prep:* 60 m | *Style:* American

Ingredients

- 6 oz Cream Cheese
- 1/3 cup Natural Creamy Peanut Butter 1/3 Less Sodium & Sugar
- 2 tbsps Xylitol
- 1 tsp Vanilla Extract
- 1 pinch Stevia
- 1 cup Heavy Cream
- 1/8 tbsp Xanthan Gum
- 3 bars Snack Caramel Double Chocolate Crunch Bar

Directions

1. Powder the xylitol before using. To do this place 2 tablespoons in a blender and pulse 3-4 times until powdered.
2. Beat softened cream cheese with a mixer on medium speed until creamy. Add peanut butter, powdered granular sugar substitute, and vanilla; beat to combine. Taste and increase sweetness if desired by adding a pinch of stevia.
3. Add 1 cup cream and 1/4 teaspoon xanthan gum (optional, helps decreases ice crystal formation when frozen); beating until light and fluffy.
4. Cut Atkins bars lengthwise into three segments then finely chop the segments; fold into mixture. Using a 2 tablespoon scoop or measure drop onto a wax paper covered baking sheet (small enough to fit in your freezer

or use a silicon mold filling each with 2 Tbsp). Place in the freezer until fully frozen; at least 4 hours. To serve, eat directly from the freezer or place 2 on a serving plate and allow to partially thaw in the refrigerator for 30 minutes. The recipe makes 24 bombs. Each serving is 2 bombs (or 4 Tbsp total).

Frozen Peppermint Pie

Servings: 8 | Prep: 20 m | Style: American

Ingredients

- 1 cup Heavy Cream
- 6 pieces Sugar Free Starlite Mints
- 1 tbsp Organic Virgin Coconut Oil
- 1/2 cup Almond Meal Flour
- 5 servings Atkins Snack Dark Chocolate Decadence Bar
- 8 servings Easy Peppermint Ice Cream

Directions

Use the Atkins recipe to make Easy Peppermint Ice Cream; you will need 1 full recipe (about 3 cups). Please note, you can use vanilla sugar free ice cream instead of the Easy Peppermint Ice Cream but it will add about 5g NC to each serving. If you choose to do this you will need 12 mints (crushed) - add half of them to the ice cream mixture and the other half to the top.

1. Allow the ice cream to sit at room temperature for about 20 minutes to soften.
2. Chop the Atkins Dark Chocolate Decadence bar into 1 inch pieces. Place in a food processor and process until it resembles fine crumbs. Add the coconut oil and almond meal and process until combined. Press into a pie place and place in the freezer while preparing the rest of the filling.
3. Whip heavy cream to firm peaks. Fold together the softened ice cream with the whipped cream and pour into the prepared pie shell. Sprinkle crushed peppermint candies on the top and place in the freezer until fully set (about 1 hour).

Ginger Flan

Servings: 6 | Prep: 180 m | Style: French | Cook: 25 m

Ingredients

- 3 large Egg Yolks
- 2 large Eggs (Whole)
- 1 1/2 cups Heavy Cream
- 1 cup Tap Water
- 8 individual packets Sucralose Based Sweetener (Sugar Substitute)
- 1 tsp Vanilla Extract
- 3 tsps Ginger

Directions

1. Heat oven to 350°F. Place a roasting pan on center shelf in oven and fill almost half way with boiling water.
2. In a blender, combine egg yolks and whole eggs, cream, water, sugar substitute, vanilla, and ginger until very smooth.
3. Pour through a sieve into a shallow 1-quart baking dish. Carefully place dish in roasting pan (water should come up halfway up sides). Bake 30-35 minutes until a knife inserted in center comes out clean.
4. Transfer to wire rack; cool to room temperature. Spray a piece of plastic wrap with cooking spray, lay directly over flan and chill 3 hours in refrigerator.
5. Remove plastic wrap and un-mold by placing a platter or plate over the top and inverting the platter onto a table so that the pan is now upside down on the platter. Remove top pan.

Ginger Ice Cream with Caramelized Pears

Servings: 10 | Prep: 180 m | Style: American | Cook: 10 m

Ingredients

- 1 small (approx 3 per lb) Pear
- 3 1/2 cups Heavy Cream

- 1/2 cup Tap Water
- 1/4 cup slices (1" dia) Ginger
- 7 large Egg Yolks
- 2 tsps Unsalted Butter Stick
- 4 tbsps Sugar Free Vanilla Syrup
- 2/3 cup Sucralose Based Sweetener (Sugar Substitute)

Directions

1. Combine cream, water and ginger in a heavy, medium saucepan over medium heat. Bring almost to a boil; remove from the heat and let stand 10 minutes.
2. Whisk egg yolks and sugar substitute in a large bowl until lightened and thick. Gradually whisk half of the hot cream into egg mixture; return mixture to pan. Cook, stirring constantly, over medium heat until mixture registers 170°F on an instant-read thermometer or is thick enough to coat the back of a spoon.
3. Strain through a fine-mesh strainer into an airtight container, pressing with a spoon to extract liquid from ginger solids. Cover and refrigerate until cold. Pour mixture into ice cream maker and churn according to manufacturer's instructions.
4. Transfer to an airtight container and freeze until ready to serve. Just before serving, melt butter in a small skillet over high heat; add pear and cook until tender and lightly browned, 3 to 4 minutes. Pour syrup into a small serving bowl; stir pear into syrup. Scoop ice cream into bowls; top with pears.

Holiday Cookies

Servings: 24 | Prep: 25 m | Style: American | Cook: 12 m

Ingredients

- 1 cup Whole Grain Soy Flour
- 3 tsps Baking Soda
- 3 tbsps Sucralose Based Sweetener (Sugar Substitute)
- 4 oz Cream Cheese
- 2 tbsps Unsalted Butter Stick
- 2 tbsps Sour Cream (Cultured)
- 1 large Egg (Whole)
- 1 tsp Vanilla Extract

Directions

1. Preheat oven to 350°F. Line a baking sheet with parchment paper and set aside.
2. In a food processor, pulse soy flour, baking soda, sugar substitute, cream cheese and butter for 30 seconds, until texture resembles a coarse meal.
3. In a small bowl, mix together sour cream, egg and vanilla extract. Add sour cream mixture to soy mix mixture and pulse until just-combined, about 15 seconds. Chill in freezer 10 minutes or until firm.
4. Roll dough out between 2 sheets of plastic wrap or waxed paper to 1/8 thickness. Using cookie cutters, cut out dough in desired shapes. Arrange cookies on prepared baking sheet and bake cookies 10-12 minutes, until lightly golden. Allow to cool completely before decorating.

Indulgent Espresso Chocolate Cake

Servings: 8 | **Prep:** 25 m | **Style:** American | **Cook:** 35 m

Ingredients

- 10 oz Sugar Free Chocolate Chips
- 10 tbsps Unsalted Butter Stick
- 1 tsp rounded Coffee (Instant Powder, Decaffeinated)
- 1 tbsp Tap Water
- 1 tsp Vanilla Extract
- 1/4 tsp Salt
- 24 tsps Erythritol
- 1 pinch Stevia
- 4 large Eggs (Whole)
- 1/3 cup Cocoa Powder (Unsweetened)

Directions

1. Preheat oven to 325°F. Grease an 8-inch round baking pan and line with parchment paper (a spring form pan works best). Set aside.
2. Melt chocolate and butter in a double boiler. Remove from heat and transfer to a large bowl. Alternatively melt chocolate with butter in a small bowl in the microwave at 30 second intervals; stirring in between. In a small cup, mix espresso powder, water, vanilla and salt; stir into chocolate. Set mixture aside to cool.

3. With an electric mixer on medium-high speed, beat eggs, 1/2 cup (24 tsp) granular sugar substitute, stevia and cocoa powder until it falls in thick ribbons when the beater is lifted, about 6 minutes. In three additions, fold eggs into the chocolate mixture.
4. Pour batter into prepared pan and smooth top. Bake 30-35 minutes, or until a toothpick inserted near middle of cake comes out with a few moist crumbs and cake is evenly raised. Cool completely on a wire rack. To remove cake, run a knife around edge of pan. Dip bottom of pan into hot water for 1 minute, then turn cake out onto cutting board. (if using a spring form pan, carefully remove sides and serve on the platter.) Turn right side up onto a serving platter. Serve with whipped cream and raspberries (Phase 2 or Atkins 40 only), if desired.

Irish Coffee

Servings: 6 | Prep: 5 m | Style: Other | Cook: 10 m

Ingredients

- 36 fl ozs Decaffeinated Coffee
- 3 tsps Sucralose Based Sweetener (Sugar Substitute)
- 9 fl oz (no ice) Whiskey
- 1/2 cup Heavy Cream

Directions

1. In a small saucepan, warm whiskey over medium-low heat (do not boil). Stir sugar substitute and whiskey into brewed coffee.
2. In the small bowl of an electric mixer, beat heavy cream on medium to soft peaks.
3. Divide coffee among 6 cups, and top each with a dollop of whipped cream.

Lemon Mousse

Servings: 8 | Prep: 180 m | Style: French | Cook: 20 m

Ingredients

- 1 package (1 oz) Gelatin Powder (Unsweetened)
- 1/4 cup Fresh Lemon Juice
- 7 large Eggs (Whole)
- 6 individual packets Sucralose Based Sweetener (Sugar Substitute)
- 1 1/2 fl oz (no ice) Brandy
- 1 1/2 cups Heavy Cream

Directions

1. For this recipe substitute Grand Marnier or orange liquor for the brandy to give it more citrus flavor. If you prefer not to consume uncooked egg whites, use a powdered egg white product (sold in the baking section of most supermarkets) instead.
2. In a medium bowl, dissolve gelatin in lemon juice. Set bowl over a saucepan of simmering water (water should not touch the bottom of the bowl). Separate the whites from the yolks; place the whites in a large bowl and place the yolks into a sauce pan.
3. Whisk together the egg yolks and sugar substitute. Cook while whisking constantly over medium-high heat until a candy thermometer registers 170°F (about 4 minutes). Remove from heat; stir in brandy or orange liqueur. Transfer to a large bowl.
4. With an electric beater, beat egg whites until stiff peaks form; set aside. In another large bowl whip the cream until stiff peaks form. Fold egg whites into yolk-gelatin mixture until combined. Gently fold in whipped cream. Taste for sweetness; adjust if necessary. Cover with foil and refrigerate until well chilled.

Low Carb Pumpkin Pecan Cheesecake

Servings: 10 | Prep: 25 m | Style: Other | Cook: 50 m

Ingredients

- 1 1/2 cup halves Pecan Nuts
- 1 tbsp Sucralose Based Sweetener (Sugar Substitute)
- 1/2 tsp Cinnamon
- 2 tbsps Unsalted Butter Stick
- 1 large Egg White
- 24 oz Cream Cheese

- 1 cup Heavy Cream
- 2/3 cup Sucralose Based Sweetener (Sugar Substitute)
- 15 oz Pumpkin (Without Salt, Canned)
- 1 tsp Vanilla Extract
- 1 tsp Pumpkin Pie Spice
- 3 large Eggs (Whole)

Directions

To make crust:

1. Heat oven to 350°F.
2. In a food processor, combine pecans, 1 tablespoon sugar substitute and cinnamon. Process until finely ground. Add the butter (melted) and egg white and pulse a few times to combine; press onto the bottom of a 9-inch springform pan, rounding up to cover the pan seam. Bake until golden and set, 8 to 10 minutes. Cool completely on a wire rack.

To make filling:

1. Reduce oven to 325°F.
2. Combine cream cheese, 2/3 cup sugar substitute and cream in a large bowl. With an electric mixer at medium speed, beat until smooth. Add pumpkin purée, vanilla and pumpkin pie spice, mixing to combine. Beat in eggs, one at a time, just until combined.
3. Pour batter over crust. Bake until just set, 45 to 50 minutes. Turn off oven and let stand 10 minutes; transfer to a wire rack and cool completely.
4. Cover and refrigerate until chilled, 4 hours or overnight. Slice and serve.

Low-Carb Chocolate Blueberry Cheesecake Tartlets

*Servings: 12 | **Prep:** 360 m | **Style:** American | **Cook:** 40 m*

Ingredients

- 2 cups Almond Meal Flour
- 4 tbsps Cocoa Powder (Unsweetened)
- 1 tbsp Sucralose Based Sweetener (Sugar Substitute)
- 1/4 cup Unsalted Butter Stick
- 6 oz Cream Cheese
- 1/2 cup Ricotta Cheese (Whole Milk)

- 2 large Eggs (Whole)
- 1/2 tsp Vanilla Extract
- 1/2 cup Sucralose Based Sweetener (Sugar Substitute)
- 1 cup Fresh Blueberries
- 1 tbsp Tap Water
- 1 large Egg Yolk

Directions

1. Preheat oven to 350°F. Liberally grease the cups of a 12-cup muffin tin, or 2 x 12 mini muffin pans or use muffin papers. In a medium bowl, whisk together almond meal, 3 tablespoons cocoa powder, and Splenda. Pour in butter and stir with fork until it forms coarse crumbs. Place one heaping tablespoon of almond crust into the bottom of each mini muffin tin or about 2 1/2 tablespoons in the regular muffin tin wells or paper cups. Using your fingers, press gently to work dough down and up the sides of the tin. Repeat until all muffin tins are filled. Place pan in oven and bake 5-7 minutes. Remove from oven and let cool.
2. Place cream cheese, ricotta cheese, eggs, vanilla, 1 tablespoon cocoa powder, and Splenda into a blender, and puree until smooth and free of lumps. Pour cream cheese mixture evenly into cooled crusts, leaving 1/4-inch rim of space at the top of each cup. Place pan back in oven and bake for 30-35 minutes for large muffin tins or 10-12 minutes for mini muffin tins, until the batter is no longer wet and firms around the edges. Remove from heat and let cool to room temperature.
3. Prepare the topping. In a small saucepan, add blueberries and water over medium heat. Bring to simmer, mashing blueberries with the back of a wooden spoon, until blueberries are hot and have released their juices. Place your egg yolk in a small bowl. Whisking swiftly and continuously, add a tablespoon of warm blueberry juice to yolks to temper. Repeat again two more times until yolk is tempered. Whisking quickly and constantly, pour tempered yolk into pan with blueberries. Stir, cooking, until blueberries are significantly thickened. Remove from heat and let cool slightly. Set aside to cool.
4. Spoon blueberry topping evenly over the tops of the cheesecake cups, spreading to cover evenly. Place muffin tin in refrigerator and let cool 4-5 hours or overnight, until chilled completely. To serve, carefully pop cheesecake cups out of muffin tin and place on serving tray. Two per person if using the mini muffin tins or 1 per person if using the regular muffin tins.

Mascarpone Parfait

*Servings: 4 | **Prep**: 15 m | **Style**: Italian*

Ingredients

- 1 cup Heavy Cream
- 8 oz Mascarpone
- 1 tbsp Sucralose Based Sweetener (Sugar Substitute)

Directions

1. In the large bowl of an electric mixer, beat heavy cream on medium-high to soft peaks.
2. Reduce speed to medium; add mascarpone and sugar substitute, beating just until smooth, 15 to 30 seconds. Divide and spoon the cream mixture into four parfait cups.
3. Garnish with mint sprigs and lemon peel, if desired.

Mexican Hot Chocolate Souffle

*Servings: 2 | **Prep**: 15 m | **Style**: French | **Cook**: 17 m*

Ingredients

- 1 tsp Unsalted Butter Stick
- 9 tsps Erythritol
- 4 tbsps Sugar Free Chocolate Chips
- 2 large Egg Yolks
- 1/2 fl oz Tap Water
- 1 tsp Vanilla Extract
- 3/4 tsp Cinnamon
- 1/8 tbsp Red or Cayenne Pepper
- 3 large Egg Whites
- 1 pinch Stevia

Directions

1. Preheat oven to 400°F. Grease the bottom and up the sides of a 2-cup deep souffle dish with butter and sprinkle 1 1/2 teaspoons granular sugar substitute (erythritol) to coat all buttered areas. Set aside.
2. Melt the chocolate in a small bowl in a microwave at 30 second intervals until melted through. Do not overheat and stir between intervals.
3. In a medium bowl whisk 2 egg yolks with 1 tablespoon warm water, 1 teaspoon vanilla, 3/4 teaspoon ground cinnamon and 1/8 teaspoon cayenne pepper (add more if more spice is desired). Add the melted chocolate and whisk until incorporated and smooth. Set aside.
4. In a medium bowl whip the egg whites with 2 1/2 tablespoons granular sugar substitute (erythritol) and a large pinch of stevia to stiff peaks. Whisk a few tablespoons of the egg whites into the chocolate mixture, then quickly but gently fold in the remaining egg whites until a lighter airy mixture results and all ingredients are blended (do not over blend or you will deflate the egg whites).
5. Pour into the souffle dish and bake on a sheet pan for 15-18 minutes. The souffle will rise over the top of the dish and it should appear slightly jiggly but not wet in the center when shaken. Serve immediately.

Mixed Berry Shortcakes

Servings: 6 | Prep: 35 m | Style: Other | Cook: 15 m

Ingredients

- 1 cup Whole Grain Soy Flour
- 1 tsp Baking Powder (Straight Phosphate, Double Acting)
- 2 2/3 tbsps Sucralose Based Sweetener (Sugar Substitute)
- 1 tsp Salt
- 6 tbsps Unsalted Butter Stick
- 1 2/3 cups Heavy Cream
- 1/4 cup Sour Cream (Cultured)
- 1 cup whole Strawberries
- 1 large Egg (Whole)
- 1 cup Blueberries
- 1 cup Raspberries
- 1/2 cup half Pecans

Directions

1. Preheat oven to 375°F.
2. In a food processor, pulse flour, baking powder, pecans, 3 tablespoons of the sugar substitute and salt until nuts are finely ground. (If you don't have a food processor, grind the nuts in a nut or coffee grinder.)
3. Add the butter and pulse until its the texture of cornmeal. In a liquid measuring cup or bowl, whisk 2/3 cup of the heavy cream, sour cream and egg. Pour evenly over the dry mixture and pulse just until combined.
4. Chill dough for 30 minutes. Separate dough into 12 equal-sized pieces (you'll need about 3 1/2 tablespoons of dough for each piece). Put each piece into a disk measuring 2 1/2 to 3-inches across. Space disks evenly on baking sheet, leaving 1 inch between biscuits to allow for spreading during the baking process.
5. Bake shortcakes about 20 minutes, until bottoms are golden brown. Cool on baking sheet set on a wire rack.
6. With an electric mixer on medium speed, beat remaining cup of heavy cream with remaining 2 teaspoons sugar substitute until soft peaks form.
7. To assemble: Dollop 1/4 cup whipped cream on 6 six shortcakes, top with 1/2 cup berries and cover with remaining shortcakes.

Mocha Granita

*Servings: 6 | **Prep:** 195 m | **Style:** Other*

Ingredients

- 1 cup Tap Water
- 1 cup (8 fl oz) Coffee (Brewed From Grounds)
- 10 individual packets Sucralose Based Sweetener (Sugar Substitute)
- 1/3 cup Cocoa Powder (Unsweetened)
- 4 tbsps Sugar Free Chocolate Syrup

Directions

1. Mix water, coffee, and sugar substitute in a heavy saucepan over medium heat. Whisk in cocoa powder and syrup. Bring mixture to a gentle boil.
2. Simmer, stirring constantly, 3 minutes. Remove from heat; pour mixture through a fine strainer into a large measuring cup. Refrigerate until cold.
3. Pour mixture into ice cube trays, filling only half way. Freeze until firm. Before serving, process chocolate cubes in a food processor until chopped and slushy.

4. Serve immediately.

Mocha-Hazelnut Ice Cream

Servings: 12 | Prep: 255 m | Style: Other | Cook: 18 m

Ingredients

- 3 1/2 cups Heavy Cream
- 3 oz Unsweetened Baking Chocolate Squares
- 1/3 cup Cocoa Powder (Unsweetened)
- 3 tsp roundeds Coffee (Instant Powder, Decaffeinated)
- 6 large Egg Yolks
- 1 cup Sucralose Based Sweetener (Sugar Substitute)
- 1 tbsp Vanilla Extract
- 1/3 cup chopped Hazelnuts or Filberts

Directions

1. In a medium saucepan, combine 3 cups of the cream, chocolate, cocoa powder and coffee granules; cook over medium-low heat, stirring occasionally, until chocolate melts and mixture just begins to simmer. Remove from heat and cool to room temperature. Whisk until smooth.
2. In a medium bowl, whisk egg yolks, remaining 1/2 cup cream and sugar substitute together until blended. Gradually whisk 1 cup of chocolate mixture into yolk mixture; add to saucepan with remaining chocolate mixture and whisk to combine.
3. Cook over medium-low heat, stirring constantly, until mixture coats the back of a spoon (175°F on a candy thermometer), about 3 minutes. Remove from heat; stir in vanilla and cool slightly.
4. Pour custard into a glass or metal bowl; cover with plastic wrap and refrigerate for 4 hours or overnight. Pour custard into ice-cream maker; freeze according to manufacturers directions.
5. During last 5 minutes, add hazelnuts. Transfer to an airtight container, cover and freeze for 4 hours or overnight. Let stand at room temperature until soft enough to scoop, about 15 minutes.

Molten Chocolate Cake

Servings: 4 | *Prep:* 5 m | *Style:* American | *Cook:* 8 m

Ingredients

- 6 tbsps Unsalted Butter Stick
- 2 oz Baking Chocolate Squares
- 2 large Egg Yolks
- 1 tbsp Whole Grain Soy Flour
- 2 large Eggs (Whole)
- 1/3 cup Sucralose Based Sweetener (Sugar Substitute)
- 1 tsp Vanilla Extract

Directions

1. Preheat oven to 375°F.
2. Generously grease four 6-ounce custard cups with butter and dust with sugar substitute. Place cups on a baking sheet.
3. Place butter and chocolate in a double boiler over medium heat and cook until just melted, about 3 minutes (or 1 minute in a microwave on high). Remove from heat and let cool to room temperature.
4. Pour chocolate mixture into a large bowl; add soy flour and stir until just combined. Set aside.
5. In a large bowl, beat eggs, egg yolks, sugar substitute and vanilla with an electric mixer on high speed until almost firm peaks form, about 4 minutes.
6. In three additions, fold egg mixture into chocolate mixture.
7. Divide batter in cups. Bake 8 -9 minutes until a toothpick inserted near edge comes out clean and inserted in center comes out with some batter.
8. Cool 3 minutes. Run knife around edge, turn upside down to release onto serving plates. Serve immediately. Makes 4 servings.

Old Fashioned Bread Pudding

Servings: 6 | *Prep:* 40 m | *Style:* Other | *Cook:* 60 m

Ingredients

- 1/2 cup Sucralose Based Sweetener (Sugar Substitute)
- 1 cup Heavy Cream
- 1 cup Tap Water
- 6 large Eggs (Whole)

- 1 tsp Vanilla Extract
- 1 tsp Cinnamon
- 8 servings Atkins Cuisine Bread

Directions

1. If you have a vanilla bean, use the seeds scraped from 1 whole bean. Instead of 1 teaspoon cinnamon substitute 1 3-inch cinnamon stick.
2. Preheat oven to 350°F. Generously butter a 9x9 -inch baking pan; set aside.
3. In a large bowl, whisk together eggs and sugar substitute.
4. In a medium saucepan over medium heat, bring cream, water, vanilla and cinnamon to a boil. Slowly whisk hot cream mixture into egg mixture. Add bread and toss well. Let stand 10 minutes, turning occasionally with a rubber spatula.
5. Transfer pudding mixture into to prepared pan. Place pan in a larger roasting pan, fill the outer pan with enough hot water to come half way up the sides of the pudding pan.
6. Bake for until set, about 55 minutes. Let cool for 15 minutes before cutting. Serve warm or chilled. Makes 6 servings.

Panna Cotta

Servings: 6 | Prep: 195 m | Style: Italian | Cook: 5 m

Ingredients

- 1 package (1 oz) Gelatin Powder (Unsweetened)
- 2 cups Heavy Cream
- 8 individual packets Sucralose Based Sweetener (Sugar Substitute)
- 1 tsp Vanilla Extract

Directions

1. Lightly oil 6 6-ounce custard cups. In small bowl sprinkle gelatin over 3 tablespoons cold water, let sit 5 minutes until softened.
2. Meanwhile, in medium saucepan combine heavy cream, 1/2 cup water, sugar substitute and scrapped out vanilla bean seeds or use vanilla extract. Bring to a boil over medium heat.

3. Remove from heat, add gelatin mixture; stir until melted. Pour mixture into prepared cups. Cover surface with plastic wrap to prevent skin from forming. Refrigerate at least 3 hours.
4. Turn out onto serving plates.

Passover Angel Food Cake with Rhubarb-Strawberry Sauce

Servings: 12 | *Prep*: 120 m | *Style*: Italian | *Cook*: 30 m

Ingredients

- 1 cup Matzo Meal
- 1 1/2 cups Sucralose Based Sweetener (Sugar Substitute)
- 1/2 tsp Salt
- 1 3/4 large Egg Whites
- 2 tsps Vanilla Extract
- 1/2 tsp Pure Almond Extract
- 12 oz Rhubarb
- 1 cup half Strawberries

Directions

For the cake: Heat oven to 375°F.

1. In a bowl, whisk cake meal, 1 1/4 cup sugar substitute and salt to combine. Place mixture in a wire sieve set over the bowl. With an electric mixer on medium, beat egg whites until stiff peaks form. Stir in extracts.
2. In three additions, sift dry ingredients over the whites, gently folding in with a rubber spatula. Transfer batter to a 10 tube pan.
3. Bake 30 minutes, until cake begins to pull away from the sides of the pan. Invert cake in pan over a funnel or bottle neck, if pan does not have feet. Cool completely, about 1 1/2 hours.
4. With narrow spatula or knife, loosen cake from sides of pan and gently shake onto serving plate.

For the sauce:

1. In a medium pot, mix rhubarb, 1/2 cup strawberries, 1/4 cup sugar substitute and 1/4 cup water. Cook over medium heat 15 minutes, until rhubarb falls apart. Reduce heat and stir frequently during the last 5 minutes of cooking time.

2. Remove from heat; transfer to a bowl and fold in remaining strawberries. Cool completely and serve with cake. Makes 12 servings.

Peach-Buttermilk Sherbert

Servings: 8 | *Prep*: 1440 m | *Style*: American | *Cook*: 20 m

Ingredients

- 3 medium (2-1/2" dia) (approx 4 per lb) Peaches
- 1/2 cup Xylitol
- 1 pinch Stevia
- 1/4 cup Fresh Lemon Juice
- 1/2 tsp Salt
- 1 cup Buttermilk (Reduced Fat, Cultured)
- 1 cup Heavy Cream

Directions

1. Coarsely dice peaches. In a medium pan combine the peaches and granular sugar substitutes; cook over medium heat for 15-20 minutes until very soft. Remove from heat and allow to cool for 10 minutes.
2. In a blender puree the peaches and cooking juices with lemon juice and salt (adjust to your taste). Add the buttermilk and cream. Mix to combine and place in the refrigerator overnight or at least 4 hours to chill.
3. Place the mixture in an ice cream maker and follow manufacturers directions. Once the sherbert is done serve immediately or pack into a freezer-safe container and place in freezer. This sherbert will keep in the freezer for up to one month. Place frozen sherbert in the refrigerator for 20-30 minutes before serving and use an ice cream scoop that has been dipped in hot water to serve more easily. Makes 1 quart; 1 serving = 1/2 cup.

Peanut Butter and Jelly Thumbprints

Servings: 18 | *Prep:* 5 m | *Style:* American | *Cook:* 20 m

Ingredients

- 1 cup Natural Creamy Peanut Butter 1/3 Less Sodium & Sugar
- 24 tsps Erythritol
- 1 large Egg (Whole)
- 1 tsp Vanilla Extract
- 1/2 tsp Baking Soda
- 1/2 tsp Salt
- 6 tbsps Sugar Free Seedless Blackberry Jam

Directions

Use Raspberry Sugar Free jam instead of the Blackberry listed in the ingredients. Strawberry is great too!

1. Preheat oven to 325°F. Prepare two cookie sheets with silpats or parchment paper.
2. In a small bowl combine the peanut butter, granular sugar substitute, egg, vanilla, baking soda and salt. Blend together with a fork until thoroughly combined, about 3 minutes.
3. Using a 2 tbsp scoop or measure, divide dough into 18 balls on two cookie sheets placing about 2 inches apart. Bake for 10 minutes, remove from oven and make an indentation with the back of a small spoon (a round teaspoon works great) then drop one teaspoon of sugar-free jam into the well. Put back in the oven for another 10 minutes. Cool on the pan for 15 minutes then place on a wire rack. Cookies will keep in an airtight container in the refriferator for 1 week.

Pear Tart

*Servings: 6 | **Prep:** 40 m | **Style:** Other | **Cook:** 30 m*

Ingredients

- 3/4 cup Whole Grain Soy Flour
- 9 tbsps Sucralose Based Sweetener (Sugar Substitute)
- 4 tbsps Unsalted Butter Stick
- 11 oz Cream Cheese
- 1 tbsp Sour Cream (Cultured)
- 2 small (approx 3 per lb) Pear
- 1 fl oz (no ice) Brandy

- 1/2 tsp Pure Almond Extract
- 1/2 tsp Ginger (Ground)
- 2 tbsps Sugar Free Apricot Preserves
- 1 large Egg (Whole)
- 2 tsps Tap Water
- 1 oz Almonds

Directions

1. Preheat oven to 350°F.
2. For crust: In a food processor, pulse flour and 2 tablespoons sugar substitute to combine, about 10 seconds. Add butter and pulse until mixture resembles a coarse meal, about 30 seconds.
3. Add 3 ounces cream cheese and the sour cream and pulse until the dough starts to come together, about 30 more seconds. Put dough on the bottom and up the sides of an ungreased 10 tart pan.
4. Prick dough about 15 times with a fork and chill in freezer while preparing filling.
5. For filling: In a small bowl, toss pear slices with 1 tablespoon of the sugar substitute, Cognac, 1/4 teaspoon of the almond extract and ginger until evenly distributed. Set aside.
6. In a large bowl with an electric mixer on high speed, beat 8 ounces cream cheese at room temperature and 1/3 cup sugar substitute until soft and creamy, about 3 minutes. Add egg and remaining 1/4 teaspoon almond extract; beat until smooth, 1 minute more (scrape down sides of bowl as necessary).
7. Pour cream cheese mixture into chilled tart shell. Arrange pears on top of cream cheese mixture in slightly overlapping concentric circles. If there is liquid left from the pears, pour it evenly over the tart.
8. Bake for 30 minutes, or until cheese mixture is just set. Remove from oven and place on a wire rack to cool.
9. Melt jam with water over medium heat. Brush over hot tart and sprinkle with almonds. Let tart cool completely before serving.

Peppermint-Chocolate Truffles

Servings: 6 | Prep: 20 m | Style: American

Ingredients

- 4 oz Sugar Free Chocolate Chips

- 2 tbsps Heavy Cream
- 1 tbsp Unsalted Butter Stick
- 10 Bob's Starlight Mints Peppermint Sugar Free Candy
- 1 tbsp Vanilla Extract

Directions

1. Sugar-free striped hard peppermint candies can be found at some grocery stores or at specialty candy stores. Unwrap them and place them in a plastic bag then crush with a rolling pin or hammer before using.
2. Place chocolate in a small microwavable bowl; set aside. Place cream and butter in another small microwavable bowl; set aside.
3. Microwave chocolate for 30 seconds on medium; repeat for another 30 seconds. Microwave the bowl of chocolate a third time, along with the bowl of cream and butter, for another 30 seconds. Remove and pour the hot cream and butter mixture over the partially melted chocolate; let sit 1 minute. Stir to completely melt the chocolate and smooth the mixture. Add extract and thoroughly mix. If the chocolate isn't completely melted, return to the microwave for an additional 20 seconds.
4. Place the bowl in the refrigerator, covered with plastic wrap, for about 1 hour or until firm.
5. Working quickly to avoid melting, form 12 equal-size balls of the chocolate mixture with your fingers, immediately roll in a small amount of unsweetened cocoa powder or roll each in the peppermint candies (optional) to coat evenly. Set on a serving plate. Serve right away or refrigerate in an airtight container for up to 5 days. 2 truffles per serving.

Pineapple-Coconut Granita

*Servings: 4 | **Prep:** 105 m | **Style:** Other | **Cook:** 5 m*

Ingredients

- 1/2 fruit Pineapple
- 1/2 cup Sucralose Based Sweetener (Sugar Substitute)
- 1/2 cup Tap Water
- 3/4 tsp Coconut Extract

Directions

1. In a food processor, pulse the pineapple until very smooth, about 2 minutes.
2. In a small saucepan over high heat, dissolve sugar substitute in water. Remove from heat. Add pineapple purée and coconut extract, stirring to combine. Pour the mixture into a 9 x13 pan.
3. Place the pan in freezer for 30 minutes or until ice crystals begin to form. Using a fork, break up ice and return to freezer. Continue breaking up ice crystals every 30 minutes until mixture is granular and completely frozen, about 1 1/2 hours.
4. Once the mixture is frozen cover the pan with plastic wrap, or if making a day ahead, place granita in a plastic storage container with a lid and store in freezer.
5. To serve, remove granita from freezer and allow to thaw for 2-3 minutes, breaking up any large ice crystals.

Pineapple-Mango Layer Cake

Servings: 8 | Prep: 50 m | Style: American | Cook: 20 m

Ingredients

- 1/2 fruit Pineapple
- 1/2 cup sliced Mangos
- 1 cup Whole Grain Soy Flour
- 1 tsp Baking Powder (Straight Phosphate, Double Acting)
- 1/4 tsp Salt
- 6 large Eggs (Whole)
- 3/4 cup Sucralose Based Sweetener (Sugar Substitute)
- 2 tsps Pure Almond Extract
- 1/4 cup Unsalted Butter Stick
- 1/2 cup Heavy Cream
- 1 tbsp Sucralose Based Sweetener (Sugar Substitute)

Directions

1. For cake: Preheat oven to 350°F. Line two 8-inch-round cake pans with parchment paper, grease and dust with soy flour. Core the pineapple (cut off green outsides) and peel the mango. Dice all or leave about half of the

pineapple in half-rings and half of the mango in slices for a decorative top; set aside.

2. In a medium bowl, whisk together soy flour, baking powder and salt. Separate the egg yolks from the whites. Set yolks aside. In a large bowl with an electric mixer on medium speed, beat whites until frothy, about 3 minutes. Slowly add 3/4 cup (12 Tbsp) sugar substitute and continue beating until stiff, but not dry, peaks form, about 4 minutes.

3. In a small bowl, whisk together yolks, almond extract and melted butter. Slowly pour yolk mixture into the beaten egg whites and continue mixing on medium speed until yolks are combined, about 1 minute. In three additions, gently fold the dry ingredients into the egg white mixture using a rubber spatula. Divide batter in prepared pans; smooth tops.

4. Bake until a toothpick inserted in centers comes out clean, about 20 minutes. Cool on wire rack for 5 minutes, then turn out to cool completely.

5. To assemble: In a small bowl with an electric mixer on medium, whip heavy cream with 1 tablespoon sugar substitute until soft peaks form, about 3 minutes. Place one cake layer on a serving plate. Spread half the whipped cream over cake and place diced pineapple and mango pieces all around. Place second layer over whipped cream. Top with remaining whipped cream and decorate top with pieces or sliced pineapple and mango.

6. For a decorative top: Starting at the edge of the cake, arrange fruit in concentric circles, alternating pineapple and mango slices. Cut into 8 servings.

Pinwheel Cookies

Servings: 28 | Prep: 45 m | Style: Other | Cook: 18 m

Ingredients

- 4 oz Cream Cheese
- 2 tbsps Unsalted Butter Stick
- 2 tbsps Sour Cream (Cultured)
- 4 tsps Sucralose Based Sweetener (Sugar Substitute)
- 1 cup Whole Grain Soy Flour
- 1 tsp Baking Powder (Straight Phosphate, Double Acting)
- 1/4 cup chopped English Walnuts
- 2 oz Sugar Free Chocolate Chips
- 1/4 tsp Cinnamon

Directions

1. Line two baking sheets with aluminum foil; set aside.
2. In a bowl, with an electric mixer on low, mix cream cheese, butter, sour cream and sugar substitute until smooth, about 4 minutes. With the mixer still on low, sift flour and baking powder together and gradually add until dough pulls away from the side. Form dough into a rectangle, cover with plastic wrap and refrigerate for 20 minutes.
3. While dough is chilling, combine walnuts, chocolate chips and cinnamon. Roll dough between two pieces of plastic wrap to a rectangle measuring 8 x11.
4. Before removing the dough from the freezer, preheat oven to 350°F. Remove top layer of plastic wrap. Sprinkle chocolate-nut filling evenly over dough, leaving a 1/2-inch border along the longer side.
5. Roll dough up jelly roll style, beginning with the long side and using bottom sheet of plastic wrap to help roll the dough into a cylinder. Place in freezer and chill for 10 minutes.
6. Using a sharp knife, cut roll into 1/2-inch slices. Arrange slices on prepared baking sheets. Bake 18 minutes, or until lightly golden and set.

Pistachio Butter Cookies

Servings: *24* | **Prep:** *20 m* | **Style:** *American* | **Cook:** *16 m*

Ingredients

- 1/2 cup Dry Roasted Pistachio Nuts (Without Salt Added)
- 1/4 cup, dry, yield Oatmeal
- 1/3 cup Sucralose Based Sweetener (Sugar Substitute)
- 1/3 cup Whole Grain Wheat Flour
- 1/3 cup Whole Grain Soy Flour
- 1/8 tsp Salt
- 1/4 tsp Baking Powder (Straight Phosphate, Double Acting)
- 1/2 cup Unsalted Butter Stick
- 1 large Egg (Whole)
- 1 tsp Vanilla Extract
- 1/3 second spray Original Canola Cooking Spray

Directions

1. Preheat oven to 375°F. Lightly grease a baking sheet with oil spray.

2. Process pistachios, oatmeal, sugar substitute, flours, salt and baking powder in a food processor until nuts and oatmeal are finely ground, about 1 minute. Add butter, egg and vanilla processing until combined, about 15 seconds, scraping down sides if necessary. Chill dough for 15 minutes, until firm.
3. Roll dough into 24 balls and place on prepared sheet. Flatten with palm of hand to about 1/8 thick. Bake cookies until bottoms and edges are deep golden, 14-16 minutes. Cool cookies on baking sheet 1 minute before transferring to wire racks to cool completely. Store in an airtight container.

Pumpkin Cheesecake

Servings: 10 | Prep: 240 m | Style: American | Cook: 45 m

Ingredients

- 24 oz Cream Cheese
- 15 oz Pumpkin (Without Salt, Canned)
- 2/3 cup Sucralose Based Sweetener (Sugar Substitute)
- 1/2 tsp Vanilla Extract
- 1/2 tsp Cinnamon
- 1/4 tsp Ginger (Ground)
- 3 large Eggs (Whole)

Directions

1. Be sure to use pure pumpkin purée, not pumpkin pie mix, which is sweetened with sugar.
2. Heat oven to 325°F. Spray an 8x3-inch deep cake pan with vegetable cooking spray. Line bottom with a round of parchment or wax paper; spray paper; set aside.
3. In a large bowl, with an electric mixer on medium, beat cream cheese until smooth. Add pumpkin purée, sugar substitute, vanilla, cinnamon and ginger; beat until smooth.
4. Beat in eggs one at a time, just until combined. Pour batter into prepared pan. Place cake pan in a deep roasting pan and carefully pour in enough boiling water into roasting pan to reach halfway up sides of cake pan. Bake 42-45 minutes, until cake is just set in center. Turn off oven, open door and let stand in oven 15 minutes. Remove cake pan from water bath and transfer to a wire rack; cool completely. Run a knife around edge of cake, cover and refrigerate until chilled (4 hours or overnight).

5.   To remove cake from pan, dip bottom of pan into hot water for just a few seconds to loosen. Place serving platter over top and invert. Remove pan and peel off paper. Garnish with mint and pecans, if desired.

Pumpkin Mousse

*Servings: 8 | **Prep:** 25 m | **Style:** American*

Ingredients

- 1 package (1 oz) Gelatin Powder (Unsweetened)
- 1/4 cup Tap Water
- 2 tsps Pumpkin Pie Spice
- 15 oz Pumpkin (Without Salt, Canned)
- 1 1/2 cups Heavy Cream
- 1/2 cup Sucralose Based Sweetener (Sugar Substitute)
- 2 tsps Vanilla Extract

Directions

1.   In small bowl, sprinkle gelatin over cool water, let sit 5 minutes until gelatin softens. Meanwhile, in a small skillet over medium heat, toast pumpkin pie spice 1 2 minutes until fragrant, stirring frequently. Reduce heat to low, stir in gelatin mixture and cook 1-2 minutes more until gelatin melts. Remove from heat; cool to room temperature.
2.   Place pumpkin purée in a large bowl.
3.   In another large bowl, with an electric mixer on high, beat cream, sugar substitute and vanilla until soft peaks form. With a rubber spatula, slowly fold in cooled gelatin mixture.
4.   In three additions, gently fold whipped cream mixture into pumpkin purée.
5.   Divide mousse into 8 dessert glasses. Chill 2 hours.

Pumpkin Pie Topped with Meringue and Toasted Nuts

*Servings: 8 | **Prep:** 15 m | **Style:** American | **Cook:** 60 m*

Ingredients

- 1/3 cup 100% Stone Ground Whole Wheat Pastry Flour
- 1/2 cup chopped Pecan Nuts
- 1 cup Sucralose Based Sweetener (Sugar Substitute)
- 6 tbsps Unsalted Butter Stick
- 1 fl oz Tap Water
- 15 oz Pumpkin (Without Salt, Canned)
- 1 tsp Cinnamon
- 3/4 tsp Ginger (Ground)
- 1/4 tsp Cloves (Ground)
- 1/4 tsp Salt
- 2 large Eggs (Whole)
- 1 1/4 cups Heavy Cream
- 3 large Egg Whites
- 1/4 tsp Cream Of Tartar
- 1/4 cup Sucralose Based Sweetener (Sugar Substitute)
- 1/2 cup chopped Pecan Nuts
- 2 servings All Purpose Low-Carb Baking Mix

Directions

Use the Atkins recipe to make All Purpose Low-Carb Baking Mix for this recipe. 1 serving =1/3 cup so you will need 2/3 cup

For pie:

1. Heat oven to 425ºF.
2. In a large bowl whisk together flour, 2/3 cup baking mix, pecans (chop finely) and 1/4 cup sugar substitute. Cut in butter with a pastry blender or two knives until butter pieces are about the size of peas. Add the ice water; stir to combine.
3. Transfer crust mixture to a 9-inch pie plate. Press along bottom and sides of pie plate to form a crust. Place in freezer to harden, about 15 minutes.
4. Cover crust with aluminum foil and bake 15 minutes; remove from oven and take off foil. Reduce oven to 375ºF.
5. In a bowl, whisk pumpkin purée, 3/4 cup sugar substitute, ground cinnamon, ginger, cloves, and salt to combine. Mix in eggs, one at a time. Add heavy cream and mix well.
6. Pour filling into partially baked pie crust. Cover crust edge with aluminum foil. Bake 40 minutes, or until filling is set but still a little jiggly in the middle. Cool on a wire rack while you make the meringue but turn the oven down to 350°F.

For meringue and toasted nut topping:

1. Whip egg whites and cream of tartar with an electric beater until frothy. Slowly add 1/4 cup granulated sugar substitute until fully incorporated then whip at high speed until stiff glossy peaks form. Top pie with meringue and then sprinkle the 1/2 cup finely chopped nuts on top. Place in the oven and continue to bake for 15-20 minutes until the nuts are toasted and browned.
2. Cool on a wire rack until ready to serve. The pie may be made up to 3 days prior to serving, but do not add the meringue until you are ready to serve. Be sure the pie has warmed to room temperature if previously chilled before adding and cooking the meringue and nuts (otherwise your pie plate may crack with the sudden change in temperature). The meringue topping will not keep more than a day once made.

Pumpkin Pie with Pecan Crust

Servings: 8 | Prep: 15 m | Style: American | Cook: 44 m

Ingredients

- 1/3 cup 100% Stone Ground Whole Wheat Pastry Flour
- 1/2 cup chopped Pecan Nuts
- 1 cup Sucralose Based Sweetener (Sugar Substitute)
- 6 tbsps Unsalted Butter Stick
- 1 fl oz Tap Water
- 15 oz Pumpkin (Without Salt, Canned)
- 1 tsp Cinnamon
- 3/4 tsp Ginger (Ground)
- 1/4 tsp Cloves (Ground)
- 1/4 tsp Salt
- 2 large Eggs (Whole)
- 1 1/4 cups Heavy Cream
- 2 servings All Purpose Low-Carb Baking Mix

Directions

Use the Atkins recipe to make All Purpose Low-Carb Baking Mix for this recipe. 1 serving =1/3 cup so you will need 2/3 cup.

1. Heat oven to 425ºF.
2. In a large bowl whisk together flour, 2/3 cup baking mix, pecans (chop finely) and 1/4 cup sugar substitute. Cut in butter with a pastry blender or

two knives until butter pieces are about the size of peas. Add the ice water; stir to combine.

3. Transfer crust mixture to a 9-inch pie plate. Press along bottom and sides of pie plate to form a crust. Place in freezer to harden, about 15 minutes.

4. Cover crust with aluminum foil and bake 15 minutes; remove from oven and take off foil. Reduce oven to 375ºF.

5. In a bowl, whisk pumpkin purée, 3/4 cup sugar substitute, ground cinnamon, ginger, cloves, and salt to combine. Mix in eggs, one at a time. Add heavy cream and mix well.

6. Pour filling into partially baked pie crust. Cover crust edge with aluminum foil. Bake 40 minutes, or until filling is set but still a little jiggly in the middle. Cook on a wire rack. Makes 8 servings.

Pumpkin Pots

Servings: 6 | *Prep*: 10 m | *Style*: American | *Cook*: 38 m

Ingredients

- 2 large Eggs (Whole)
- 2 large Egg Yolks
- 1 14 oz can Coconut Cream
- 1 tsp Vanilla Extract
- 15 oz Pumpkin (Without Salt, Canned)
- 1/4 cup Xylitol
- 1 pinch Stevia
- 1/4 cup Sugar Free Maple Flavored Syrup
- 1 tsp Ginger (Ground)
- 1 tsp Cinnamon
- 1/4 tsp Nutmeg (Ground)
- 3/4 tsp Salt

Directions

1. For this recipe, add or delete spices as desired (the combination given is generally a pumpkin pie spice mixture). Add the stevia sparingly, taste the recipe before baking if you are unsure and add more stevia or sugar-free maple syrup if more sweetness or maple flavor is desired; whisk in any additional thoroughly. Additionally, this recipe can easily be made by substituting heavy cream for the coconut milk; add 1.3g NC per serving.

2. Preheat oven to 400°F. Lightly grease 6 ramekins; set aside. You will also need a pan big enough to accommodate all the ramekins and deep enough to hold 1-inch of water without spilling into the ramekins.
3. Whisk the whole eggs and yolks with the coconut milk and vanilla in a medium bowl. Set aside.
4. In a medium sauce pot combine the pumpkin, granular sugar substitutes, maple syrup, ginger, ground cinnamon, nutmeg and salt. Cook over medium-high heat until reduced slightly, fragrant and shiny; about 15 minutes stirring often to prevent burning on the bottom of the pan. Remove from heat and quickly whisk in the egg mixture.
5. Divide mixture into 6 ramekins (do not overfill) and place in a deep sided pan. Fill the pan with hot water until it reaches about 1-inch up the side of the ramekins. Place in oven and bake for 10 minutes at 400°F then reduce heat to 300°F and cook an additional 25-30 minutes or until the centers jiggle only slightly in the center. Remove from oven and allow to sit in the water bath to cool to room temperature. These are wonderful eaten warm about 20 minutes after baking or cold after being refrigerated for at least 3 hours or up to 2 days. Store leftovers in the refrigerator covered with plastic wrap and eat within 1 week. Top with a dollop of whipped cream just before serving if desired.

Pumpkin-Spice Brownies

Servings: 16 | Prep: 10 m | Style: American | Cook: 30 m

Ingredients

- 2 oz Unsweetened Baking Chocolate Squares
- 1/2 cup Unsalted Butter Stick
- 1 tbsp Cocoa Powder (Unsweetened)
- 24 tsps Erythritol
- 2 tsps Vanilla Extract
- 4 large Eggs (Whole)
- 4 tbsps Organic High Fiber Coconut Flour
- 1/4 tsp Baking Soda
- 1/4 tsp Salt
- 1/2 tsp Cinnamon
- 8 oz Cream Cheese
- 1/3 cup Sucralose Based Sweetener (Sugar Substitute)
- 2/3 cup Pumpkin (Without Salt, Canned)
- 1 1/2 tsps Pumpkin Pie Spice

Directions

You will need 4 oz or 1/2 cup erythritol for this recipe. Powdered pure erythritol may be purchased from specialty stores or online. Granulated erythritol is more easily found in health food stores and may also easily be powdered by placing it in a blender and pulsing for 5 seconds. Be sure to use powdered erythritol and measure after it is powdered. 4oz = 1 cup powdered erythritol. Sucralose may be used for the brownie (use 1 full cup) and add 1.5g NC to each serving total; some people find the combination of chocolate and sucralose to be bitter.

1. Preheat an oven to 350°F. Grease an 8x8-inch pan.
2. Melt the butter and chocolate in a small bowl at 30 second intervals in the microwave until melted. Thoroughly blend the chocolate and butter together then add in the cocoa powder and powdered erythritol (1 cup made from 1/2 cup granulated) and continue to blend until smooth. Add 1 teaspoon vanilla and 3 eggs; whisk until incorporated. Combine the coconut flour, baking soda, salt and cinnamon in a small bowl. Add to the chocolate mixture and stir until thickened. Set the brownie mixture aside.
3. Using a hand blender cream the cream cheese with the sucralose in a small bowl. Add 1 egg, pumpkin purée, pumpkin spice blend and 1 teaspoon vanilla; beat until smooth.
4. Spread 2/3 of the brownie mixture into the prepared pan. Then pour the cream cheese mixture over the top. Drop the remaining 1/3 of the brownie batter by spoonfuls over the cream cheese mixture and then take a knife and gently swirl the layers together. Bake for 30 minutes until a tooth pick inserted in the center comes out clean. Allow to cool before cutting. Best served at room temperature but keep refrigerated in an airtight container for up to 1 week.

Raspberry Parfait

Servings: 2 | Prep: 5 m | Style: American

Ingredients

- 1/2 cup Heavy Cream
- 4 oz Mascarpone
- 2 individual packets Sucralose Based Sweetener (Sugar Substitute)
- 1/2 cup Raspberries

Directions

1. Beat 1/2 cup heavy crem until soft peaks form.
2. Add 4 oz mascarpone and 2 pakcets of sweetener. Beat just until smooth.
3. Using 1/2 cup raspberries, layer with the dairy mixture in 2 parfait glasses.

Root Beer Float

*Servings: 1 | **Prep:** 5 m | **Style:** American*

Ingredients

- 1 can Diet Root Beer
- 2 tbsps Heavy Cream

Directions

1. Combine half of the root beer can with 7 ice cubes and cream in a blender. Purée until smooth.
2. Add the remaining root beer can; pulse to incorporate. Enjoy!

Snickerdoodle Cupcakes

*Servings: 8 | **Prep:** 25 m | **Style:** American | **Cook:** 22 m*

Ingredients

- 3/4 cup Unsalted Butter Stick
- 1/4 cup Sucralose Based Sweetener (Sugar Substitute)
- 2 large Eggs (Whole)
- 2 tsps Vanilla Extract
- 3 tbsps Heavy Cream
- 1 fl oz Tap Water
- 4 tbsps Organic High Fiber Coconut Flour
- 3/4 cup Almond Meal Flour
- 3/4 tsp Baking Powder (Straight Phosphate, Double Acting)
- 1/8 tsp Salt

- 2 tsps Cinnamon
- 2 large Egg Whites
- 1/3 cup Xylitol

Directions

This recipe is suitable for all phases except for the first two weeks of Induction due to the nuts. This recipe uses xylitol for the frosting. Be sure to measure it first and then powder it in a blender before use.

Cupcakes:

1. Preheat oven to 350°F. Prepare a muffin tin with 8 foil or paper liners. Beat 1/4 cup softened butter and sucralose until light and fluffy. Add 2 whole eggs, 1 tsp vanilla, heavy cream, 2 Tbsp water and coconut flour.
2. In a separate bowl whisk to combine the almond flour, baking powder, salt and 2 tsp cinnamon. Combine the almond mixture with the egg mixture and blend until smooth. Fill the muffin wells and bake for 20-25 minutes until cooked through. Allow to sit in the muffin tin for 5 minutes then remove to a baking rack to cool. Frost once cooled.

Buttercream Frosting:

1. Prepare a pan with simmering water fitted with another pan over the top (Bain Marie). Do not allow the surface of the water to touch the bottom of the top pan. To the top pan (a metal mixing bowl works great for this purpose) add 2 egg whites (be sure there are no yolks), a dash of cream of tartar, 1 tsp water and 1/3 cup xylitol (it is not necessary to powder it). Whisk this mixture continuously for 5-10 minutes over the water bath until all the xylitol has dissolved.
2. Pour this mixture into a separate bowl and whip with a blender until stiff fluffy peaks form. Add 1 tsp vanilla, blend to incorporate. The frosting may be used, as is, immediately (it does not store well) as a marshmallow frosting - dust the cupcakes with cinnamon as a garnish.

For butter cream:

1. To the marshmallow frosting, continue to beat on medium speed, begin adding about 1/2 cup butter 1 tablespoon at a time (allow to beat for 1 minute between each addition of butter). The frosting may break down and get soupy looking, continue to add butter and beat until it comes together (more butter may be necessary, 1 tablespoon at a time).
2. Add 1-2 tsp cinnamon (to taste, optional) and blend to combine. Buttercream should be used immediately by piping onto the cooled cupcake with a pastry bag and fancy tip or by simply cutting the corner of a plastic bag. Buttercream frosted cupcakes may be refrigerated in an

airtight container for up to 5 days. Serve at room temperature dusted with cinnamon.

Spiced Coconut Bark

Servings: 12 | *Prep:* 15 m | *Style:* American |

Ingredients

- 7 oz Sugar Free Chocolate Chips
- 1 tsp Cinnamon
- 1/8 tsp Chili Powder
- 1/4 tsp Coarse Kosher Salt
- 5 tbsps Dried Coconut

Directions

1. Melt chocolate in the microwave at 30 second intervals (about 3 times) until it begins to melt. Stir in between and do not over heat.
2. Stir in ground cinnamon and chipotle pepper (as deisred for taste, amounts given are delicious but feel free to play with different levels to your taste). Stir in 2 tablespoons shredded coconut. Pour onto parchment paper, spread out evenly into a 6x8-inch rectangle and sprinkle remaining 3 tablespoons shredded coconut on top. Sprinkle coarse Kosher salt on top as well (optional).
3. Place in the refrigerator for 10-15 minutes to firm up then divide into 12 equal portions (squares of 2x2 inches are best for portioning).

Spiced Snack Cake

Servings: 9 | *Prep:* 25 m | *Style:* Other | *Cook:* 25 m

Ingredients

- 1 tsp rounded Coffee (Instant Powder, Decaffeinated)
- 1/4 cup Tap Water

- 4 tbsps Heavy Cream
- 1 cup Whole Grain Soy Flour
- 2 tsps Cinnamon
- 1/4 tsp Cloves (Ground)
- 1 1/2 tsps Baking Powder (Straight Phosphate, Double Acting)
- 1 tsp Cocoa Powder (Unsweetened)
- 1 tbsp Ginger (Ground)
- 1/2 tsp Allspice Ground
- 1/4 tsp Salt
- 2 large Eggs (Whole)
- 1/2 cup Unsalted Butter Stick
- 2 tsps Vanilla Extract
- 1/2 cup Sucralose Based Sweetener (Sugar Substitute)

Directions

1. Heat oven to 350°F. Lightly butter an 8-inch square baking pan and line bottom with parchment paper; set aside.
2. Combine coffee and hot water in a cup; stir until coffee is dissolved. Cool. Stir in cream; set aside.
3. In a medium bowl, combine soy flour, ginger, cinnamon, baking powder, cocoa powder, allspice, cloves and salt; set aside.
4. In a large bowl, with electric mixer on low, beat butter just until creamy. Increase speed to medium-high and beat butter until smooth and light in color, 1 1/2 to 2 minutes.
5. Gradually beat in sugar substitute. Add eggs one at a time, beating well after each addition and scraping sides of bowl as necessary. Beat in vanilla. Reduce speed to medium-low.
6. Add dry mixture in three additions, alternating with the coffee-cream mixture and beginning and ending with dry mix. Beat just until combined. Scrape down sides of bowl and beat 10 seconds more.
7. Spoon batter into prepared pan and smooth top. Bake until a toothpick inserted in center of cake comes out clean, about 25 minutes. Cool on a wire rack. Run a knife around edge of pan, and invert onto wire rack; peel off parchment paper.
8. Invert again onto a cutting board. Using a serrated knife, cut into 9 squares. Dust with cinnamon, and serve warm or at room temperature.

Star Spangled Berry Trifle

Servings: *12* | **Prep:** *180 m* | **Style:** *American*

Ingredients

- 1 fl oz Fresh Lemon Juice
- 1 fl oz Tap Water
- 2 1/2 tsps Vanilla Extract
- 1 tsp Pure Almond Extract
- 9 tbsps Xylitol
- 2 pinches Stevia
- 1/2 cup Organic High Fiber Coconut Flour
- 1/2 tsp Salt
- 2 large Eggs (Whole)
- 2 cups Heavy Cream
- 1 cup Coconut Milk Unsweetened
- 12 large Egg Whites
- 1 tsp Thick-It-Up
- 3 cup sliceds Strawberries
- 3 cups Blackberries

Directions

1. Preheat oven to 350°F. Prepare a large sheet pan with with parchment paper. Set aside.
2. Beat egg whites until frothy. Add the lemon juice and water. Continue to beat and slowly add in 4 tablespoons xylitol, a pinch of stevia, and 1 teaspoon each of vanilla and almond extracts. Fold in the coconut flour and salt until just incorporated. Place mixture on top of the parchment and smooth out with a spatula, making sure it stays on the parchment.. Bake for 15-20 minutes, remove and allow to cool 5 minutes on the pan. Quickly turn the cake over and gently lift the parchment off of the cake, set the cake aside to cool.
3. While the cake is baking make pastry cream. Place 1 cup heavy cream and 1 cup coconut milk into a 1 quart pan. Add 2 tablespoons xylitol and a pinch of stevia along with a pinch of salt. Heat over medium high heat until bubbles just start to appear around the edges of the pan.
4. In a small bowl combine the eggs, Thick-It-Up and 2 tablespoons xylitol. Whisk to combine. Continue whisking and slowly add about half of the hot cream mixture to the eggs. Return egg mixture to the rest of the cream in the pan. Cook for 5-10 minutes until the mixture has boiled for about 1-2 minutes and thickened; stir continuously. Strain through a mesh strainer into a bowl , place plastic wrap on the surface and set aside. Allow to cool to room temperature (speed this up by placing over an ice water bath); about 30 minutes, add in 1 teaspoon vanilla extract, and place into the refrigerator to cool for at least 2 hours.

5. Whip the cream with 1 tablespoon xylitol and 1/2 teaspoon vanilla until fully whipped. Fold whipped cream into cold pastry cream. Additional stevia may be added to taste.

6. Assemble Trifle. Cut out stars or other designs from the cake; set aside. Cut up the remaining pieces and gently mix into the pastry cream. Start by layering the strawberries on the bottom. Add 1/2 of the pastry cream mixture then place the blackberries on top of the pastry cream. Top it off with a final layer of pastry cream and decorate top with the reserved cake stars. If desired, place a few reserved stars along the inside of the bowl as you layer the ingredients up. The serving size is about 1 cup.

Strawberries and Cream Cupcakes

*Servings: 10 | **Prep:** 10 m | **Style:** American | **Cook:** 20 m*

Ingredients

- 7 oz Unsalted Butter Stick
- 1/4 cup Xylitol
- 3 large Eggs (Whole)
- 1 tsp Vanilla Extract
- 1/3 cup Organic High Fiber Coconut Flour
- 1/4 cup Heavy Cream
- 1 1/2 fl ozs Tap Water
- 1 cup Almond Meal Flour
- 1 tsp Baking Powder (Straight Phosphate, Double Acting)
- 1/4 tsp Salt
- 8 oz Cream Cheese
- 1/2 cup Sucralose Based Sweetener (Sugar Substitute)
- 2 tbsps Sugar Free Strawberry Jam
- 10 small (1" dia) Strawberries

Directions

Xylitol usually comes in granular form. Please measure first and then powder in a blender before using in this recipe. You may substitute granular sucralose 1:1 for the xylitol in the cupcakes but please add 0.6g NC per serving to the total g NC.

Cupcakes:

1. Preheat oven to 350°F. Line a muffin tin with 10 paper or foil liners. Beat 1/3 cup (about 3oz) softened butter and the powdered xylitol until light and fluffy, about 3 minutes. Add one egg at a time until incorporated, then the vanilla.
2. Add the coconut flour and blend until incorporated. Add the heavy cream and water and continue to blend until smooth.
3. Combine the almond flour, baking powder and 1/4 tsp salt. Add to the egg mixture forming a thickened batter.
4. Divide equally into the 10 muffin liners and bake for 20-25 minutes until golden brown on top and baked through. Allow to cool.

Frosting:

1. Beat 1/2 cup (about 4 oz) butter, cream cheese and a dash of salt for about 2 minutes. Add the sucralose and 2 tablespoons sugar-free strawberry jam. 2-3 drops of red food coloring may be added for a pinker color.
2. Using a piping bag and fancy tip or simply a quart-sized plastic bag with a corner cut off, pipe the frosting onto the cupcakes and garnish with a strawberry.
3. The cupcakes can be kept in an airtight container refrigerated for up to one week. Serve at room temperature.

Strawberries with French Cream

*Servings: 4 | **Prep:** 10 m | **Style:** French*

Ingredients

- 1/2 cup Heavy Cream
- 1 tbsp Sucralose Based Sweetener (Sugar Substitute)
- 3 tbsps Sour Cream (Cultured)
- 4 pint as purchased, yields Strawberries

Directions

1. With an electric mixer on high speed, beat cream and sugar substitute until soft peaks form, about 4 minutes.
2. Beat in sour cream until well-mixed. Serve with berries.

Strawberry Granita

*Servings: 6 | **Prep:** 120 m | **Style:** Italian*

Ingredients

- 16 oz Strawberries
- 1 cup Tap Water
- 3/4 cup Sucralose Based Sweetener (Sugar Substitute)
- 1 tbsp Fresh Lemon Juice

Directions

1. In a food processor fitted with a steel blade, purée the strawberries. Add water, sugar substitute and lemon juice. Pulse to combine.
2. Pour mixture into a 9 by 13-inch baking pan. Place in freezer. Freeze 30 minutes.
3. Stir with fork. Freeze an additional 1 1/2 to 2 hours, scraping with a fork every 30 minutes (mixture should be granular) and breaking up any large pieces.
4. Serve in dessert bowls and garnish with mint sprigs, if desired.

Strawberry Shortcake Trifle

*Servings: 12 | **Prep:** 100 m | **Style:** American | **Cook:** 20 m*

Ingredients

- 1 1/2 cups Almond Meal Flour
- 1 tsp Baking Powder (Straight Phosphate, Double Acting)
- 4 tbsps Sucralose Based Sweetener (Sugar Substitute)
- 3 tbsps Unsalted Butter Stick
- 2 large Eggs (Whole)
- 2 cups Heavy Cream
- 1 individual packet Sucralose Based Sweetener (Sugar Substitute)
- 4 tsps Vanilla Extract
- 8 oz Cream Cheese
- 4 tbsps Sugar Free Apricot Preserves

- 2 cup sliceds Strawberries
- 1 oz Almonds

Directions

1. Preheat oven to 350°F. Spray a sheet pan with non-stick spray and set aside.
2. In a food processor, pulse the almond flour, baking powder and 2 teaspoons sugar substitute until mixed. Add the cold butter and pulse until it becomes crumbly. Add the eggs and 3 tablespoons of cream and pulse until the mixture is thoroughly combined, about 30 seconds.
3. Drop about 2 tablespoons mixture onto the sheet pan making 12 rounded biscuits. Bake for 20 minutes until tops crack and are golden on the edges. Allow to cool.
4. In a medium bowl beat the remaining cream, 2 tablespoons sugar substitute and 2 teaspoons vanilla extract until soft peaks form, about 3 to 4 minutes. Place one-third of the whipped cream in a small bowl and set aside.
5. Whisk 2 tablespoons sugar substitute and 2 teaspoons vanilla extract into cream cheese. With a rubber spatula, gently fold cream cheese into the remaining two-thirds of the whipped cream until well combined. Set aside.
6. Cut biscuits in half. Spread each with about 1 teaspoon jam, then cut into 1-inch pieces.

To assemble:

1. Spread one-third of the biscuit pieces on the bottom of a 2-quart glass dessert dish.
2. Spread half of the cream cheese mixture over biscuit pieces and top with 1 cup strawberries. Repeat.
3. Scatter remaining biscuit pieces over last layer of berries. Cover with reserved whipped cream. Top with remaining berries and scatter the toasted almonds on top. Chill for 1 hour for flavors to blend.

Strawberry-Rhubarb Pie

Servings: 8 | *Prep:* 135 m | *Style:* American | *Cook:* 15 m

Ingredients

- 4 stalks Rhubarb

- 1/2 cup Tap Water
- 1/3 cup Sucralose Based Sweetener (Sugar Substitute)
- 3 1/2 cup halves Strawberries
- 1/2 tsp Thick-It-Up
- 1/2 tsp Fresh Lemon Juice
- 1/8 tsp Salt
- 8 servings Atkins Cuisine Pie Crust

Directions

Use the Atkins recipe to make Atkins Cuisine Pie Crust for this recipe.

1. Prepare pie crust according to recipe. Pre-bake the pie shell.
2. Chop rhubarb into 1-inch pieces and place it in a medium saucepan over medium heat with the water and sugar substitute. Bring to a boil. Reduce the heat and simmer until rhubarb is very soft, about 10 to 15 minutes. Turn heat down to low.
3. Add berries, thickener, lemon juice and salt and stir until thickened, about 3 minutes. Pour filling into prepared pie shell.
4. Chill until set, about 2 hours. Serve with sweetened whipped cream, if desired. Makes 8 servings.

Sweet Potato-Pumpkin Purée

Servings: 12 | **Prep:** 20 m | **Style:** American | **Cook:** 65 m

Ingredients

- 3 large Egg Whites
- 5 tbsps Sucralose Based Sweetener (Sugar Substitute)
- 15 oz Pumpkin (Without Salt, Drained, Cooked, Boiled)
- 1/2 cup half Pecan Nuts
- 1 1/2 lbs Sweet Potato
- 1/2 cup Heavy Cream
- 1/2 tsp Salt
- 1/2 tsp Pumpkin Pie Spice
- 1/2 tsp Cinnamon
- 1/4 cup Unsalted Butter Stick

Directions

1. Heat oven to 250°F. Lightly butter a baking sheet.
2. Place egg whites in a medium mixing bowl; beat with an electric mixer at high speed until foamy. Gradually add sugar substitute and continue mixing just until soft peaks form. Spoon onto prepared baking sheet and spread with a spatula to ¼-inch thickness. Bake 35 minutes. Turn oven off; let meringue stand in oven for 45 minutes. Crush meringue and place in a bowl. Add pecans and toss gently to combine. Set aside.
3. While meringue is resting, place sweet potatoes in a medium saucepan. Cover with water to 2 inches above potatoes and bring to a boil. Cook until tender, about 20 minutes, and drain. Return saucepan to medium-high heat. Add potatoes, butter, cream sugar substitute, salt, cinnamon, pumpkin pie spice and pumpkin puree. Stir to combine. Mash with a potato masher until smooth. Heat through, about 1 minute.
4. Transfer potato mixture to a serving dish and cover with meringue topping.

Tiramisu Cupcakes

*Servings: 6 | **Prep**: 25 m | **Style**: Italian | **Cook**: 15 m*

Ingredients

- 3 tbsps Unsalted Butter Stick
- 3 large Eggs (Whole)
- 1/4 cup Sucralose Based Sweetener (Sugar Substitute)
- 4 tsps Vanilla Extract
- 1 /4 cup Organic High Fiber Coconut Flour
- 1/4 tsp Baking Powder (Straight Phosphate, Double Acting)
- 1/4 tsp Salt
- 4 oz Mascarpone
- 5 tbsps Xylitol
- 1 1/4 tsp dries Coffee (Instant Powder)
- 1/2 cup Heavy Cream
- 1/2 fl oz Tap Water

Directions

Xylitol is used in combination with sucralose in this recipe to provide a more rounded sweetness. Xylitol usually comes granulated but is better incorporated if it is powdered before use. Please measure first then powder in a blender.

Cupcakes:

1. Preheat oven to 375°F. Prepare a muffin tin with paper or foil cups.
2. Using an electric mixer blend together the butter and sucralose until light and fluffy; about 2 minutes. Add eggs, 1 tsp vanilla, coconut flour, baking powder and salt. Blend until smooth then fill 6 muffin cups and bake for 15 minutes or until cooked through. Allow to sit for 5 minutes in the tin then place on a cooling rack.
3. Soaking syrup: combine 2 tsp vanilla, 2 Tbsp xylitol, 1 tsp espresso powder and 1 1/2 Tbsp water. Prick cupcakes with a tooth pick and pour 1 tsp soaking syrup per cupcake over the top.

Mascarpone Frosting:

1. Beat together the mascarpone cheese, 3 Tbsp xylitol, 1 tsp vanilla and 1/4 tsp espresso powder until smooth.
2. In a separate bowl whip the heavy creamy until stiff peaks form.
3. Fold the whipped cream into the mascarpone mixture until combined. Place mixture in a pastry bag fitted with a fancy tip or simply use a plastic sandwich bag with a corner cut off. Pipe the frosting onto the cooled cupcakes. Best if served the same day or they may be refrigerated overnight in an airtight container. Serve at room temperature dusted with cocoa powder and topped with crushed espresso beans if desired.

Tropical Raspberry Smoothie

*Servings: 1 | **Prep:** 5 m | **Style:** Other*

Ingredients

- 1/2 cup Coconut Cream
- 4 oz Firm Silken Tofu
- 1/2 cup Red Raspberries
- 2 tsps Sucralose Based Sweetener (Sugar Substitute)
- 1/8 tsp Coconut Extract

Directions

1. Combine coconut milk, tofu, 1/2 cup raspberries, sugar substitute (if desired) and coconut extract in a blender; blend until smooth. (If you want

to remove the seeds, you can strain the mixture through a sieve, then return it to the blender).

2. With the machine running, add 3 ice cubes, one at a time, and blend until smooth.
3. Pour into a tall glass, and garnish with whipped cream and raspberries, if desired. Serve immediately.

Truly Coconut Cake

Servings: 16 | Prep: 20 m | Style: American | Cook: 37 m

Ingredients

- 2 cups Unsalted Butter Stick
- 13 tbsps Xylitol
- 2 tsps Vanilla Extract
- 3 tsps Coconut Extract
- 6 large Eggs (Whole)
- 3 /4 cups Organic High Fiber Coconut Flour
- 1 tsp Baking Powder (Straight Phosphate, Double Acting)
- 1 tsp Salt
- 1 cup Coconut Milk Unsweetened
- 1 cup Dried Coconut
- 16 oz Cream Cheese

Directions

Xylitol is used in this recipe to decrease the net carbs. Please measure first 8 Tbsp and then 5 Tbsp; keeping them separate and then powder each in a blender and set aside in separate bowls. The granules tend to be large and don't dissolve as readily as regular sugar or other granular sugar substitutes. Sucralose may be substituted by decreasing each of the amounts used by about 1/4 cup (add 2g NC to the total net carb count per serving. Please note this will make it too high in NC for Phase 1.)

1. Preheat oven to 325°F. Prepare two 9-inch round pans with oil spray, cut out parchment paper to fit into the bottom of each pan, place the paper in the pan and spray it with oil. Set aside.
2. With an electric mixer beat 1 cup butter and then the 8 Tbsp of xylitol that was powdered until light and fluffy, about 3 minutes. Add the vanilla and 2 tsp coconut extract; blend to combine. Add the eggs one at a time blending after each addition; the mixture may separate a bit at this point.

3. Sift together 3/4 cup coconut flour, baking powder and salt. Add to butter mixture and mix until thoroughly combined. Add in the coconut milk and 1/2 cup shredded coconut, blend until incorporated. Scoop into prepared pans and spread evenly with a spatula.
4. Bake for 35-40 minutes until cakes begin to pull away from the pans and are fully set in the center. Cool for 10 minutes in the pan, remove from pan and then cool on a rack. The cakes will be a little fragile so be careful handling them. Place cooled cakes in the refrigerator until ready to frost and serve. Frost just before serving.
5. Frosting: with an electric mixer blend the cream cheese and 1 cup butter until smooth. Add the 5 Tbsp of xylitol that was powdered and 1 teaspoon coconut extract; blend until light and fluffy. Use 1/3 of the frosting to frost between the layers and the remaining to frost the top and the sides of the cake.
6. Toast the remaining 1/2 cup shredded coconut in the oven at 350°F for 5 minutes until lightly browned. Sprinkle coconut on top of the cake and along sides if desired. Refrigerate any remaining cake for up to one week.

Vanilla Mousse with Rhubarb Sauce

Servings: 2 | Prep: 15 m | Style: American | Cook: 10 m

Ingredients

- 2 stalks Rhubarb
- 1/4 cup Tap Water
- 1 tbsp Sugar Free Strawberry Jam
- 1/2 cup Heavy Cream
- 4 oz Greek Yogurt - Plain (Container)
- 3 tsps Sucralose Based Sweetener (Sugar Substitute)

Directions

1. For the rhubarb sauce: In a small saucepan, combine the rhubarb, water and strawberry jam; bring to a simmer over medium heat. Reduce heat to medium-low; cover and simmer, stirring occasionally, until rhubarb is a sauce-like consistency, about 10 minutes. Set aside to cool.
2. For the vanilla mousse: In a mixing bowl, with an electric mixer on medium-high speed, beat together the cream, 4 oz yogurt, and sugar substitute to semi-firm peaks. Reserve 1/4 cup mousse for topping.

3. To assemble: Set out two martini glasses or wineglasses. Spoon 1/4 cup mousse in the bottom of each glass and spread evenly. Top each with 1 1/2 tablespoons rhubarb sauce. Divide the remaining mousse between the glasses, then top with the remaining rhubarb. Top with the reserved 1/4 cup mousse, dividing evenly.

Vanilla-Almond Butter Cookies

Servings: 24 | Prep: 10 m | Style: American | Cook: 10 m

Ingredients

- 1/2 cup Blanched & Slivered Almonds
- 3/4 cup dry Whole Grain Soy Flour
- 3 tsps Baking Powder (Straight Phosphate, Double Acting)
- 3/4 cup Sucralose Based Sweetener (Sugar Substitute)
- 1 large Egg (Whole)
- 1 large Egg Yolk
- 2 tsps Vanilla Extract
- 1/4 cup Unsalted Butter Stick

Directions

This recipe is suitable for all phases except for the first two weeks of Induction due to the nuts.

1. Preheat oven to 375°F. In a food processor, finely grind the almonds with the soy flour, baking powder, and sugar substitute.
2. In a separate bowl, with an electric mixer on medium, beat whole egg and egg yolk, vanilla and butter until well incorporated (mixture will not attain a smooth consistency). With a rubber spatula, fold in soy mixture just until combined.
3. Form dough into 24 small balls; arrange on an ungreased baking sheet. Lightly flatten them with a fork to silver dollar size.
4. Bake 8 to 10 minutes, until set. Cool on baking sheets before transferring to a wire rack.

Vanilla-Bean Biscotti

*Servings: 24 | **Prep:** 90 m | **Style:** Italian | **Cook:** 50 m*

Ingredients

- 1/3 cup Unsalted Butter Stick
- 1/2 cup Sucralose Based Sweetener (Sugar Substitute)
- 2 tsps Vanilla Extract
- 2 large Eggs (Whole)
- 2 tbsps Sour Cream (Cultured)
- 3/4 cup dry Whole Grain Soy Flour
- 1 tsp Baking Powder (Straight Phosphate, Double Acting)

Directions

1. Preheat oven to 350°F. In a bowl with an electric mixer, cream butter with sugar substitute and vanilla seeds until light and fluffy, about 3 minutes.
2. Add eggs one at a time, mixing well between each addition. Scrape down sides of bowl with spatula.
3. Add sour cream and beat to combine. Scrape down sides of bowl again.
4. Add the soy flour, baking powder and beat on low speed until just combined. Chill dough for 1 hour.
5. On an ungreased baking sheet, form dough into a 12 by 2 inch log, shaping with moist fingertips if necessary. Bake log until almost firm, about 30-35 minutes. Transfer baking sheet to rack and cool for 10 minutes.
6. Using a serrated knife, carefully cut log crosswise into -inch-thick slices. Arrange slices, cut side down, on baking sheet. Bake at 325° for 17-20 minutes, until firm and crisp. Cool completely on baking sheet on wire rack.

Vanilla-Coconut Ice Cream

*Servings: 8 | **Prep:** 240 m | **Style:** Italian | **Cook:** 5 m*

Ingredients

- 1 cup Dried Coconut
- 6 large Egg Yolks
- 3/4 cup Sucralose Based Sweetener (Sugar Substitute)
- 2 cups Heavy Cream

- 1 14 oz can Coconut Cream
- 2 tsps Coconut Extract
- 1 tsp Vanilla Extract
- 1/4 tsp Salt

Directions

1. Toast coconut in an over at 350°F for 5-7 minutes - stirring halfway though. Remove from oven and set aside.
2. In a medium bowl, whisk yolks and sugar substitute to combine.
3. In a medium pot, bring heavy cream to a simmer over medium-high heat. Slowly pour one cup cream into yolk mixture, whisking constantly. Pour yolk mixture back into pot. This process is known as tempering.
4. Cook, stirring constantly over medium heat, until mixture is thick enough to coat the back of a spoon, approximately 3-5 minutes. Remove from heat. Stir in coconut milk, coconut and vanilla extracts, and salt. Chill 4 hours.
5. Pour ice cream mix into ice cream maker. Process according to manufacturer's directions. About 5 minutes before ice cream is finished, add the toasted coconut.

Vegan Coconut-Vanilla Shake

Servings: 4 | Prep: 5 m | Style: American

Ingredients

- 1 14 oz can Coconut Cream
- 3 heaping scoops Soy Protein Powder
- 1/2 tsp Vanilla Extract

Directions

1. Combine coconut milk, soy protein powder, and extract in a blender and blend until smooth.

Walnut Blondies

Servings: 12 | *Prep:* 20 m | *Style:* American | *Cook:* 14 m

Ingredients

- 1 cup chopped English Walnuts
- 1 cup Unsalted Butter Stick
- 1 cup Sucralose Based Sweetener (Sugar Substitute)
- 1 tsp Vanilla Extract
- 1 cup Whole Grain Soy Flour
- 1/2 cup 100% Stone Ground Whole Wheat Pastry Flour
- 1 oz Vital Wheat Gluten
- 3 large Eggs (Whole)
- 1 1/2 tsps Baking Powder (Straight Phosphate, Double Acting)
- 1/2 tsp Cinnamon
- 1 square Unsweetened Baking Chocolate Squares

Directions

1. Heat oven to 325°F. Toast walnuts on a sheet pan for 8-10 minutes, cool and then coarsely chop. Set aside.
2. Line a 13-by-9-inch baking pan with aluminum foil extending 2 inches over both short sides of pan. Grease foil, and set aside.
3. Whisk butter, sugar substitute, eggs and vanilla extract together in a large bowl. In another bowl whisk flours, gluten, baking powder and cinnamon together; stir into butter mixture until well combined. Stir in walnuts. Spread evenly into prepared pan. Bake until puffed and set, and a toothpick inserted in center comes out clean (top will not be browned), 12 to 14 minutes.
4. Cool completely in pan on a wire rack. Drizzle chocolate in thin lines over entire surface of blondies. Let stand until set, about 1 hour. (The recipe can be prepared up to this point, covered with plastic wrap and stored at room temperature overnight.)
5. Firmly gripping the foil on both ends, lift blondies out of pan, and place on work surface. Cut into 12 pieces, and serve.

Walnut Brownies

Servings: 16 | *Prep:* 15 m | *Style:* American | *Cook:* 25 m

Ingredients

- 1/2 second spray Original No-Stick Cooking Spray
- 1 cup Unsalted Butter Stick
- 3 tbsps Sucralose Based Sweetener (Sugar Substitute)
- 4 large Eggs (Whole)
- 1/2 cup dry Whole Grain Soy Flour
- 1/2 cup Tap Water
- 4 oz Sugar Free Chocolate Chips
- 2 tsps Vanilla Extract
- 1 cup chopped English Walnuts

Directions

1. Preheat oven to 350°F. Line an 8 square baking pan with aluminum foil and spray with cooking spray.
2. Melt chocolate over a double boiler or in the microwave and set aside to cool.
3. With an electric mixer on medium, beat butter and sugar substitute until light and creamy, about 4 minutes. Turn speed down to low and beat in eggs, one at a time. Add melted chocolate and blend well. Add soy flour, water, sugar substitute and extracts (3 Tbsp chocolate extract is optional); mix until just combined. Fold in nuts. Transfer batter to prepared pan.
4. Bake 20 to 25 minutes, until a tester inserted in the center comes out with just a few crumbs. Cool and cut into 16 squares.

Chapter 3: Entree Recipes

***

Almond-Raspberry Cupcakes

Servings: 10 | Prep: 15 m | Style: American | Cook: 25 m

Ingredients

- 2 large Eggs (Whole)
- 1/4 cup Unsalted Butter Stick
- 1/3 cup Sucralose Based Sweetener (Sugar Substitute)
- 2 tbsps Heavy Cream
- 1 fl oz Tap Water
- 1/2 tsp Fresh Lemon Juice
- 1 tsp Vanilla Extract
- 2 tsps Pure Almond Extract
- 2 1/2 cups Almond Meal Flour
- 1/2 tsp Baking Powder (Straight Phosphate, Double Acting)
- 1/2 tsp Salt
- 3 1/3 tbsps Sugar Free Red Raspberry Preserves

Directions

1. Preheat oven to 350°F. Place 10 paper cups in a muffin pan and set aside. In a small bowl beat the egg yolks with 1/4 cup sucralose, butter, cream, water, lemon juice or vinegar and extracts until fully combined. Set aside.
2. In another bowl beat the egg whites until frothy, add the remaining 2 tablespoons of sucralose and continue to beat until stiff peaks form. Gently fold the egg whites into the egg yolk mixture.
3. In a separate bowl, combine the almond meal, baking powder and salt. Gently fold into the egg mixture. Divide this batter equally between the muffin cups then drop 1 teaspoon of raspberry jam into the center.
4. Bake for 20-30 minutes until a toothpick inserted in the center comes out clean. Allow to cool in the pan for 20 minutes. Enjoy warm or at room temperature. Refrigerate remaining cupcakes in an airtight container for up t0 one week and serve at room temperature. These may also be frozen for up to 1 month.

Apricot-Glazed Brisket

*Servings: 8 | **Prep:** 10 m | **Style:** American | **Cook:** 210 m*

Ingredients

- 4 lbs Beef Brisket (Whole, Lean Only)
- 2 tsps Salt
- 2 tsps Paprika
- 1 tsp Black Pepper
- 3 tbsps Sugar Free Apricot Preserves

Directions

1. Heat oven to 475F. Season brisket with salt, paprika and pepper.
2. Place brisket fat side down in a Dutch oven. Scatter onions and carrots around the beef. Cook 15 minutes.
3. Turn brisket fat side up and add 1/2 cup water. Cover tightly. Reduce oven temperature to 375°F. Cook 3 to 4 hours, until brisket is fork tender.
4. Heat broiler. Remove brisket from Dutch oven and place on a broiler pan. Spread jam over brisket. Broil 6 from heat source 5 minutes, until jam is lightly browned in spots. While brisket is broiling, remove onions and carrots from cooking juices.
5. Cover brisket with foil and allow to rest 15 minutes before serving. Remove surface fat with a spoon and serve with degreased cooking juices.

Artichokes with Lemon-Butter

*Servings: 4 | **Prep:** 10 m | **Style:** American | **Cook:** 15 m*

Ingredients

- 4 medium Artichokes (Globe or French)
- 4 fruit (2-1/8" dia) Lemon
- 2 tbsps Coriander Seed
- 2 tbsps Salt
- 1/2 cup Unsalted Butter Stick

Directions

1. Bring 4 quarts of water to a boil in a large pot. Trim the stems of the artichokes to about 2 inches.
2. Halve 3 lemons and squeeze juice into water. Add lemon halves, coriander seeds and salt. Place artichokes in the cooking liquid, and cover with a heavy plate to keep them from floating. Boil 15 minutes, until a paring knife, inserted where the stem meets the bottom, comes out easily. Remove and drain excess water.
3. In a small bowl, melt butter in a microwave or saucepan. Mix in juice of remaining lemon, salt and pepper.
4. Serve each person one whole artichoke, accompanied by a ramekin of butter sauce and a large bowl for discarded leaves. Season with freshly ground salt and pepper to taste.

Arugula, Pear and Hazelnut Salad

*Servings: 4 | **Prep:** 10 m | **Style:** American*

Ingredients

- 10 oz Arugula (Rocket)
- 1/2 cup crumbled Gorgonzola Cheese
- 2 servings Maple-Dijon Vinaigrette
- 1 medium (approx 2-1/2 per lb) Pears
- 40 nuts Hazelnuts or Filberts

Directions

1. Use the Atkins recipe to make Maple-Dijon Vinaigrette for this recipe. You will need 4 Tbsp. This salad is delicious served with salmon.
2. Toast hazelnuts in a dry skillet for about 15 minutes or toast on a sheet pan in an oven at 350°F (stir 2-3 times for both methods); allow to cool and gently rub off outer skin, coarsely chop, and set aside.
3. Make the Maple-Dijon Vinaigrette and toss 4 tablespoons with the arugula and Gorgonzola cheese. Transfer to serving plates.
4. Arrange the pear slices in a fan on top and sprinkle with hazelnuts.

Asian Beef Salad with Edamame

*Servings: 1 | **Prep**: 720 m | **Style**: Asian | **Cook**: 5 m*

Ingredients

- medium (4-1/8" long) Scallions or Spring Onions
- 1/4 tsp Garlic
- 1/2 tbsp Tamari Soybean Sauce
- 1/4 tbsp Sodium and Sugar Free Rice Vinegar
- 1/4 tsp Toasted Sesame Oil
- 1/8 tsp Sucralose Based Sweetener (Sugar Substitute)
- 4 1/4 oz Beef Top Sirloin (Trimmed to 1/8" Fat, Choice Grade)
- 1/8 tsp Curry Powder
- 1/16 tsp Ginger (Ground)
- 1/2 tbsp Canola Vegetable Oil
- 3/4 cup Spring Mix Salad
- 1/4 medium (approx 2-3/4" long, 2-1/2" dia) Red Sweet Pepper
- 2 oz Waterchestnuts
- 1/2 cup Shelled Edamame

Directions

Note: Because only half of the marinade is used in this recipe for the salad dressing and the rest is used as a marinade and discarded, please double the first six ingredients. (The nutritionals shown are correct.) For added flavor, use dark (toasted) sesame oil instead of regular sesame oil.

1. Mix green onions, garlic, soy sauce, rice wine vinegar, sesame oil and sugar substitute in a small bowl. Pour half into a resealable plastic bag; add steak and marinate overnight in the refrigerator.
2. To remaining soy sauce mixture, add curry powder and ground ginger. Heat canola oil in a large skillet over high heat until very hot.
3. Drain beef and discard marinade; quickly stir-fry beef 2 to 3 minutes in hot oil. Transfer to a large mixing bowl. Add salad greens, bell pepper, water chestnuts, edamame and reserved soy dressing. Toss to coat.

Asian Beef Salad with Sesame Seeds

Servings: 1 | *Prep:* 720 m | *Style:* Asian | *Cook:* 5 m

Ingredients

- 1/4 tsp Garlic
- 1/2 tbsp Tamari Soybean Sauce
- 1/8 tbsp Sodium and Sugar Free Rice Vinegar
- 1/4 tsp Sesame Oil
- 1/8 tsp Sucralose Based Sweetener (Sugar Substitute)
- 1/8 tsp Curry Powder
- 1/16 tsp Ginger (Ground)
- 4 1/4 oz Beef Top Sirloin (Trimmed to 1/8" Fat, Choice Grade)
- 1 cup Spring Mix Salad
- 1/2 tbsp Canola Vegetable Oil
- 1/4 large (2-1/4 per lb, approx 3-3/4" long, 3" dia) Sweet Red Peppers
- 2 oz Waterchestnuts
- 1 tbsp Dried Whole Sesame Seeds
- 1 large Scallions or Spring Onion

Directions

Note: Because only half of the marinade is used in this recipe for the salad dressing and the rest is used as a marinade and discarded, please double the first six ingredients. (The nutritionals shown are correct.) For added flavor, use dark (toasted) sesame oil instead of regular sesame oil.

1. Mix green onions, garlic, soy sauce, rice wine vinegar, sesame oil and granular sugar substitute in a small bowl. Pour half into a resealable plastic bag; add steak and marinate overnight in the refrigerator.
2. To remaining soy sauce mixture, add curry powder and ginger. Heat canola oil in a large skillet over high heat until very hot.
3. Drain beef and discard marinade; quickly stir-fry beef 2 to 3 minutes in hot oil for medium doneness. Transfer to a large mixing bowl. Add salad greens, bell pepper, water chestnuts and reserved soy dressing. Toss to coat. Sprinkle with sesame seeds.

Asian Lobster Salad

Servings: 2 | *Prep:* 15 m | *Style:* Asian

Ingredients

- 3/4 lb Northern Lobster
- 2 cups shredded Chinese Cabbage (Bok-Choy, Pak-Choi)
- 1/2 small Sweet Red Pepper
- 4 medium (4-1/8" long) Scallions or Spring Onions
- 1 tbsp Dried Whole Sesame Seeds
- 2 tbsps Sodium and Sugar Free Rice Vinegar
- 2 tbsps Tamari Soybean Sauce
- 1 tbsp Canola Vegetable Oil
- 1 tsp Sesame Oil
- 1 tsp Ginger

Directions

1. For the salad: In a large serving bowl, combine lobster, cabbage, bell pepper, scallions and sesame seeds.
2. For the dressing: In a small bowl, whisk the rice vinegar, Tamari soy sauce, ginger and sesame and canola oils together.
3. Pour dressing over salad and toss gently to coat. Season with fresh ground black pepper and salt.

Asian Marinade

Servings: 6 | Prep: 5 m | Style: Asian

Ingredients

- 8 tbsps Tamari Soybean Sauce
- 2 tbsps Sodium and Sugar Free Rice Vinegar
- 2 tbsps Xylitol
- 1 tbsp Ginger
- 1 tsp Garlic
- 2 tsps Toasted Sesame Oil
- 2 tbsps Canola Vegetable Oil

Directions

Try this simple marinade with chicken kebabs, salmon or tuna steaks, pork chops or beef tenderloin. Marinate chicken and meat for up to 24 hours in the refrigerator, fish for up to 2 hours. Each serving is 2 Tbsp.

1. Combine tamari, vinegar, sugar substitute, ginger, garlic and sesame oil in a bowl. Slowly whisk in canola oil until combined.

Asian Steak Salad

Servings: 2 | Style: Asian | Cook: 45 m

Ingredients

- clove Garlic
- 2 large Young Green Onions
- 1/4 oz Ginger
- 1 medium (approx 2-3/4" long, 2-1/2" dia) Red Sweet Pepper
- 1 tbsp Organic Tamari
- 1/2 tbsp Unseasoned Rice Wine Vinegar
- 1/2 tsp Sesame Oil
- 1/4 tsp No Calorie Sweetener
- 8 oz Beef Top Sirloin (Trimmed to 1/8" Fat)
- 1/4 tsp Curry Powder
- 1 tbsp Vegetable Oil
- 5 oz Baby Spinach

Directions

1. Finely chop the garlic and place in a medium bowl. Finely chop the green onions and add to the garlic. Peel and grate the ginger and place in a small bowl. Remove the stem, pith and seeds from the red bell pepper and discard. Cut into ¼-inch thin strips; set aside.
2. To the medium bowl with the garlic and green onions, add tamari sauce, rice wine vinegar, sesame oil and sugar substitute and stir until well combined. Pour HALF of the tamari mixture into the ziplock bag; set aside.
3. Pat dry the sirloin steak with paper towels and cut into ⅛-inch slices. Place in the bag with the marinade. Seal the bag tightly and place in the refrigerator to marinate. To the tamari mixture remaining in the medium bowl add the curry powder and the ginger; hold for step 5.
4. Heat 1 tablespoon of canola oil in a large sauté pan over medium-high heat. When the pan is hot, remove the steak from the marinade, and quickly stir-fry for 2 to 3 minutes until the beef is cooked through (Discard the marinade). Transfer the steak to a large bowl,

5. Add the red pepper, baby spinach the reserved tamari mixture. Toss to coat all ingredients well.
6. Divide the Asian Beef Salad between two plates and enjoy!

Asian Tuna Kebabs

Servings: 8 | Prep: 25 m | Style: Asian | Cook: 8 m

Ingredients

- 5 1/3 tbsps Tamari Gluten Free Soy Sauce
- 2 2/3 fl ozs Rice Wine
- 1 tbsp Toasted Sesame Oil
- 1 tbsp Ginger
- 3 tsps Garlic
- 2 tsps Sucralose Based Sweetener (Sugar Substitute)
- 32 oz boneless Tuna
- 3 large Scallions or Spring Onions
- 1 large (2.25 per pound, approx 3-3/4" long, 3" dia) Red Sweet Pepper
- 3/4 lb Eggplant

Directions

You'll need 8 bamboo skewers, which should be soaked in water for 15 minutes before cooking. Or use metal skewers. Chinese eggplants are thinner and less bitter than Italian ones and can be found in Asian markets or well-stocked produce sections of most supermarkets.

1. Heat grill to high.
2. Combine soy sauce, rice wine, sesame oil, ginger, garlic and sugar substitute in a large bowl.
3. Add tuna, scallions and red pepper and toss to coat. Marinate for 15 minutes in the refrigerator. Remove tuna, scallions and red pepper from marinade and set aside.
4. Toss eggplant in marinade and let sit for 3 minutes. Remove eggplant and set aside with other ingredients. Discard marinade.
5. Thread skewers, alternating 3 pieces of tuna, 2 pieces of scallions, 2 pieces of red pepper and 3 pieces of eggplant on each. Eggplant should be skewered through both skin sides of the rounds.
6. Grill for 3 -4 minutes per side tuna will be rare in the center.

Asian Vegetable Bowl

Servings: 6 | **Prep:** 10 m | **Style**: Asian | **Cook:** 10 m

Ingredients

- 3 cups chopped Scallions or Spring Onions
- 2 cups Mushroom Pieces and Stems
- 4 tbsps Tamari Soybean Sauce
- 3 tsps Ginger
- 1 clove Garlic
- 1 pepper Serrano Pepper
- 1 cup chopped or sliced Red Tomato
- 6 oz Firm Silken Tofu
- 1 carrot (7-1/2") Carrots
- 1/2 oz Cilantro (Coriander)
- 2 cups shredded Chinese Cabbage (Bok-Choy, Pak-Choi)
- 6 cups Chicken Broth, Bouillon or Consomme

Directions

1. To make this soup suitable for earlier phases, simply omit the carrot. Also vegetable broth may be substituted for the chicken broth to make it appropriate for Vegetarians and Vegans.
2. In a large saucepan, bring broth and tamari to a boil.
3. Reduce heat; add bok choy, mushrooms, ginger, garlic (minced) and chili. Simmer for 5 minutes, until bok choy is tender but still crisp and mushrooms are softened.
4. Add tomatoes, green onions, tofu and carrot. Heat through for 1 minute.
5. Stir in cilantro just before serving.

Asian Veggie and Pork Bowl

Servings: 2 | **Prep:** 10 m | **Style:** Asian | **Cook:** 45 m

Ingredients

- 4 medium (4-1/8" long) Young Green Onions
- 1/4 oz Cilantro (Coriander)
- 4 oz Brown Mushrooms (Crimini Italian)
- 1/4 oz Ginger
- 1 clove Garlic
- 1/2 pepper Serrano Pepper
- 5 oz Chinese Cabbage (Bok-Choy, Pak-Choi)
- 1 italian Tomato
- 8 oz Pork Loin (Tenderloin)
- 1 cube Chicken Stock Cubes (Dry, Dehydrated)
- 1 tbsp Organic Tamari
- 1 tbsp Vegetable Oil

Directions

1. Slice the green onions into ¼-inch pieces on a bias; set aside. Remove the stems from the crimini mushrooms and discard stems. Cut the mushrooms into ¼-inch slices; set aside. Remove the cilantro leaves from the stems and discard stems. Roughly chop the cilantro and set aside.
2. Peel the ginger and finely chop; set aside. Finely chop the garlic cloves; set aside. Remove the stem, pith and seeds from only HALF of the Serrano chile and discard. Finely chop and set aside. Remove the end of the baby bok choy and cut into very thin slices lengthwise; set aside. Cut the tomato in half lengthwise. Cut each half into three wedges; set aside.
3. Pat dry the pork tenderloin with paper towels. Cut into ¼-inch thin slices. Heat a medium sauté pan with 1 tablespoon of canola oil over medium-high heat. When hot, add the pork tenderloin slices and sear for 2 to 3 minutes until browned and cooked through. Remove the pork from the pan and set aside.
4. Bring the chicken stock concentrate, tamari sauce and 2 cups of water to a boil in a large sauce pot over high heat. Reduce the heat to medium-high, add the mushrooms, ginger, garlic, serrano and the baby bok choy. Simmer for 5 minutes, until the bok choy is tender but still crisp and the mushrooms are softened.
5. Add the tomatoes, green onions and the pork to the sauce pot. Heat through for 1 minute. Remove from heat and stir in the cilantro.
6. Ladle the soup into two bowls. Enjoy!

Asian-Style Coleslaw

Servings: 6 | *Prep:* 15 m | *Style:* Asian

Ingredients

- 1 large (7-1/4" to 8-1/2" long) Carrots
- 1 cup chopped Snowpeas (Pea Pod)
- 12 oz Chinese Cabbage (Bok-Choy, Pak-Choi)
- 2 tbsps Extra Virgin Olive Oil
- 1 tbsp Toasted Sesame Oil
- 2 tbsps Sodium and Sugar Free Rice Vinegar
- 1 tbsp Tamari Soybean Sauce
- 2 tsps Ginger
- 1 tsp Sucralose Based Sweetener (Sugar Substitute)

Directions

1. To make this suitable for earlier phases, simply eliminate the carrot.
2. Place cabbage in a large bowl; grate carrot into cabbage. Mix in snow peas.
3. In a small bowl, mix oils, vinegar, tamari, ginger and sugar substitute.
4. Pour dressing over salad; toss to coat. Season to taste with salt.

Asparagus and Leek Soup

Servings: *4 |* ***Prep:*** *15 m |* ***Style:*** *Other |* ***Cook:*** *15 m*

Ingredients

- 2 tbsps Unsalted Butter Stick
- 1 leek Leeks
- 3/4 lb Asparagus
- 1 tsp Garlic
- 1 14.5 oz can Chicken Broth, Bouillon or Consomme
- 1/3 cup Heavy Cream

Directions

1. Melt butter in a large pot over medium-high heat. Add leeks and sauté for 3 minutes. Add asparagus and cook 1 minute more. Add garlic and sauté for 30 more seconds.
2. Add broth to pot and bring to a boil.

3. Lower heat, cover and simmer 8 to 10 minutes, until asparagus is tender.
4. Mix in cream, salt and pepper. Blend soup in a food processor or blender until smooth.
5. Return to pot to heat through before serving (if necessary). Season with salt and freshly ground black pepper to taste.

Asparagus in Vinaigrette with Walnuts

Servings: 4 | Prep: 10 m | Style: American | Cook: 10 m

Ingredients

- 1 lb Asparagus
- 1/4 small Onion
- 2 tbsps White Wine Vinegar
- 1 tsp Dijon Mustard
- 1/2 individual packet Sucralose Based Sweetener (Sugar Substitute)
- 1/2 tsp Salt
- 1/4 tsp Black Pepper
- 1/4 cup Extra Virgin Olive Oil
- 4 cups Spring Mix Salad
- 1/4 cup chopped English Walnuts

Directions

1. To toast nuts, place them on a baking sheet in a preheated 325°F oven, turning them after 3 minutes. Bake for another 3 to 6 minutes, checking frequently to avoid burning. You can substitute almonds for walnuts, if you prefer. To make this dish suitable for Induction, simply eliminate the walnuts.
2. Steam asparagus until crisp-tender, about 4-7 minutes, depending upon size. Drain, and pat dry with paper towels. Set aside.
3. Combine white onion, vinegar, mustard, sugar substitute, salt and pepper in a mixing bowl. Gradually whisk in oil.
4. Divide lettuce on 4 plates; arrange asparagus on top and drizzle with vinaigrette. Sprinkle with walnuts and additional salt and pepper, if desired.

Asparagus Tarragon Cream Soup

*Servings: 8 | **Prep:** 25 m | **Style:** Other | **Cook:** 30 m*

Ingredients

- 1 tbsp Extra Virgin Olive Oil
- 3 14.5 oz cans Chicken Broth, Bouillon or Consomme
- 2 lbs Asparagus
- 3 stalk medium (7-1/2" - 8" long) Celery
- 1/4 tsp Salt
- 1/4 tsp Black Pepper
- 1 small Onion
- 1/2 tbsp leaf Tarragon
- 3/4 cup Heavy Cream

Directions

1. Heat oil in a large pot over medium-high heat. Add white onion and cook 5 minutes, until softened but not browned.
2. Add broth, asparagus, celery, salt, pepper and half of the tarragon to the pot. Bring to a boil.
3. Lower heat, cover and simmer 20 minutes, until asparagus is very tender.
4. In a blender, puré soup in batches until smooth. Return to pot. Add cream and remaining tarragon and heat soup through over medium heat. Season with salt and freshly ground black pepper.

Asparagus Wrapped in Chili Spiced Bacon

*Servings: 4 | **Prep:** 20 m | **Style:** American | **Cook:** 12 m*

Ingredients

- 1 tsp Chili Powder
- 1/2 tsp Sucralose Based Sweetener (Sugar Substitute)
- 4 slices Bacon
- 24 spears Asparagus

Directions

1. Soak 16 wooden toothpicks in warm water for 20 minutes.
2. Preheat grill. Place a sheet of wax paper on a sheet pan and set aside. Combine the chili powder and sugar substitute in a small bowl.
3. Cut bacon strips in 1/2. Lay them on the sheet pan and dust with the chili powder mixture.
4. Wrap three asparagus spears together with one slice of bacon (with the dusted side facing towards the asparagus); securing each end with a toothpick. You should have 8 packets.
5. Grill uncovered over medium-low heat for 12 minutes turning halfway through or until bacon is crisp.
6. Discard toothpicks and serve immediately. Each serving is 2 wraps.

Asparagus, Mushrooms and Peas

Servings: 6 | Prep: 15 m | Style: American | Cook: 25 m

Ingredients

- 3 tbsps Unsalted Butter Stick
- 3 medium (4-1/8" long) Scallions or Spring Onions
- 1 tsp Garlic
- 1 or 3oz Portobello Mushroom Cap
- 1/4 cup Vinegar (Cider)
- 1 cup Tap Water
- 1 lb Asparagus
- 1/2 cup Green Peas
- 2 tbsps Heavy Cream
- 8 leaves Basil
- 1/4 dash Salt
- 1/4 tsp Black Pepper

Directions

1. In a large skillet, melt 2 tablespoons butter over medium-high heat. Reduce heat to medium. Add scallions, and cook until green portion is wilted, about 3 minutes.
2. Add garlic (minced), and cook for 30 seconds.

3. Add remaining tablespoon butter; when melted, add mushrooms. Cook, stirring occasionally, until mushrooms are softened, about 5 minutes.
4. Add vinegar, and cook for 2 minutes.
5. Pour the water into skillet. Add asparagus, and bring to boil over medium-high heat. Reduce heat to medium, and simmer for 5 minutes.
6. Add peas, and cook for 2 minutes.
7. Add heavy cream, and continue to simmer until sauce thickens, about 2 minutes.
8. Transfer to a serving bowl, stir in basil, and season to taste with salt and pepper.
9. Sprinkle with Parmesan, if desired. Serve immediately.

Atkins Chocolate Slushies

Servings: 4 | Prep: 120 m | Style: American | Cook: 10 m

Ingredients

- 1 cup Heavy Cream
- 1/2 cup Tap Water
- 2 tbsps Cocoa Powder (Unsweetened)
- 8 tbsps Sugar Free Chocolate Syrup
- 1 tsp Vanilla Extract

Directions

1. In a medium saucepan combine cream, water, cocoa powder and 1/2 cup unsweetened chocolate syrup.
2. Bring to a boil over medium heat. Reduce heat to low; cook, stirring occasionally, 5 minutes. Remove from heat and stir in vanilla.
3. Pour mixture into two ice cube trays. Freeze 2 hours.
4. Before serving transfer cubes into a food processor. Pulse until mixture is finely chopped and slushy.

Atkins Cinnamon Pie Crust

Servings: 8 | Prep: 10 m | Style: American

Ingredients

- 1/4 tsp Salt
- 1 tsp Sucralose Based Sweetener (Sugar Substitute)
- 1 tsp Cinnamon
- 1/2 cup Unsalted Butter Stick
- 3 3/4 servings All Purpose Low-Carb Baking Mix
- 2 tbsps Tap Water

Directions

Use the Atkins recipe to make All Purpose Low-Carb Baking Mix. You will need 1 1/4 cups to make one pie crust.

1. Pulse the baking mix, salt, sugar substitute, and cinnamon in a food processor to incorporate; add butter and pulse until mixture resembles a coarse meal, about 30 seconds. Pulse in water until dough just comes together, about 30 seconds (add up to 1 more tablespoon if necessary).
2. Transfer dough to a sheet of plastic wrap; form into a a disk about 6 inches in diameter. Wrap tightly in plastic; refrigerate until firm, about 30 minutes.
3. Roll and bake as directed in pie recipe. Makes 1 pie crust.

Atkins Coconut Layer Cake

*Servings: 12 | **Prep**: 30 m | **Style**: American | **Cook**: 22 m*

Ingredients

- large Eggs (Whole)
- 1 1/2 cups Sucralose Based Sweetener (Sugar Substitute)
- 3 tsps Coconut Extract
- 2/3 cup Whole Grain Soy Flour
- 1 tsp Baking Powder (Straight Phosphate, Double Acting)
- 6 large Egg Whites
- 2 cups Unsalted Butter Stick
- 1/4 tsp Salt
- 2/3 cup Dried Coconut

Directions

1. Heat oven to 350°F. Grease two 8-inch cake pans; line bottoms with parchment paper; then grease the paper. Melt 1/2 cup butter and set aside. Place remaining butter (1 1/2 cups) on a plate, cut it into 1 Tbsp portions, and keep it at room temperature.
2. With an electric mixer on high, beat whole eggs, 3/4 cup sugar substitute and 1 tbsp coconut extract until ribbons form, about 5 minutes.
3. In three additions cup sift soy flour, baking power and salt over egg mixture; fold in with a rubber spatula to combine.
4. Fold in 1/2 cup melted butter. Then pour batter into prepared pans.
5. Bake for 22 minutes until cake springs back in middle when lightly touched. Cool in pans on wire racks 5 minutes. Line racks with paper towels and invert cake layers. Gently peel off parchment and cool completely.
6. For frosting: in a double boiler or a bowl placed over simmering water, whisk egg whites, 3/4 cup sugar substitute and salt until temperature reaches 130°F. Transfer whites to mixing bowl and beat on high speed until cool and fully whipped. Reduce speed to medium and beat in 1 1/2 cups room temperature butter 1 tablespoon at a time until well combined, thick and creamy, about 10 minutes - do not rush the process.
7. Place one cake layer on serving plate. Mix 1 cup frosting with half the coconut (1/3 cup); frost bottom layer. Place top cake layer over bottom layer. Cover top and sides with remaining frosting and pat remaining 1/3 cup coconut over frosting. Optional: toast coconut (3-5 minutes at 350°F). Makes 12 servings.

Atkins Cuisine Brownies

Servings: 25 | Prep: 15 m | Style: American | Cook: 30 m

Ingredients

- 4 oz Unsweetened Baking Chocolate Squares
- 1/2 cup Unsalted Butter Stick
- 1/2 cup Heavy Cream
- 5 large Eggs (Whole)
- 1 cup Sucralose Based Sweetener (Sugar Substitute)
- 2 tsps Baking Powder (Straight Phosphate, Double Acting)
- 4 1/2 servings All Purpose Low-Carb Baking Mix

Directions

1. Use the Atkins recipe to make All Purpose Low-Carb Baking Mix to use in this recipe. You will need 1 1/4 cups.
2. Pre-heat oven to 325°F.
3. Place the unsweetened chocolate and butter together in a bowl and microwave on high power for approximately 2 minutes until chocolate is melted. Whisk in heavy cream.
4. In a separate bowl, add the eggs and 1 cup of granular sugar substitute. Beat together using an electric mixer until mixture is just blended. Reduce mixer to low speed and then blend in the chocolate mixture.
5. With a wooden spoon, mix in the baking powder and 1 1/4 cups low-carb baking mix.
6. Coat 8 x 8 inch pan with non-stick vegetable oil spray and spread batter evenly into pan.
7. Bake at 325°F for 30-35 minutes or until done (toothpick inserted in the center comes out clean). (Do not over-bake or brownies will be dry and hard.)
8. Once cooled, cut into 5 rows by 5 rows to make 25 brownies.

Atkins Cuisine Cookies

*Servings: 36 | **Prep:** 20 m | **Style:** American | **Cook:** 10 m*

Ingredients

-   1 tsp Baking Powder (Straight Phosphate, Double Acting)
-   1/2 tsp Salt
-   1 cup Salted Butter Stick
-   1 cup Sucralose Based Sweetener (Sugar Substitute)
-   2 tsps Vanilla Extract
-   2 large Eggs (Whole)
-   6 servings All Purpose Low-Carb Baking Mix
-   6 oz Sugar Free Chocolate Chips

Directions

Use the Atkins recipe to make All Purpose Low-Carb Baking Mix for this recipe; you will need 2 cups but the recipe makes 3. Save any remaining in an airtight container in the refrigerator.

1. Preheat oven to 375°F.
2. Blend all dry ingredients together in a small mixing bowl, set aside.
3. Mix melted butter, sugar substitute and vanilla at medium speed with an electric mixer until well blended. Add eggs one at a time, mixing well after each addition. Gradually add dry ingredient mixture, beating until blended. Gently mix in chocolate chips with a wooden spoon or spatula.
4. Spoon rounded teaspoonfuls of cookie dough onto a cookie sheet coated with non-stick vegetable oil spray. Gently flatten cookies by pressing with hand or spatula.
5. Cook at 375° F for 10 to 12 minutes or until done or until lightly browned. Remove from baking sheet and place cookies on a wire rack to cool. (Do not overbake cookies or they will be dry and hard.)

Atkins Cuisine Pizza with Sausage, Bell Peppers and Onions

*Servings: 8 | **Prep:** 20 m | **Style:** American | **Cook:** 30 m*

Ingredients

- 1 1/2 tsps Baking Powder (Straight Phosphate, Double Acting)
- 1/2 tsp Salt
- 1 individual packet Sucralose Based Sweetener (Sugar Substitute)
- 1 cup Tap Water
- 3 tbsps Extra Virgin Olive Oil
- 1/2 cup Tomato Sauce
- 1 cup shredded Whole Milk Mozzarella Cheese
- 1 link (5" long) Italian Sausage
- 1/2 medium (approx 2-3/4" long, 2-1/2" dia) Green Sweet Pepper
- 1/2 medium (approx 2-3/4" long, 2-1/2" dia) Red Sweet Pepper
- 1 small Red Onion
- 6 servings All Purpose Low-Carb Baking Mix

Directions

Use the Atkins recipe to make All Purpose Low-Carb Baking Mix for this recipe. You will need 2 cups.

1. Preheat oven to 425°F.
2. Blend together baking mix, baking powder, salt and sugar substitute in a large mixing bowl.

3. Add water and oil. Using a wooden spoon or a spatula, combine into a dough. Using a spatula, remove the dough from the bowl and place on a clean surface lightly coated with olive oil spray.
4. Coat rolling pin with oil spray and roll the dough out to fit the pizza pan or stone. Or use your hands to pat the dough into shape.
5. Bake the crust for 10 minutes and remove from oven.
6. Spread tomato sauce evenly over the pizza. Sprinkle with mozzarella and top with sausage rounds, green and red bell pepper slices and onions. Sprinkle with salt and pepper to taste.
7. Return to the oven and continue baking for 10-15 minutes. Cut into 8 slices.

Atkins Cuisine Pizza-Barbecue Chicken Supreme

Servings: 8 | Prep: 20 m | Style: American | Cook: 30 m

Ingredients

- 1 1/2 tsps Baking Powder (Straight Phosphate, Double Acting)
- 1/2 tsp Salt
- 1 individual packet Sucralose Based Sweetener (Sugar Substitute)
- 1 cup Tap Water
- 1 small Red Onion
- 1 cup cooked, diced Chicken Breast
- 2 servings Barbecue Sauce
- 1/2 medium (approx 2-3/4" long, 2-1/2" dia) Green Sweet Pepper
- 6 servings All Purpose Low-Carb Baking Mix
- 1 cup shredded Whole Milk Mozzarella Cheese
- 3 tbsps Extra Virgin Olive Oil

Directions

Using barbecue sauce instead of tomato sauce spices up the chicken topping. You can substitute other vegetable and meat toppings for variety.

1. Heat oven to 425°F.
2. Blend together baking mix (2 cups), baking powder, salt and sugar substitute in a large mixing bowl.
3. Add water and oil. Using a wooden spoon or a spatula, combine into a dough. Using a spatula, remove the dough from the bowl and place on a clean surface lightly coated with olive oil spray.

4. Coat rolling pin with oil spray and roll the dough out to fit the pizza pan or stone. Or use your hands to pat the dough into shape.
5. Bake the crust for 10 minutes and remove from oven.
6. Spread Barbecue Sauce (about 1/2 cup) evenly over the pizza. Sprinkle with mozzarella and top with chicken pieces, bell pepper slices and onions. Sprinkle with salt and pepper, to taste.
7. Return to the oven and continue baking for 10-15 minutes. Cut into 8 slices.

Atkins Yorkshire Pudding

*Servings: 9 | **Prep**: 5 m | **Style**: Other | **Cook**: 35 m*

Ingredients

- 1/2 cup Whole Grain Soy Flour
- 2 oz Vital Wheat Gluten
- 3 large Eggs (Whole)
- 1 cup Whole Milk
- 1 tsp Salt
- 1/3 cup Canola Vegetable Oil
- 1 tsp Baking Powder (Straight Phosphate, Double Acting)

Directions

1. Preheat oven to 450° F.
2. Whisk together soy flour, gluten, eggs, milk and salt.
3. Pour drippings or oil into an 8-inch square baking dish, and place on center rack in oven for 5 minutes, until drippings or oil is smoking hot. Then add batter and bake 15 minutes.
4. Lower temperature to 350° F and bake for 15 to 20 minutes more, until lightly browned. Serve piping hot.

Avocado Gazpacho Smoothie

*Servings: 1 | **Prep**: 5 m | **Style**: Mexican*

Ingredients

- 1 cup Tap Water
- 1 fruit without skin and seed California Avocado
- 1 oz Goat Cheese (Soft)
- 1 tbsp Heavy Cream
- 2 tsp choppeds Chives
- 2 tsps Fresh Lime Juice
- 1/8 tsp Salt

Directions

1. Place cut-up avocado in a blender. Add remaining ingredients, and blend until smooth. If needed, add additional water, 1 tablespoon at a time, to reach desired consistency.
2. Pour into a tall glass, and garnish with chives and an avocado slice, if desired. Serve immediately.

Avocado Zucchini Soup

Servings: 4 | Prep: 10 m | Style: American | Cook: 15 m

Ingredients

- 1 fruit without skin and seed California Avocado
- 2 tbsps Extra Virgin Olive Oil
- 4 medium (4-1/8" long) Scallions or Spring Onions
- 1 tsp Ginger
- 1 clove Garlic
- 2 medium Zucchinis
- 29 oz Bouillon Vegetable Broth
- 1 cup Tap Water
- 1/2 tsp Salt
- 1/2 tsp Black Pepper
- 1 tbsp Fresh Lemon Juice
- 1/16 cup chopped Sweet Red Peppers

Directions

1. Heat oil in a large saucepan over medium heat. Add 2/3 of the green onions and cook 3 minutes; stir in ginger and garlic and cook, stirring, 1 minute more. Add broth, water, zucchini, salt, and pepper.
2. Cover and cook 10 minutes, until zucchini is very soft. Cool slightly. Then, stir in avocado.
3. Puree soup in batches in a food processor or blender. Return to pan to heat through and stir in lemon juice.
4. Garnish with red pepper and remaining green onions.

Baby Greens with Grapefruit and Red Onion

Servings: 4 | Prep: 15 m | Style: Mexican

Ingredients

- 1 fruit (3-3/4" dia) Grapefruit (Pink and Red)
- 1 fruit (3-3/4" dia) White Grapefruit
- 1/4 tsp Yellow Mustard Seed
- 3 tbsps Extra Virgin Olive Oil
- 1 tsp Tarragon
- 3 3/4 cups Spring Mix Salad
- 1/2 small Red Onion

Directions

If you don't have a grapefruit knife to easily remove the segments, use this method: Slice off just enough of the top and bottom of each grapefruit so they can stand upright on a cutting board. Using a sharp chefs knife and working from the top, circle the entire fruit, peeling the skin off and leaving very little of the bitter white pith behind. Using a smaller paring knife, cut out each segment from the white membrane. Squeeze out any remaining juice from fruit when done. Reserve 1 tablespoon of juice for the dressing and save the additional juice for another use.

1. Section grapefruits.
2. Add reserved grapefruit juice to a mixing bowl. Add mustard. Slowly drizzle in olive oil, whisking well, until well combined.
3. Stir in tarragon; add salt and freshly ground black pepper to taste, set aside.

4. Add greens and toss gently with grapefruit sections, red onion and salad dressing.

Baby Spinach, Pickled Beets and Tomato Salad

Servings: 1 | Prep: 5 m | Style: American

Ingredients

- 1 1/2 cups Baby Spinach
- 1/4 cup sliced Pickled Beets
- 5 Cherry Tomatoes

Directions

1. Place the spinach leaves in a bowl. Add beets and tomatoes and gently toss with low-carb salad dressing of your choice.
2. Season to taste with salt and freshly ground black pepper.

Bacon and Goat Cheese Salad

Servings: 6 | Prep: 25 m | Style: Other | Cook: 15 m

Ingredients

- 2 cups chopped Endive
- 3 tbsps chopped Chives
- 8 oz Goat Cheese (Soft)
- 2 tbsps Extra Virgin Olive Oil
- 1 large Egg (Whole)
- 1 1/2 tbsps Red Wine Vinegar
- 1 tbsp Dijon Mustard
- 1 1/2 servings Atkins Cuisine Bread
- 3/4 tsp Black Pepper
- 4 cups shredded Cos or Romaine Lettuce
- 6 medium slice (yield after cooking) Bacon

Directions

1. FOR SALAD: Cook bacon in a large nonstick skillet over medium heat, turning once, until crisp, about 6 to 7 minutes. Transfer with a slotted spoon to paper towels. Reserve 1 tablespoon of bacon drippings.
2. In a large bowl, combine romaine, endive, and chives; set aside.
3. In a food processor or blender, process bread to make crumbs; spread crumbs on a plate. Place goat cheese slices cut side down on work surface and press lightly to flatten. Dip each slice in egg; let excess drip off. Place on crumbs, pressing to coat evenly and completely.
4. Wipe out bacon skillet with a paper towel; add oil and heat over medium heat. Add goat-cheese patties and cook until browned, about 2 minutes per side (reduce heat if browning occurs too fast or cheese is melting). Transfer to a plate lined with paper towels. Remove skillet from heat.
5. DRESSING: Add reserved bacon drippings, olive oil, vinegar, mustard and pepper to skillet. Whisk to combine. Add warm dressing and bacon to bowl with greens. Toss to combine. Arrange salad on individual serving plates and top each with a goat-cheese patty.

Bacon Wrapped Filet with Blue Cheese Butter Sauce

Servings: 2 | Style: American | Cook: 45 m

Ingredients

- 2 medium (4-1/8" long) Young Green Onions
- 4 oz Portobello Mushroom Cap
- 3 Cherry Tomatoes
- 12 oz Beef Tenderloin (Lean Only, Trimmed to 1/8" Fat)
- 2 slices Bacon
- 1 tbsp Unsalted Butter Stick
- 3 oz Blue Cheese
- 1/3 tbsp Red Wine Vinegar
- 8 oz Baby Spinach
- 2 tsps Olive Oil
- 1/4 tsp Salt
- 1/4 tsp Black Pepper

Directions

1. Preheat the oven to 425ºF. Finely dice the green part of the green onions and place in a small bowl. Dice the white part of the onion and set aside. Remove the cap from the mushroom and discard the stem. Chop the mushroom into ¼-inch pieces; set aside.
2. Pat dry the beef with paper towels. Slice the tenderloin in half widthwise and press down on the halves slightly into filet mignon steaks. Season each filet with ⅛ teaspoon each of salt and pepper. Wrap the outer edge of each steak with a bacon slice. Set aside.
3. Add the butter and 1 ounce of the blue cheese to the bowl with the green onions and stir until well combined. Pour the red wine vinegar into another small bowl, add ¼ teaspoon each of salt and pepper and slowly whisk in 1 tablespoon of olive oil; hold.
4. Heat 2 teaspoons of olive oil in a large non-stick sauté pan over medium-high heat. When the oil is hot, add the steaks and sear on all sides, turning frequently with tongs until browned, about 3 minutes. Transfer to a sheet pan lined with foil and roast for 6 to 8 minutes, or until desired doneness.
5. Meanwhile, in the same sauté pan over medium-high heat, add the mushrooms and the white part of the onion, season with ⅛ teaspoon each of salt and pepper and reduce the heat to low. Saute while stirring until the mushrooms are tender, about 4 minutes. Place the baby spinach in a large bowl and add the remaining 2 ounces of blue cheese. Drizzle the vinaigrette over the spinach. Toss until well combined.
6. Spoon the mushrooms evenly onto two plates. Top with a filet and a dollop of the blue cheese butter. Arrange the salad next to steak and enjoy!

Bacon-Egg Salad Flatout Wrap

*Servings: 1 | **Prep**: 10 m | **Style**: American*

Ingredients

- 2 large Boiled Eggs
- 1 tbsp Real Mayonnaise
- 1/2 tsp or 1 packet Yellow Mustard
- 1 flatbread Light Original Flatbread
- 1 1/2 oz cooked Turkey Bacon

Directions

1. Mix together chopped eggs, mayonnaise and mustard. Add salt and pepper to taste.
2. Spread mixture on one rounded end of Flatout. Top with cooked crumbled bacon.
3. Roll up and cut in half.

Bahian Halibut

Servings: 4 | Prep: 10 m | Style: Other | Cook: 10 m

Ingredients

- 2 tbsps Extra Virgin Olive Oil
- 2 tbsps Fresh Lime Juice
- 2 lbs Atlantic and Pacific Halibut
- 4 tbsps chopped Onions
- 1 cup chopped Green Sweet Pepper
- 1 pepper Serrano Pepper
- 1 tsp Garlic
- 1 tsp Salt
- 1/2 cup Coconut Cream
- 1 small whole (2-2/5" dia) Red Tomato

Directions

1. The state of Bahia in Brazil borders the Caribbean and includes what is known as the Coconut Coast and was first settled by the Portuguese. This heat of this well-seasoned fish dish is tamed with coconut milk.

2. With a fork, whisk 1 tablespoon oil and all the lime juice on large platter, add fish, and turn to coat. Dice the onion, bell pepper and the serrano pepper (be sure to use gloves to protect your hands from the heat of the pepper - do not include the seeds or ribs if you want to reduce the heat). Mince the garlic and add to a bowl with the onions and peppers. Chop the tomatoes, place in a small bowl and set aside.
3. Heat remaining tablespoon oil in a 12-inch nonstick skillet over medium heat. Add garlic and the diced onion and peppers. Cook 6 minutes until onion is translucent and peppers are just tender.

4. Sprinkle 1/2 teaspoon of salt over fish and add fish to skillet; pour coconut milk over fish and add tomato. Reduce heat to medium-low and simmer 8 to 9 minutes, turning fish halfway through cooking time.
5. Stir remaining salt into sauce, spoon over fish a few times, and serve immediately.

Baked Artichoke-Parsley Cheese Squares

Servings: 8 | Prep: 10 m | Style: American | Cook: 35 m

Ingredients

- 2 tbsps Extra Virgin Olive Oil
- 3 medium (4-1/8" long) Scallions or Spring Onions
- 3 tsps Garlic
- 1 package (9 oz) Artichokes (Globe or French, Unprepared, Frozen)
- 1/2 tsp Oregano
- 1/4 tsp Crushed Red Pepper Flakes
- 4 large Eggs (Whole)
- 1 cup shredded Monterey Jack Cheese
- 1/8 cup dry Whole Grain Soy Flour
- 2 tbsps Parsley
- 1/2 tsp Salt
- 1/4 tsp Black Pepper

Directions

1. Preheat oven to 325°F.
2. In a medium skillet over medium-high heat, heat oil and sauté green onion until softened, about 4 minutes. Add garlic and sauté until aroma is released, about 30 seconds. Add artichokes, oregano and pepper flakes and cook until artichokes are warmed through, about 2 minutes. Allow to cool slightly, about 5 minutes.
3. In a large bowl, gently whisk eggs, cheese, soy flour, parsley, salt and pepper until well-combined. Using a wooden spoon, stir in artichoke mixture.
4. Pour artichoke batter into an 8 square baking dish and bake 30 minutes, until set and slightly golden on top. Cool slightly before cutting into squares.

Baked Catfish with Broccoli and Herb-Butter Blend

*Servings: 1 | **Prep:** 5 m | **Style:** American | **Cook:** 15 m*

Ingredients

- 6 oz Channel Catfish (Farmed)
- 1 cup chopped Broccoli
- 1 serving Herb-Butter Blend

Directions

1. Cooking fish in an aluminum-foil packet makes for easy cleanup and works especially well for single portions. Add a vegetable and you have a complete quick meal. Use any compound butter or use 1 tablespoon of the Atkins recipe: Herb-Butter Blend.
2. Preheat oven to 350°F.
3. Place the catfish on a 12-inch square piece of foil. Sprinkle fish with salt and freshly ground pepper to taste. Arrange broccoli florets around fish.
4. Fold up the sides of the foil and crimp tightly to form a sealed packet.
5. Bake for 10 15 minutes until fish is flaky and broccoli is tender.
6. Transfer to a dish, open foil and top with a tablespoon of Herb-Butter Blend.

Baked Chicken with Artichokes

*Servings: 4 | **Prep:** 20 m | **Style:** American | **Cook:** 40 m*

Ingredients

- 8 oz Mushroom Pieces and Stems
- 1/2 tsp Salt
- 1/2 cup chopped Onions
- 20 oz boneless (yield after cooking) Chicken Thigh
- 4 1/2 tsps Garlic
- 4 fl ozs Sauvignon Blanc Wine
- 1 tsp Rosemary
- 1/4 tsp Crushed Red Pepper Flakes

- 1 1/2 tsp grounds Oregano
- 3 tbsps Extra Virgin Olive Oil
- 1 package (9 oz), yield Artichokes (Globe or French) (with Salt, Frozen, Drained, Cooked, Boiled)
- 1/2 tsp Black Pepper
- 3/4 serving All Purpose Low-Carb Baking Mix

Directions

1. Use the Atkins recipe to make All Purpose Low-Carb Baking Mix for this recipe. Dredging chicken in flour before sautéing seals in the juices and give it a nice color.
2. Preheat oven to 350°F. Place 1/4 cup baking mix, salt and pepper in a shallow plate and mix well. Dredge chicken in the mixture, turning to coat evenly and then tapping to remove any excess.
3. In large skillet, heat oil over medium-high heat. Cook chicken until lightly browned, turning once, about 4 minutes. Transfer to baking dish.
4. Add onion to skillet and sauté until softened, about 2 minutes. Add mushrooms and sauté until lightly golden, about 3 more minutes. Add garlic and sauté until aroma is released, about 30 seconds. Stir in wine, artichokes, rosemary and red pepper flakes and bring to a simmer.
5. Pour artichoke mixture over chicken in the baking dish, cover and bake 40 minutes, until chicken is tender and cooked through. Season with additional salt and pepper, if desired, and stir in oregano before serving.

Baked Fennel au Gratin

*Servings: 6 | **Prep:** 5 m | **Style:** French | **Cook:** 50 m*

Ingredients

- 2 bulbs Fennel Bulk
- 1/2 tsp Salt
- 1/4 tsp Black Pepper
- 1 cup Heavy Cream
- 1/2 cup shredded Gruyere Cheese
- 2 tbsps Parmesan Cheese (Grated)
- 1/2 serving All Purpose Low-Carb Baking Mix
- 1/4 cup Unsalted Butter Stick

Directions

1. Use the Atkins recipe to make All Purpose Low-Carb Baking Mix for this recipe.
2. Preheat oven to 375°F.
3. Grease a shallow 2-quart baking dish with 1 teaspoon butter and set aside.
4. Trim fennel leaving 1 stalks, Quarter bulbs and remove center core. Cut crosswise into 1/4 slices. Place fennel in a saucepan and cook in lightly salted water over medium heat until just tender, about 10 minutes. Drain fennel and season with salt and pepper. Transfer fennel to dish, pressing down to form an even layer. Set aside.
5. In a medium saucepan melt butter over medium heat. Stir in 3 Tbsp baking mix and cook 2 minutes.
6. Add cream and bring to a boil. Cook, whisking constantly, until slightly, about 5 minutes. Turn off heat and stir in Gruyere until melted.
7. Pour sauce evenly over fennel and sprinkle dish with Parmesan cheese.Cover with foil and bake 15 minutes; uncover and bake 15-20 minutes more until golden brown and bubbly.

Baked Goat Cheese and Ricotta Custards

Servings: 4 | Style: Italian | Cook: 50 m

Ingredients

- 1 1/3 second sprays Original Canola Cooking Spray
- 1 cup Ricotta Cheese (Whole Milk)
- 6 oz Goats Cheese (Semisoft)
- 3 tbsps Parmesan Cheese (Grated)
- 1/4 cup chopped English Walnuts
- 12 leaves Spinach
- 2 large Eggs (Whole)
- 1/8 tsp Salt
- 1/8 tsp Black Pepper
- 2 tbsps Basil

Directions

1. Heat oven to 350°F. Spray cooking spray onto four 5-ounce ramekins or custard cups.

2. Combine ricotta, goat cheese, Parmesan, walnuts, basil, egg, salt, and pepper in a bowl and mix well.
3. Line each ramekin with 3 spinach leaves. Divide cheese mixture; fill full. Bake 30 minutes. Cool 5 minutes.
4. To serve, run a knife around the rim of each custard. Invert onto small plates.Salt and pepper to taste.

Baked Meatballs

Servings: 4 | Prep: 8 m | Style: American | Cook: 35 m

Ingredients

- 1 tbsp Extra Virgin Olive Oil
- 1/2 large Scallions or Spring Onion
- 1 1/2 tsps Garlic
- 1/2 lb Ground Veal
- 1/2 lb Ground Beef (80% Lean / 20% Fat)
- 1/2 lb Ground Pork
- 1/2 cup Parmesan Cheese (Grated)
- 2 large Eggs (Whole)
- 1/2 tsp Salt
- 1/4 tsp Black Pepper

Directions

If possible, have the butcher grind together the three different meats. Be sure to wash your hands thoroughly after handling raw pork.

1. Heat oven to 375°F.
2. In a skillet, over high heat, heat oil, cook onion 5 minutes, stirring frequently, until softened. Add garlic (minced) and cook 1 minute more.
3. Transfer to a bowl and mix in ground meats, cheese, eggs, salt, and pepper. Roll into golf ball-size meatballs. Place on a jelly roll pan.
4. Bake 20- 25 minutes, until browned and cooked through.

Baked Quesadillas

*Servings: 4 | **Prep:** 10 m | **Style:** Mexican | **Cook:** 10 m*

Ingredients

- 2 tbsps Light Olive Oil
- 2 tbsps chopped Onions
- 16 oz Pork Chops or Roasts (Center Rib, Bone-In)
- 8 slice (1 oz) Monterey Jack Cheese
- 1/4 cup Green Tomato Chile Sauce (Salsa Verde)
- 1 Jalapeno Pepper
- 1/4 cup Cilantro (Coriander)
- 1/2 tsp Black Pepper
- 1/4 tsp Salt
- 1 tortilla Low Carb Tortillas

Directions

1. Make sure the tortillas contain no more than 3 grams of Net Carbs each. Serve with sour cream and additional red or green salsa, if desired.
2. Heat oven to 450°F.
3. Heat 1 tablespoon of the oil in large skillet over medium-high heat. Cook chopped white onion 5 minutes, until softened.
4. Transfer to a bowl. Add pork, cheese, green salsa, chopped jalapeño, cilantro, pepper and salt. Mix well.
5. Brush one side of each tortilla with remaining oil.
6. Spoon one-sixth of pork mixture over half of non-oiled side of each tortilla and fold in half over filling.
7. Place on a baking sheet. Bake 5 minutes, until crisp and golden.

Baked Red Bell Peppers Filled with Cherry Tomatoes and Feta

*Servings: 4 | **Prep:** 10 m | **Style:** American | **Cook:** 45 m*

Ingredients

- 2 medium (approx 2-3/4" long, 2-1/2" dia) Sweet Red Peppers
- 2 oz Feta Cheese
- 8 Cherry Tomatoes
- 1/2 tsp ground Thyme (Dried)

- 2 tbsps Basil
- 1 tbsp Extra Virgin Olive Oil

Directions

1. Preheat oven to 400°F.
2. Cut peppers in half lengthwise. Remove stems, ribs and seeds.
3. Gently combine feta, tomatoes, thyme and basil. Fill pepper halves with the mixture.
4. Place in a baking dish and drizzle with olive oil.
5. Bake, covered with aluminum foil, for 30 minutes. Remove foil and bake an additional 15 minutes until the tomatoes burst and cheese is golden-brown.

Baked Salmon with Bok Choy and Mixed Greens

*Servings: 1 | **Prep**: 15 m | **Style**: American | **Cook**: 10 m*

Ingredients

- 3/4 cup chopped Snowpeas (Pea Pod)
- 1/16 tsp Salt
- 8 oz Chinese Cabbage (Bok-Choy, Pak-Choi)
- 2 oz Pickled Okra
- 3 oz Cooked Red Peppers
- 1/16 tsp Black Pepper
- 1/2 oz Salsa
- 1/2 tbsp Extra Virgin Olive Oil
- 1 tbsp Reserva Sherry Vinegar
- 1/4 tbsp Unsalted Butter Stick
- 6 oz Atlantic Salmon (Farmed)
- 1 cup shredded or chopped Mixed Salad Greens

Directions

1. Use the Atkins recipe for Sherry Vinaigrette for the salad.
2. Preheat oven to 475° F. Place olive oil and butter in a skillet large enough to hold fish in a single layer.
3. Place skillet with just the olive oil and butter into the oven for 3 minutes, until butter is melted. Season fish with salt and pepper. Place fish flesh

side down in prepared skillet. Bake 10 minutes, turning carefully once halfway through cooking time, until just cooked through.

4. Remove from skillet; tent with foil. Add bok choy and lemon peel to skillet. Stir to coat with pan's oil. Place in oven 1 minute, until leaves are wilted and stems are warmed through.
5. To make puree, blend peppers and salsa in a blender 30 seconds.
6. Top bok choy with fish and dollop with the purée.
7. Toss the greens, okra, peppers and snow peas with the Sherry Vinaigrette. Serve with the salmon and bok choy.

Baked Salmon with Bok Choy and Red Bell Pepper Purée

Servings: 4 | Prep: 10 m | Style: American | Cook: 10 m

Ingredients

- 3/4 cup chopped Snowpeas (Pea Pod)
- 1/16 tsp Salt
- 8 oz Chinese Cabbage (Bok-Choy, Pak-Choi)
- 2 oz Pickled Okra
- 3 oz Cooked Red Peppers
- 1/16 tsp Black Pepper
- 1/2 oz Salsa
- 1/2 tbsp Extra Virgin Olive Oil
- 1 tbsp Reserva Sherry Vinegar
- 1/4 tbsp Unsalted Butter Stick
- 6 oz Atlantic Salmon (Farmed)
- 1 cup shredded or chopped Mixed Salad Greens

Directions

1. Use the Atkins recipe for Sherry Vinaigrette for the salad.
2. Preheat oven to 475° F. Place olive oil and butter in a skillet large enough to hold fish in a single layer.
3. Place skillet with just the olive oil and butter into the oven for 3 minutes, until butter is melted. Season fish with salt and pepper. Place fish flesh side down in prepared skillet. Bake 10 minutes, turning carefully once halfway through cooking time, until just cooked through.
4. Remove from skillet; tent with foil. Add bok choy and lemon peel to skillet. Stir to coat with pan's oil. Place in oven 1 minute, until leaves are wilted and stems are warmed through.

5. To make puree, blend peppers and salsa in a blender 30 seconds.
6. Top bok choy with fish and dollop with the purée.
7. Toss the greens, okra, peppers and snow peas with the Sherry Vinaigrette. Serve with the salmon and bok choy.

Baked Tamari-Lemon Pork Chops

Servings: 4 | Prep: 15 m | Style: Asian | Cook: 40 m

Ingredients

- 8 tbsps Tamari Soybean Sauce
- 2 tbsps Worcestershire Sauce
- 2 tsps Garlic
- 1 fl oz Fresh Lemon Juice
- 1/2 tsp Black Pepper
- 1 tsp Canola Vegetable Oil
- 1 1/2 lbs Pork Chops or Roasts (Center Loin, Bone-In)

Directions

1. If you want to serve a dipping sauce with the chops, rather than boiling the marinade, make a fresh batch.
2. In a shallow dish, combine tamari, Worcestershire sauce, garlic (minced), lemon juice, pepper and oil. Add pork chops and turn to coat evenly.
3. Cover, and refrigerate for at least 1 hour or overnight.
4. Preheat oven to 375°F. Remove chops from marinade and pat dry.
5. Place in a roasting pan and bake for 35 40 minutes.

Baked Tofu with Asian Marinade

Servings: 4 | Prep: 5 m | Style: Asian | Cook: 30 m

Ingredients

- 6 oz Firm Silken Tofu

- 1 serving Asian Marinade

Directions

1. Use 2 tablespoons of the Atkins recipe: Asian Marinade.
2. Drain and pat tofu dry with a paper towel. Cut into 1/4 inch strips. Coat with marinade in a shallow dish. Marinate for 30 minutes or more if desired.
3. Preheat oven to 375°
4. Bake on a greased flat pan for 15 minutes, turn over and bake an additional 15 minutes till golden brown and slightly crispy.

Baked Tofu with Cajun Rub

Servings: 4 | Prep: 5 m | Style: Asian | Cook: 30 m

Ingredients

- 6 oz Firm Silken Tofu
- 1 serving Cajun Rub
- 1 tsp Extra Virgin Olive Oil

Directions

1. Use 1 tablespoon of Atkins recipe: Cajun Rub.
2. Drain and pat tofu dry with a paper towel. Cut into 1/4 inch strips. Rub seasoning and oil onto tofu allow to marinate for 30 minutes if desired. Or rub seasoning into tofu and cook immediately.
3. Preheat oven to 375°
4. Bake on a greased flat pan for 15 minutes, turn over and bake an additional 15 minutes till golden brown and slightly crispy.

Baked Tofu with Chipotle Marinade

Servings: 1 | Prep: 5 m | Style: Mexian | Cook: 30 m

Ingredients

- 6 oz Firm Silken Tofu
- 1 serving Chipotle Marinade

Directions

1. Use the Atkins recipe to make Chipotle Marinade for this recipe. You will need 2 Tbsp.
2. Drain and pat tofu dry with a paper towel. Cut into 1/4-inch strips. Marinate tofu for 30 minutes (or more if desired) in Chipotle Marinade.
3. Remove from marinade and pat dry. Preheat oven to 375°F.
4. Bake on a greased flat pan for 15 minutes; turn over and bake another 15 minutes until golden brown and slightly crispy.

Baked Tofu with Latin Marinade

*Servings: 1 | **Prep:** 5 m | **Style:** Mexian | **Cook:** 30 m*

Ingredients

- 6 oz Firm Silken Tofu
- 1 serving Latin Marinade

Directions

1. Use 2 tablespoons of the Atkins recipe: Latin Marinade.
2. Drain and pat tofu dry with a paper towel. Cut into 1/4 inch strips and coat with marinade.
3. Preheat oven to 375° 3. Marinate tofu for 30 minutes or more if desired.
4. Bake on a greased flat pan for 15 minutes, turn over and bake an additional 15 minutes till golden brown and slightly crispy. Serve immediately or store in refridgerator for up to 3 days for use on a salad or reheat for a warm dish.

Baked Tofu with Mediterranean Marinade

*Servings: 1 | **Prep:** 5 m | **Style:** Mediterranean / Greek | **Cook**: 30 m*

Ingredients

- 6 oz Firm Silken Tofu
- 1 serving Mediterranean Marinade

Directions

1. Drain and pat tofu dry with a paper towel. Cut into 1/4 inch strips.
2. Preheat oven to 375°
3. Marinate tofu in Mediterranean Marinade for 30 minutes or more if desired.
4. Bake on a greased flat pan for 15 minutes, turn over and bake an additional 15 minutes till golden brown and slightly crispy.

Baked Tofu with Moroccan Rub

*Servings: 1 | **Prep:** 5 m | **Style:** Middle Eastern | **Cook:** 30 m*

Ingredients

- 6 oz Firm Silken Tofu
- 1 serving Moroccan Rub
- 1 tsp Extra Virgin Olive Oil

Directions

1. Use the Atkins recipe for Moroccan Rub. You will need 1 Tbsp.
2. Drain and pat tofu dry with a paper towel. Cut into 1/4 inch strips. Rub 1 Tbsp seasoning combined with 1 tsp oil onto tofu allow to marinate for 30 minutes if desired. Or rub seasoning into tofu and cook immediately.
3. Preheat oven to 375°F.
4. Bake on a greased flat pan for 15 minutes, turn over and bake an additional 15 minutes till golden brown and slightly crispy.

Baked Tofu with Red Bell Pepper, Broccoli and Peanut Sauce

Servings: 4 | *Prep:* 10 m | *Style:* American | *Cook:* 22 m

Ingredients

- 28 oz Firm Silken Tofu
- 2 tbsps Canola Vegetable Oil
- 3 tbsps Soy Sauce Tamari
- 2 medium (approx 2-3/4" long, 2-1/2" dia) Sweet Red Peppers
- 2 cups chopped Broccoli
- 4 tbsps Natural Creamy Peanut Butter 1/3 Less Sodium & Sugar
- 1 1/2 fl ozs Lime Juice
- 3 tsps Chili Garlic Sauce
- 2 tsps Sucralose Based Sweetener (Sugar Substitute)
- 1/4 cup Cilantro (Coriander)

Directions

1. Preheat oven to 450°.
2. Combine 2 Tbsp tamari soy sauce and 2 Tbsp oil, set aside.
3. Cut tofu into 6 rectangles, brush with soy and oil mixture. Place on baking pan.
4. Add peppers and broccoli to baking pan and brush with soy and oil mixture. Bake for 10 minutes, turn tofu pieces over and continue to bake for an additional 12 minutes till tofu is browned and vegetables are softened.
5. While tofu and vegetable are baking, combine, peanut butter, lime juice, 1 Tbsp tamari, chili garlic sauce and sugar substitute in a sauce pan over low heat until warmed through.
6. Toss baked tofu and vegetables with sauce and serve immediately with cilantro on top.

Balsamic Pork Loin and Cauliflower

Servings: 2 | *Prep:* m | *Style:* American | *Cook:* 45 m

Ingredients

- 28 oz Firm Silken Tofu
- 2 tbsps Canola Vegetable Oil
- 3 tbsps Soy Sauce Tamari
- 2 medium (approx 2-3/4" long, 2-1/2" dia) Sweet Red Peppers
- 2 cups chopped Broccoli
- 4 tbsps Natural Creamy Peanut Butter 1/3 Less Sodium & Sugar
- 1 1/2 fl ozs Lime Juice
- 3 tsps Chili Garlic Sauce
- 2 tsps Sucralose Based Sweetener (Sugar Substitute)
- 1/4 cup Cilantro (Coriander)

Directions

1. Preheat oven to 450°.
2. Combine 2 Tbsp tamari soy sauce and 2 Tbsp oil, set aside.
3. Cut tofu into 6 rectangles, brush with soy and oil mixture. Place on baking pan.
4. Add peppers and broccoli to baking pan and brush with soy and oil mixture. Bake for 10 minutes, turn tofu pieces over and continue to bake for an additional 12 minutes till tofu is browned and vegetables are softened.
5. While tofu and vegetable are baking, combine, peanut butter, lime juice, 1 Tbsp tamari, chili garlic sauce and sugar substitute in a sauce pan over low heat until warmed through.
6. Toss baked tofu and vegetables with sauce and serve immediately with cilantro on top.

Barbecue Rub

Servings: 12 | Prep: 5 m | Style: American

Ingredients

- 2 tbsps Garlic Powder
- 2 tbsps Onion Powder
- 6 tsps Xylitol
- 1 1/2 tbsps Chili Powder
- 2 tbsps Cumin
- 1 1/2 tbsps Black Pepper

- 1 tsp Salt
- 1 tsp Yellow Mustard Seed
- 1 tsp Allspice Ground

Directions

1. Use this simple rub to spice up meats before grilling and roasting. Its flavor pairs beautifully with the Atkins recipe for Barbecue Sauce. Rub this on ribs before cooking and then baste the ribs with the sauce during the last 10-20 minutes of grilling or cooking. Each serving is 1 Tbsp.
2. Combine cumin, garlic powder, onion powder, xylitol, chili powder, pepper, salt, mustard and allspice in a bowl and mix well.
3. Rub onto ribs or other meats and marinate for at least an hour before grilling or baking. Remove rub before cooking and pat dry.
4. Rub lasts for up to a month in sealed container.

Barbecue Sauce

Servings: 10 | Prep: 25 m | Style: American

Ingredients

- 1 tbsp Extra Virgin Olive Oil
- 1/4 cup chopped Onions
- 2 tbsps Tomato Paste
- 1 tsp Chili Powder
- 1 tsp Cumin
- 3/4 tsp Garlic Powder
- 3/4 tsp Yellow Mustard Seed
- 1/4 tsp Allspice Ground
- 1/8 tsp Red or Cayenne Pepper
- 1 1/2 cups Unsweetened Ketchup
- 1 tbsp Vinegar (Cider)
- 2/3 tbsp Worcestershire Sauce
- 2 tsps Sucralose Based Sweetener (Sugar Substitute)
- 1/4 tsp dry Coffee (Instant Powder)

Directions

1. Most commercial barbecue sauces are full of sugar or high-fructose corn syrup. Feel free to customize the sauce to your preferences or to the recipe you'll use this sauce with. For example, you can use more or less cayenne pepper or more or less vinegar as well as other spice combinations. Each serving is 2 scant Tbsp.
2. Heat oil in a medium saucepan over medium-high heat. Add onion and sauté until soft,
3. about 3 minutes.
4. Add tomato paste, chili powder, cumin, garlic powder, mustard, allspice and cayenne pepper, cook until fragrant, about 1 minute.
5. Stir in ketchup, vinegar, Worcestershire sauce, sugar substitute and coffee; simmer, stirring occasionally, until very thick, about 8 minutes.
6. Serve warm or at room temperature, or refrigerate in an airtight container for up to 3 days.

Barbecued Glazed Ham

Servings: 10 | Prep: 25 m | Style: American | Cook: 90 m

Ingredients

- 80 oz boneless (yield after cooking) Fresh Ham
- 1 tbsp Chili Powder
- 1 tbsp Paprika
- 1 tsp Cumin
- 1/2 tsp Cinnamon
- 1/4 tsp Cloves (Ground)
- 1 tbsp Sucralose Based Sweetener (Sugar Substitute)
- 5 tbsps Sugar Free Apricot Preserves

Directions

1. Prepare the grill for indirect heat. Place a disposable aluminum drip pan in center of bottom grate or floor of grill. For a closed gas grill, heat on high for 10 to 15 minutes, then turn off heat source directly under pan, leaving the other one or two burners on. Adjust heat to register between 375°F and 425°F on an oven thermometer. For a charcoal grill, build two equal piles of briquettes on either side of drip pan. Burn coals about 25 minutes, until they are covered with gray ash.

2. Place ham onto grill and close lid. Grill 45 minutes. Turn ham over (adding more briquettes if necessary), and grill 45 to 60 minutes more, until an instant-read thermometer inserted in center of ham (away from bone) registers 140°F.
3. Combine chili powder, paprika, cumin, cinnamon, cloves and sugar substitute in a cup. Score top and sides of ham with a sharp knife in a crisscross pattern. Sprinkle rub over all sides.
4. Place ham on prepared grill over pan. Spoon or brush jam over ham. Cover and grill 5 minutes more. Let stand 15 minutes before carving.

Basic Custard Ice Cream

Servings: 8 | Prep: 20 m | Style: American | Cook: 240 m

Ingredients

- 3 cups Heavy Cream
- 3 large Egg Yolks
- 1 large Egg (Whole)
- 3/4 cup Sucralose Based Sweetener (Sugar Substitute)
- 1/8 tsp Salt
- 1/2 tsp Vanilla Extract

Directions

1. In a medium heavy saucepan, heat cream until bubbles form just around the edge of the pan. Meanwhile, whisk together yolks, eggs, sugar substitute and salt.
2. Very slowly whisk the hot cream into the eggs. Pour the mixture back into the pan. Place over medium-low heat and cook, stirring constantly, just until the mixture thickens enough to coat the back of a spoon, 1 to 2 minutes.
3. Immediately remove from the heat and pour into a clean bowl. Stir in vanilla.
4. Cover the surface of the custard with plastic wrap and refrigerate until well chilled, about 4 hours. Freeze according to the directions for your ice cream maker.

Basic Egg Salad

Servings: 4 | Prep: 5 m | Style: American

Ingredients

- 8 large Boiled Eggs
- 1/2 cup Real Mayonnaise
- 3 tsps Dijon Mustard
- 1/2 tsp Salt
- 1/4 tsp Black Pepper
- 2 stalk medium (7-1/2" - 8" long) Celery

Directions

1. Chop eggs roughly, or push them through the large-holed side of a four-sided box grater.
2. In a large mixing bowl, mix eggs with mayonnaise, mustard, salt and pepper with a wooden spoon. Stir in chopped celery.
3. Serve over lettuce or use low-carb bread or a tortilla to make a sandwich if you are in the correct phase and remember to add the extra grams to the total Net Carb count

Basic Steamed Lobster with Drawn Butter

Servings: 4 | Prep: 5 m | Style: American | Cook: 15 m

Ingredients

- 4 lobsters Northern Lobster
- 3/4 cup Unsalted Butter Stick
- 1/2 fruit (2-1/8" dia) Lemon

Directions

1. Bring 10 quarts of salted water to a boil (you may need to use two pots).

2. Plunge lobsters directly into the boiling water, making sure they are completely covered. Bring the water back up to a boil. Cover and cook for 20 minutes from the time the water returns to a boil.
3. Remove lobsters from water with tongs; drain on paper towels.
4. Serve with butter in small dipping cups and lemon wedges.

Basic Tomato Sauce

Servings: 6 | Prep: 10 m | Style: Italian | Cook: 30 m

Ingredients

- 1/4 cup Extra Virgin Olive Oil
- 1 medium (2-1/2" dia) Onions
- 1/2 stalk medium (7-1/2" - 8" long) Celery
- 2 cloves Garlic
- 1 tsp leaf Basil (Dried)
- 28 oz Crushed Tomatoes (Canned)

Directions

1. This versatile sauce is great not just with meatballs or on a low-carb or shirataki pasta, but also on sautéed zucchini, onions or peppers. Each serving is 1/2 cup.
2. Heat oil in a medium saucepan over medium heat. Dice the white onion, celery and garlic; add to pan and saute until the vegetables are very soft, about 6 minutes. Add basil and cook, stirring, 30 seconds.
3. Stir in tomatoes. Bring to a boil; reduce heat to medium-low and simmer, partially covered, until thickened, about 30 minutes. Season with salt and pepper. Serve hot

Basil Pesto

Servings: 4 | Prep: 10 m | Style: Italian

Ingredients

- 6 oz Basil
- 1/3 cup Dried Pine Nuts
- 1/3 cup Parmesan Cheese (Grated)
- 1/2 tsp Garlic
- 1/2 tsp Salt
- 1/3 cup Extra Virgin Olive Oil

Directions

1. For this recipe you will need 3 cups of chopped basil. Despite its low carb content, this recipe is not appropriate for Induction because it contains nuts. Toasting the nuts enhances the flavor. Add more garlic if you prefer. Mix pesto with mayonnaise or cream cheese for a quick dip or thick sauce to spoon over fish, chicken, beef or steamed vegetables. It's also great atop slices of tomato and mozzarella. See variation below. Each servings is 1/4 cup.
2. Combine basil, pine nuts, Parmesan, garlic and salt in a food processor or blender; pulse until finely chopped.
3. Add oil in a slow and steady stream with machine running; process until fairly smooth but not puréed.
4. Serve immediately or refrigerate in an airtight container for up to 3 days or freeze for up to 1 month.
5. Arugula-Walnut Pesto: Prepare Basil Pesto according to directions, substituting arugula for the basil and walnuts for the pine nuts.

Bearnaise Sauce

Servings: 8 | Prep: 10 m | Style: French | Cook: 10 m

Ingredients

- 2 tbsps chopped Shallots
- 1/2 tsp Tarragon
- 5 tbsps White Wine Vinegar
- 2 large Egg Yolks
- 1/2 cup Unsalted Butter Stick
- 1/8 tsp Salt
- 1/8 tsp Black Pepper

Directions

1. To make sauce: In a double boiler (or heatproof bowl set over, but not touching, a sauce pot of simmering water), combine shallot, tarragon, and vinegar. Cook 5 minutes, until most of the vinegar has evaporated.
2. Whisk in egg yolk mixture.Whisk continuously until egg yolks have thickened, about 5 minutes. Whisk in butter gradually, piece by piece, until incorporated (sauce should have the texture of mayonnaise).
3. Remove from heat. Season to taste with salt and pepper.

Béchamel Sauce

Servings: 6 | Prep: 10 m | Style: French | Cook: 20 m

Ingredients

- 1 cup Heavy Cream
- 1 cup Tap Water
- 2 tbsps chopped Onions
- 1 tsp Salt
- 1/8 tsp Black Pepper
- 1/8 tsp Nutmeg (Ground)
- 3 tsps Thick-It-Up
- 1 tbsp Unsalted Butter Stick

Directions

1. Béchamel is a mild sauce that can be used in soufflés or simmered with finely chopped vegetables or meats. Traditionally thickened with a mixture of flour and fat, our version uses heavy cream and a low-carb thickener instead. Each serving is 1/4 cup.
2. Combine cream, water, white onion, salt, pepper and nutmeg in a small saucepan over medium heat; bring to a simmer. Remove from heat; let stand for 15 minutes.
3. Strain cream mixture; return to saucepan over medium heat. Whisk in 1 tablespoon Thick-It-Up thickener; cook until sauce thickens, about 3 minutes.
4. Remove from heat; swirl in butter until melted. Use immediately

Beef and Vegetable Stew

Servings: 6 | *Prep:* 10 m | *Style:* American | *Cook:* 165 m

Ingredients

- 1 1/2 lbs Beef Chuck (Mock Tender Steak, Lean Only, Trimmed to 1/4" Fat)
- 1 tsp leaf Dried Thyme Leaves
- 1 tsp leaf Oregano
- 1 tsp Rosemary (Dried)
- 1 tsp Paprika
- 2 tsps Salt
- 1 tsp Black Pepper
- 2 tbsps Extra Virgin Olive Oil
- 2 tbsps Unsalted Butter Stick
- 1 cup White Pearl Onions
- 2 cloves Garlic
- 16 fl ozs Merlot Wine
- 1 lb Green Snap Beans
- 1 medium Carrot
- 2 tbsps Thick-It-Up

Directions

1. Heat oven to 325°F.
2. Toss beef with thyme, oregano, rosemary, paprika, salt and pepper. Heat half the oil in a Dutch oven over medium-high heat. Brown half the beef; transfer to a bowl. Repeat with remaining oil and beef. Set aside.
3. Melt butter in Dutch oven or crock pot. Add onions; cook 7 8 minutes until onions begin to brown. Add garlic during last 2 minutes of cooking time.
4. Add reserved meat and accumulated juices, wine and 2 cups water. Bring to a boil. Cover Dutch oven and place in oven. Cook 2 hours, until beef is tender.
5. Add green beans and carrots; cook 15 minutes more, just until beans and carrots are tender.
6. Transfer Dutch oven to stove top over medium-high heat. Stir in thickener; cook 2 minutes more, stirring, until sauce thickens.
7. Adjust seasonings to taste and serve immediately.

Beef Bolognaise with Parmesan

Servings: 6 | Prep: 10 m | Style: Italian | Cook: 25 m

Ingredients

- 1 1/2 lbs Beef Chuck (Mock Tender Steak, Lean Only, Trimmed to 1/4" Fat)
- 1 tsp leaf Dried Thyme Leaves
- 1 tsp leaf Oregano
- 1 tsp Rosemary (Dried)
- 1 tsp Paprika
- 2 tsps Salt
- 1 tsp Black Pepper
- 2 tbsps Extra Virgin Olive Oil
- 2 tbsps Unsalted Butter Stick
- 1 cup White Pearl Onions
- 2 cloves Garlic
- 16 fl ozs Merlot Wine
- 1 lb Green Snap Beans
- 1 medium Carrot
- 2 tbsps Thick-It-Up

Directions

1. Heat oven to 325°F.
2. Toss beef with thyme, oregano, rosemary, paprika, salt and pepper. Heat half the oil in a Dutch oven over medium-high heat. Brown half the beef; transfer to a bowl. Repeat with remaining oil and beef. Set aside.
3. Melt butter in Dutch oven or crock pot. Add onions; cook 7 8 minutes until onions begin to brown. Add garlic during last 2 minutes of cooking time.
4. Add reserved meat and accumulated juices, wine and 2 cups water. Bring to a boil. Cover Dutch oven and place in oven. Cook 2 hours, until beef is tender.
5. Add green beans and carrots; cook 15 minutes more, just until beans and carrots are tender.
6. Transfer Dutch oven to stove top over medium-high heat. Stir in thickener; cook 2 minutes more, stirring, until sauce thickens.
7. Adjust seasonings to taste and serve immediately.

Beef Burger with Feta and Tomato

*Servings: 4 | **Prep:** 10 m | **Style:** American| **Cook:** 12 m*

Ingredients

- 1 lb Ground Beef (80% Lean / 20% Fat)
- 1 large Scallions or Spring Onion
- 1/2 cup Baby Spinach
- 1/4 cup chopped or sliced Red Tomatoes
- 1/4 cup crumbled Feta Cheese
- 1 1/2 tsps fresh Dill
- 1/2 tsp Salt
- 1/2 tsp Black Pepper

Directions

1. Combine ground beef, scallion, spinach, tomato, feta, 1.5 tsp fresh dill (or 1/2 tsp dried), salt and pepper. Form into 4 patties.
2. Grill or pan-fry over medium-high heat for 6 minutes per side for medium doneness.

Beef Carpaccio with Arugula and Caper Vinaigrette

*Servings: 6 | **Prep:** 15 m | **Style:** Italian*

Ingredients

- 1 lb Ground Beef (80% Lean / 20% Fat)
- 1 large Scallions or Spring Onion
- 1/2 cup Baby Spinach
- 1/4 cup chopped or sliced Red Tomatoes
- 1/4 cup crumbled Feta Cheese
- 1 1/2 tsps fresh Dill
- 1/2 tsp Salt
- 1/2 tsp Black Pepper

Directions

1. Combine ground beef, scallion, spinach, tomato, feta, 1.5 tsp fresh dill (or 1/2 tsp dried), salt and pepper. Form into 4 patties.
2. Grill or pan-fry over medium-high heat for 6 minutes per side for medium doneness.

Beef Fajitas with Peppers

Servings: 6 | **Prep**: 10 m | **Style**: Mexian | **Cook**: 10 m

Ingredients

- 1 1/2 tsps Garlic
- 1 tsp Salt
- 1 Jalapeno Pepper
- 2 tsps Cumin
- 3/4 cup Green Tomato Chile Sauce (Salsa Verde)
- 2 tbsps Extra Virgin Olive Oil
- 1 tbsp Canola Vegetable Oil
- 1 medium (approx 2-3/4" long, 2-1/2" dia) Red Sweet Pepper
- 1 small Red Onion
- 1 medium (approx 2-3/4" long, 2-1/2" dia) Green Sweet Pepper
- 1/4 cup Cilantro (Coriander)
- 12 tortillas Low Carb Tortillas
- 3/4 cup Sour Cream (Cultured)
- 1 fl oz Fresh Lime Juice
- 32 oz boneless (yield after cooking) Steak

Directions

1. Make marinade: In a large bowl or resealable plastic bag, combine garlic, salt, lime juice, jalapeno, cumin and olive oil; whisk together. Add steak pieces to marinade; coat well. Marinate, refrigerated at least 1 hour, preferably over night for the flavors to blend.
2. Heat oven to 350° F. Wrap tortillas in foil; place in oven to warm 15 minutes before serving.
3. Remove steak from marinade; discard marinade. Grill 5 inches over hot coals (or over medium-high heat) 3 to 4 minutes per side for medium-rare; set aside.

4. In a large skillet over medium-high heat, heat canola oil. Cook bell peppers and onion 5 minutes, until vegetables are softened.
5. Slice steak thinly across the grain.
6. To assemble fajitas, spread tortillas with salsa, top with steak slices and vegetable mixture, sour cream, and cilantro. Fold over and serve.

Beef Fillet with Bacon and Gorgonzola Butter

*Servings: 2 | **Prep:** 15 m | **Style:** American | **Cook:** 20 m*

Ingredients

- 1 1/2 tsps Garlic
- 1 tsp Salt
- 1 Jalapeno Pepper
- 2 tsps Cumin
- 3/4 cup Green Tomato Chile Sauce (Salsa Verde)
- 2 tbsps Extra Virgin Olive Oil
- 1 tbsp Canola Vegetable Oil
- 1 medium (approx 2-3/4" long, 2-1/2" dia) Red Sweet Pepper
- 1 small Red Onion
- 1 medium (approx 2-3/4" long, 2-1/2" dia) Green Sweet Pepper
- 1/4 cup Cilantro (Coriander)
- 12 tortillas Low Carb Tortillas
- 3/4 cup Sour Cream (Cultured)
- 1 fl oz Fresh Lime Juice
- 32 oz boneless (yield after cooking) Steak

Directions

1. Make marinade: In a large bowl or resealable plastic bag, combine garlic, salt, lime juice, jalapeno, cumin and olive oil; whisk together. Add steak pieces to marinade; coat well. Marinate, refrigerated at least 1 hour, preferably over night for the flavors to blend.
2. Heat oven to 350° F. Wrap tortillas in foil; place in oven to warm 15 minutes before serving.
3. Remove steak from marinade; discard marinade. Grill 5 inches over hot coals (or over medium-high heat) 3 to 4 minutes per side for medium-rare; set aside.
4. In a large skillet over medium-high heat, heat canola oil. Cook bell peppers and onion 5 minutes, until vegetables are softened.

5. Slice steak thinly across the grain.
6. To assemble fajitas, spread tortillas with salsa, top with steak slices and vegetable mixture, sour cream, and cilantro. Fold over and serve.

Beef Fondue

Servings: 2 | Style: French | Cook: 25 m

Ingredients

- 3/4 lb Beef Tenderloin (Lean Only, Trimmed to 1/4" Fat, Prime Grade)
- 1 cup floweret Broccoli Flower Clusters
- 1 fruit (2-1/8" dia) Lemon
- 2 tbsps Sour Cream (Cultured)
- 2 tbsps Real Mayonnaise
- 1 1/2 tbsps Dijon Mustard
- 1 tbsp Canola Vegetable Oil

Directions

1. For this recipe you will need to fill your fondue pot with canola oil. Be sure to have enough on-hand for this purpose.
2. Trim away all fat from your meat and cut it into 3/4-inch cubes. Arrange meat, broccoli, and lemon wedges on a platter; cover and refrigerate.
3. In a small bowl, stir together sour cream, mayonnaise and mustard; cover and refrigerate.
4. Pour oil to come up 1 1/2 inches into your fondue pot (about 4 cups for an 8-inch, 2-quart pot). Pour the oil into a saucepan and place over high heat on your stove top. Heat oil to 300°F on deep-fry thermometer; oil should bubble energetically when a piece of meat is lowered in.
5. Carefully pour hot oil back into your fondue pot and set over high heat. Using fondue forks, cook meat and broccoli in the hot oil, garnishing with your choice of lemon, salt or mustard sauce.
6. If the temperature of the oil dips below 280°F the meat will cook sluggishly. Carefully pour the oil back into the pot and reheat to 300°F on the stove. Pour back into pot and continue to cook (you will probably have to do this at least once during your meal).

Beef Sautéed with Green Bell Pepper and Onions Topped with Cheese

Servings: 1 | Prep: 5 m | Style: American | Cook: 10 m

Ingredients

- 1/4 cup chopped Onions
- 1 tbsp Extra Virgin Olive Oil
- 1/2 cup chopped Green Sweet Pepper
- 1/2 cup shredded Cheddar Cheese
- 5 oz Ground Beef (80% Lean / 20% Fat)

Directions

1. Sauté ground beef in a skillet over medium-high heat with small amount of cooking oil for 1-2 minutes. Add green bell pepper and white onions.
2. Sauté until beef is browned and the peppers and onions are soft. Add salt and pepper to taste.
3. Drain off any excess fat and put onto a serving plate. Sprinkle cheese on top and allow to melt. Serve immediately.

Beef Sauteed with Vegetables Over Romaine

Servings: 6 | Prep: 10 m | Style: American | Cook: 35 m

Ingredients

- 1 1/2 lbs Ground Beef (80% Lean / 20% Fat)
- 1/4 cup chopped Onions
- 1/4 cup chopped Green Sweet Pepper
- 15 oz Tomato Sauce (Canned)
- 4 tbsps Tomato Paste
- 3 tsps Sucralose Based Sweetener (Sugar Substitute)
- 6 cups shredded Cos or Romaine Lettuce
- 6 oz Cheddar Cheese

Directions

1. Brown the beef in a non-stick skillet over medium-high heat. Add the onions and peppers during the last few minutes of browning.
2. Drain off excess fat from the skillet and add the tomato sauce, tomato paste and granular sugar substitute and season with salt and freshly ground black pepper. Allow to simmer over low heat for 30 minutes.
3. Serve immediately over shredded Romaine topped with Cheddar.

Beef Stroganoff

Servings: 4 | Prep: 15 m | Style: Other | Cook: 25 m

Ingredients

- 3 oz Mushroom Pieces and Stems
- 20 oz Beef Inside Skirt Steak (Trimmed to 1/4" Fat)
- 1/2 cup chopped Onions
- 1/8 tsp Black Pepper
- 2 tbsps Canola Vegetable Oil
- 1 tbsp Unsalted Butter Stick
- 2 oz Red Table Wine
- 1 cup Beef Broth, Bouillon or Consomme
- 1/4 cup Sour Cream (Cultured)
- 1 tsp Dijon Mustard
- 1/8 tsp Salt

Directions

1. Heat oven to warm setting. Sprinkle meat with salt and pepper.
2. In a large nonstick skillet heat oil over medium-high heat. Brown meat in batches, about 1 minute per side. Transfer to a platter and place in oven.
3. Melt butter in skillet; add yellow onion and cook 3 minutes, until softened. Add mushrooms. Cook 10 minutes, stirring occasionally, until mushroom liquid evaporates.
4. Add wine; cook 5 minutes. Stir in beef broth and cook 10 minutes, until mushrooms are coated with a thick sauce. Stir in sour cream and mustard. Add meat and accumulated juices.

5. Reduce heat to low and cook 2-3 minutes, until meat is heated through. Season to taste with salt and pepper.

Beef Tenderloin

Servings: 8 | Prep: 20 m | Style: American | Cook: 30 m

Ingredients

- 4 lbs Beef Tenderloin (Trimmed to 1/4" Fat, Prime Grade)
- 1 1/2 tbsps Extra Virgin Olive Oil
- 1 tsp Salt
- 1/2 tsp Black Pepper

Directions

1. Heat oven to 425°F.
2. Place beef in a jelly-roll pan. Rub with oil, salt and pepper. Insert a meat thermometer. Roast 30 to 35 minutes for medium-rare doneness. Thermometer should register 125°F.
3. Transfer to a cutting board; loosely tent with foil and let rest 10 minutes before slicing.

Beef, Scallions and Red Bell Pepper Sauté

Servings: 1 | Prep: 10 m | Style: American | Cook: 10 m

Ingredients

- 5 oz Steak
- 1/4 cup chopped Scallions or Spring Onions
- 1/2 cup chopped Sweet Red Peppers
- 1/4 cup shredded Mozzarella Cheese (Whole Milk)

Directions

1. Sauté beef that has been cut into strips in oil in a small skillet over medium-high heat for 1-2 minutes.
2. Add scallions and red bell pepper. Sauté until beef is browned and peppers are soft. Add salt and pepper to taste. Drain any excess fat.
3. Place meat mixture on a plate. Immediately sprinkle with cheese and allow to melt.

Bittersweet Chocolate Brownie Drops

Servings: 12 | Prep: 15 m | Style: American | Cook: 10 m

Ingredients

- 1/8 cup 100% Stone Ground Whole Wheat Pastry Flour
- 2 tbsps Whole Grain Soy Flour
- 1/4 tsp Baking Powder (Straight Phosphate, Double Acting)
- 3 oz Unsweetened Baking Chocolate Squares
- 6 tbsps Heavy Cream
- 2 tbsps Unsalted Butter Stick
- 2 large Eggs (Whole)
- 3/4 cup Sucralose Based Sweetener (Sugar Substitute)

Directions

1. Preheat oven to 375°F. Line a baking sheet with parchment paper or aluminum foil.
2. In a large bowl, whisk 2 tbsp flour, soy flour and baking powder.
3. In a microwave-safe bowl, melt chocolate, cream and butter for 1 to 2 minutes, until butter is melted and chocolate has softened. Let stand 2 minutes and stir until smooth. You can also do this step on the stovetop.
4. With an electric mixer on medium speed, beat eggs and sugar substitute until light and fluffy, about 3 minutes. Gradually beat the slightly warm chocolate mixture into the egg mixture until well-blended, about 1 minute. Turn mixer speed down to low and mix in flour mixture just combined.
5. Drop slightly rounded teaspoonfuls of dough onto prepared sheet. Bake 5 to 6 minutes, until just set but still soft on top. Transfer to a wire rack to cool completely.

Blackberry Clafouti

Servings: 8 | Prep: 10 m | Style: Italian | Cook: 45 m

Ingredients

- 1 pinch Stevia
- 6 oz Blackberries
- 1/4 cup Unsalted Butter Stick
- 1/2 tsp Pure Almond Extract
- 1/2 cup Almond Meal Flour
- 1 tsp Vanilla Extract
- 1/4 tsp Salt
- 1/2 tsp Cinnamon
- 4 large Eggs (Whole)
- 1 cup Heavy Cream
- 1/3 cup Xylitol

Directions

1. Please note lemon zest is not included in the ingredients but does add a nice flavor to the dish.
2. Preheat oven to 325°F. Grease a 1-quart shallow baking dish with butter. Arrange blackberries in the baking dish and set aside.
3. Whisk together the eggs, granular sugar substitutes, salt and almond flour. Add the cream, 1/4 cup melted butter, 1 teaspoon vanilla, 1/2 teaspoon almond extract, 1 tsp lemon zest (optional), and ground cinnamon; whisk to combine.
4. Pour this mixture over the blackberries. Bake for 35-45 minutes until puffed, golden and set in the center. Cool 20 minutes then serve warm or refrigerate up to 3 days.

Blackberry Spinach Salad with Goat Cheese Medallions

Servings: 6 | Prep: 20 m | Style: American | Cook: 10 m

Ingredients

- 1 large Egg (Whole)
- 6 oz Goat Cheese (Soft)
- 1/4 cup half Pecans
- 1/4 medium slice (1/8" thick) Red Onions
- 2 tbsps Extra Virgin Olive Oil
- 3/4 tsp Cinnamon
- 1 tbsp Xylitol
- 12 oz Blackberries
- 1 1/3 tbsps Balsamic Vinegar
- 9 cups Baby Spinach
- 30 Cherry Tomatoes

Directions

1. Preheat oven to 350°F. Or a sauté pan may be used to cook the goat cheese medallions for about 5 minutes per side over medium-high heat. Chop the pecans and onions and set them aside in separate bowls.
2. Whisk egg in a small shallow bowl. Cut the goat cheese into twelve 1/2-inch rounds, or roll into 12 equal balls and flatten. Dip each round into the whisked egg and then roll in the chopped pecans, pressing them into the cheese if necessary. Place the rounds onto a sheet pan and bake for ten minutes. Remove from oven and allow to cool slightly.
3. In a sauté pan over medium heat cook the onion in 2 tablespoons oil with the ground cinnamon and granular sugar substitute; about 3 minutes. Add 6 oz (half) of the blackberries and smash each with a fork. Continue to cook for 3-4 minutes then add balsamic vinegar and season with salt and black pepper. Cook for another 2 minutes, remove from heat and allow to cool. May be used either warm or placed in the refrigerator to cool further; this is a very thick dressing, thin with either lemon juice or water if a thinner consistency is desired.
4. Combine the spinach, tomatoes and blackberries. Toss with half of the dressing then place the goat cheese medallions on top. Serve with the remaining dressing on the side. This salad is delicious topped with either chicken, salmon or shrimp.

Blackened Salmon with Cucumber Relish and Cauliflower

Servings: 4 | Prep: 10 m | Style: American | Cook: 20 m

Ingredients

- 4 cups Cauliflower
- 1 tsp leaf Basil (Dried)
- 1 tbsp leaf Thyme (Dried)
- 2 tbsps Paprika
- 1 tsp leaf Oregano
- 1 tsp Red or Cayenne Pepper
- 1 tsp Salt
- 20 oz boneless Salmon
- 3 tbsps Light Olive Oil
- 1 cup slice Cucumber (with Peel)
- 1 fl oz Fresh Lime Juice
- 1 tbsp Extra Virgin Olive Oil
- 1/2 tsp Sucralose Based Sweetener (Sugar Substitute)
- 1/2 tsp Dill (Dried)

Directions

1. Steam cauliflower for 10 minutes or until tender. While cauliflower cooks prepare salmon.
2. Combine all spices (except dill weed) and 1 tsp salt for the blackening rub. Brush each piece of salmon with 2 tablespoons light olive oil and then coat evenly with the blackening rub. Prepare a heavy skillet with 1 tablespoon olive oil over medium high heat. Place the the salmon flesh side down and cook for 2-3 minutes until blackened. Flip over and continue to cook for 5-6 minutes until the skin is crispy and the fish flakes easily with a fork.
3. For the relish: finely dice the cucumber. Add lime juice, 1 tbsp extra virgin olive oil, granular sugar substitute, and dill weed then season with 1/4 tsp salt and 1/4 tsp pepper.
4. Mash the cooked cauliflower with and the final tablespoon of olive oil. Spoon onto four plates. Serve the salmon over the cauliflower and top with 1/4 cup cucumber relish.

Blender Mayonnaise

*Servings: 4 | **Prep:** 10 m | **Style:** American*

Ingredients

- 1 large Egg Yolk

- 2 tsps Fresh Lemon Juice
- 1 tsp Dijon Mustard
- 1/2 tsp Salt
- 1/8 tsp Black Pepper
- 1/2 cup Extra Virgin Olive Oil

Directions

1. Store-bought mayonnaise may be convenient, but it's usually made with soybean oil (high in omega-6s) and often with added sugar. In addition to using mayonnaise in tuna and other salads, it is delicious over steamed vegetables. Use canola oil instead of olive oil, if you prefer. Both are good sources of omega-3s. Each serving is 2 Tbsp.
2. Combine egg, lemon juice, mustard, salt and pepper in a blender and pulse to combine.
3. With the blender running on low speed, pour in the oil in a thin, steady stream. If the mixture becomes too thick and the oil is no longer incorporating, pulse the blender.

Blue Cheese and Bacon Soup

Servings: 6 | Prep: 10 m | Style: American | Cook: 25 m

Ingredients

- 6 medium slice (yield after cooking) Bacon
- 3 tbsps Unsalted Butter Stick
- 2 leeks Leeks
- 2 cups Mushroom Pieces and Stems
- 1 1/2 cups Cauliflower
- 2 14.5 oz cans Chicken Broth, Bouillon or Consomme
- 1/2 cup Tap Water
- 2 1/2 oz Blue or Roquefort Cheese

Directions

1. To cook bacon: heat a skillet over medium-high heat, add bacon 3-4 strips at a time (do not over crowd pan). Cook until crispy on one side then flip over and cook until crispy throughout. Remove strips from pan and place

on a paper towel to draw off remaining fat. Repeat with remaining bacon until all are cooked. When cool, crumble an set aside.
2. Melt butter in a large soup pot over medium heat. Add leeks, mushrooms and cauliflower. Cover and cook 5 minutes, stirring occasionally. Add chicken broth and water; bring to a boil. Lower heat, cover and simmer for 10 minutes, until vegetables are very tender.
3. Puree soup in batches in a blender or food processor. Return pureed soup to the soup pot. Add the blue cheese to last batch of soup and puree until smooth. Heat through over low heat, if necessary. Top with crumbled bacon just before serving.

Blue Cheese Dressing

Servings: 14 | Prep: 10 m | Style: American

Ingredients

- 1 cup crumbled, not packed Blue Cheese
- 1/2 cup Real Mayonnaise
- 1/2 cup Sour Cream (Cultured)
- 1/3 cup Heavy Cream
- 1/2 fl oz Fresh Lemon Juice
- 1/2 tsp Dijon Mustard
- 1/2 tsp Black Pepper

Directions

1. Drizzle this thick and creamy dressing over iceberg lettuce or other salad greens, or serve as a dip for fresh vegetables or Buffalo chicken wings or atop cold roast beef. If you can, make the dressing ahead to let the flavors develop. Homemade mayonnaise produces scrumptious results. See the Atkins recipe for Mayonnaise. Each serving is 2 Tbsp.
2. Combine cheese, mayonnaise, sour cream, heavy cream, lemon juice, mustard and pepper in a medium bowl, mashing with a fork to break up the cheese.
3. Use right away or refrigerate in an airtight container for up to 3 days.

Blueberry-Cucumber Chiller

*Servings: 1 | **Prep**: 10 m | **Style**: American*

Ingredients

- 1/2 cup pared, chopped Cucumber (Peeled)
- 2 tbsps Fresh Lemon Juice
- 1 oz Blueberries
- 1/2 tsp Sweetener
- 1 tsp Rosemary
- 4 ice cubes Tap Water
- 1 fl oz (no ice) Gin
- 3 oz Club Soda

Directions

This recipe was tested with Truvia brand sweetener; sucralose may also be used. This recipe may be made nonalcoholic by replacing the gin with 1 additional ounce of club soda.

1. Peel, remove seeds and coarsely chop the cucumber. Measure out 1/2 cup and place into a blender.
2. Add the lemon juice, blueberries and granular sugar substitute - Truvia® is recommended (if using sucralose use 4 tsp and add 2g NC to the total). Blend on high until thoroughly blended.
3. Add the rosemary and pulse 1-2 times just to chop up the rosemary to release it's flavor. Strain with a fine mesh strainer and press on the pulp to release all the liquid into a glass. Discard the pulp.
4. Add ice to the glass then the gin and club soda. Stir to combine.

Blueberry-Turkey Burgers

*Servings: 6 | **Prep**: 10 m | **Style**: American | **Cook**: 20 m*

Ingredients

- 1 1/4 lbs Ground Turkey
- 1 tbsp Light Olive Oil
- 3 tbsps Peppermint (Mint)
- 1 1/2 tsps Fennel Seed

- 1 1/2 tsps Cumin
- 1/2 tsp Salt
- 1/2 tsp Black Pepper
- 1/2 cup chopped Red Sweet Pepper
- 3/4 cup crumbled Feta Cheese
- 3/4 cup Blueberries

Directions

Ground turkey can be dry, adding additional olive oil is optional but the bell pepper and blueberries may pop out more easily. Use ground lamb for a different flavor.

1. Using your hands combine the ground turkey, olive oil, chopped mint, ground fennel, ground cumin, salt and pepper in a medium bowl.
2. Add the chopped red bell peppers, feta cheese and blueberries gently combining and then form into 6 equal burgers. The blueberries or peppers may need to be popped back into the burgers. Simply push them gently into place on the top side. Season with additional salt and freshly ground black pepper.
3. Grill or pan fry over medium-high heat until the internal temperature reaches 165°F and the meat is no longer pink in the center and the juices run clear. Serve immediately. Pairs well with Raita; see the Atkins recipe.

Bok Choy and Green Onions

Servings: 4 | Prep: 10 m | Style: American | Cook: 5 m

Ingredients

- 4 medium (4-1/8" long) Scallions or Spring Onions
- 1 fl oz Tap Water
- 1 tsp Sucralose Based Sweetener (Sugar Substitute)
- 1 tbsp Canola Vegetable Oil
- 1 tsp Sesame Oil
- 8 heads Chinese Cabbage (Bok-Choy, Pak-Choi)
- 1 1/2 tsps Garlic
- 1/8 tsp Crushed Red Pepper
- 1 cup in shell, edible yield Peanuts (with Salt, Boiled, Cooked)
- 2 tbsps Tamari Soybean Sauce

Directions

1. In a small bowl, mix tamari, water and sugar substitute; set aside.
2. In a wok or large, deep skillet, heat canola and sesame oils over medium-high heat. Add bok choy, green onions, garlic, soy sauce mixture and pepper flakes to taste. Stir-fry just until bok choy is wilted, about 3 minutes.
3. Stir in peanuts and serve immediately.

Bones-to-Be Chicken Wingettes

Servings: 8 | *Prep*: 10 m | *Style*: American | *Cook*: 35 m

Ingredients

- 2 tbsps Chili Powder
- 1 tsp Red or Cayenne Pepper
- 2 tsps Yellow Mustard Seed
- 2 tsps Salt
- 1/2 serving All Purpose Low-Carb Baking Mix
- 32 oz, with bone (yield after cooking, bone removed) Chicken Wing

Directions

Use the Atkins recipe to make All Purpose Low-Carb Baking Mix for this recipe. You will need half of a 1/3 cup (about 3 Tbsp) = half of a serving.

1. Heat oven to 450°F. Line a jelly-roll pan with foil, and spray with nonstick cooking spray.
2. Combine chili powder, 2 Tbsp baking mix, cayenne, mustard and salt in a large resealable bag. Add half of the wingettes, and shake to coat. Transfer to pan, and repeat with remaining wingettes.
3. Bake, turning occasionally, until crisp, browned and cooked through, 30 to 35 minutes. Transfer to a platter, and serve.

Bouillabaisse

Servings: 4 | *Prep*: 20 m | *Style*: French | *Cook*: 35 m

Ingredients

- 2 tbsps Extra Virgin Olive Oil
- 1 tbsp Unsalted Butter Stick
- 2 cloves Garlic
- 1/2 cup Leeks
- 1/2 cup sliced Fennel Bulk
- 1 cup chopped Celery
- 1/2 tsp leaf Dried Thyme Leaves
- 1/4 tsp Saffron
- 1 tbsp Tomato Paste
- 16 tbsps All Natural Clam Juice
- 1 1/2 cups Chicken Broth, Bouillon or Consomme
- 6 fl ozs White Table Wine
- 1 14.5 oz can Diced Tomato
- 1/2 tsp Salt
- 1/4 tsp Red or Cayenne Pepper
- 12 medium Clams (Mixed Species)
- 1 lb Atlantic and Pacific Halibut
- 1/2 lb Shrimp
- 1 cup raw, yield cooked Scallops
- 2 tbsps Parsley

Directions

1. Heat olive oil and butter in a large saucepan over medium heat. Add garlic (minced), leeks, fennel, celery, thyme and saffron. Sauté over medium heat for 4 to 5 minutes, or until vegetables are softened.
2. Add tomato paste, clam juice, chicken broth and wine. Stir. Add the tomatoes and juice, and season with salt and cayenne. Bring to a boil, reduce the heat and simmer for 15 minutes.
3. Add clams and cook for 3 minutes. Add fish, then the shrimp and scallops. Tuck seafood into broth, cover, and cook for 5 minutes until the fish is opaque and the clams have opened.
4. Sprinkle with fresh parsley and ladle into four large serving bowls.

Braised Leeks and Fennel

Servings: 8 | Prep: 15 m | Style: French | Cook: 45 m

Ingredients

- 4 Leeks
- 1 Fennel Bulb
- 1 cup Chicken Broth, Bouillon or Consomme
- 1 tsp Salt
- 1/2 tsp Black Pepper
- 3 tbsps Unsalted Butter Stick
- 1 tbsp Fresh Lemon Juice
- 1/3 cup Parsley

Directions

1. Preheat oven to 450°F.
2. Place leeks, fennel, broth, salt and pepper in a 11- by 9-inch pan. Dot with butter and cover pan with aluminum foil.
3. Bake 15 minutes. Uncover, stir lightly and bake uncovered until vegetables are very tender and liquid is almost all gone, about 20 minutes.
4. Mix in lemon juice and parsley.

Bratwurst with Onions and Sauerkraut

*Servings: 1 | **Prep:** 5 m | **Style:** American | **Cook:** 10 m*

Ingredients

- 1 tsp Extra Virgin Olive Oil
- 1/2 cup Sauerkraut (Solid and Liquids, Canned)
- 1 stick (3 oz) Bratwurst
- 1/2 cup sliced Onions

Directions

1. In a small skillet, heat oil over medium-high heat. Add white onions and sauté about 3 minutes. Add bratwurst and sauerkraut.
2. Continue to cook until bratwurst is browned on all sides and heated through. Serve immediately.

Bratwurst with Sauerkraut

Servings: 1 | Prep: 5 m | Style: American | Cook: 10 m

Ingredients

- 1 stick (3 oz) Bratwurst
- 1/2 cup Sauerkraut (Solid and Liquids, Canned)

Directions

1. Preheat grill or broiler.
2. Grill or broil bratwurst, turning several times until browned on all sides. Or microwave for 1 -2 minutes.
3. Meanwhile, heat sauerkraut in microwave oven.
4. Serve bratwurst with warm saurkraut.

Chapter 4: Sides Recipes

***

Baked Meatballs and Green Beans

Servings: 2 | *Style:* American | *Cook:* 45 m

Ingredients

- 6 oz Green String Beans
- 1 fruit (2-1/8" dia) Lemon
- 1 large Young Green Onion
- 1 clove Garlic
- 1 large Egg
- 8 oz Ground Pork
- 8 oz Ground Beef (85% Lean / 15% Fat)
- 1 1/2 tbsps Olive Oil
- 1/4 cup Parmesan Cheese (Grated)
- 1/4 tsp Salt
- 1/4 tsp Black Pepper

Directions

1. Preheat the oven to 375ºF. Remove the ends from the greens beans and discard; set the green beans aside. Zest the lemon; set zest aside. Juice the lemon into a small bowl, discarding seeds. Slice the green onions into ¼-inch diced pieces; set aside. Finely chop the garlic clove and set aside. Crack the egg into another small bowl and whisk with a fork; set aside.
2. Heat ½ tablespoon of olive oil in a large sauté pan over medium-high heat. When the oil is hot, add the green onion and cook for 5 minutes, stirring, until softened. Add the garlic and cook for 1 minute more. Transfer to a large bowl and let cool slightly.
3. Pat dry the ground pork and the ground beef with paper towels. Place in the large bowl with the green onions and garlic; add the Parmesan cheese, egg, and ⅛ teaspoon salt and ⅛ teaspoon black pepper. Mix until all ingredients are well combined
4. Form the beef/ pork mixture into golf ball-size meatballs and place on a sheet pan lined with foil. Bake for 20 to 25 minutes until browned and cooked through.
5. Heat 1 tablespoon of olive oil in a medium sauté pan over medium-high heat. Add the green beans and sauté for 3 to 5 minutes, until crisp-tender. Add the lemon juice, lemon zest and ¼ teaspoon each of salt and pepper. Toss to combine.

6. Divide the green beans between two plates, place the meatballs next to the green beans and enjoy!

Balsamic and Thyme Pearl Onions

Servings: 8 | Prep: 5 m | Style: American | Cook: 25 m

Ingredients

- 2 tsps Olive Oil
- 16 oz Cooked Pearl Onions (from Frozen)
- 1 tsp Xylitol
- 1/3 tbsp Balsamic Vinegar
- 1 1/2 tsps Thyme

Directions

1. Heat oil over medium-high heat in a medium skillet. Add thawed onions (be sure to pat them dry after thawing), season with salt and freshly ground black pepper, and saute until they begin to brown.
2. Sprinkle the onions with xylitol and the balsamic vinegar. Stir and continue to cook for 1 minute.
3. Add 2/3 cup water and thyme. Continue to cook over low heat until the onions are tender and the liquid has evaporated; about 20 minutes. Serve immediately. One serving is about 1/8 cup (5-6 onions).

Broccoli Florets with Lemon Butter Sauce

Servings: 8 | Prep: 10 m | Style: American | Cook: 15 m

Ingredients

- 1 lb Broccoli Flower Clusters
- 2 tbsps chopped Shallots
- 1 fl oz Sauvignon Blanc Wine
- 1 tbsp Fresh Lemon Juice

- 4 tbsps Unsalted Butter Stick
- 1/8 tsp Salt
- 1/8 tsp White Pepper

Directions

1. Cook florets in a large pot of lightly salted water 5-7 minutes, until tender. Drain; return to pot to keep warm while you prepare sauce.
2. Place shallots, 2 tbsp wine and 1 tablespoon lemon juice in a small saucepan over medium heat. Simmer until reduced to 1 tablespoon. Reduce heat to very low; stir in a few small pieces of butter, swirling with a wire whisk until mostly melted.
3. Gradually add the remaining butter, whisking constantly until sauce is smooth. Season with 1/8 tsp salt, 1/8 tsp white pepper and remaining lemon juice to taste. Do not allow sauce to boil. Pour sauce over broccoli. Enjoy!

Broccoli Rabe Parmigiano

Servings: 6 | *Prep:* 15 m | *Style:* Italian | *Cook:* 10 m

Ingredients

- 2 tbsps Extra Virgin Olive Oil
- 2 cloves Garlic
- 1/4 tsp Crushed Red Pepper Flakes
- 2 lbs Broccoli
- 1/4 cup Tap Water
- 2 tbsps Fresh Lemon Juice
- 2 tbsps Lemon Peel
- 1/8 tsp Salt
- 1/8 tsp Black Pepper
- 1/2 cup Parmesan Cheese (Grated)

Directions

Broccoli rabe has 6- to 9-inch stalks and scattered clusters of tiny broccoli-like buds. It has a more bitter taste than its more familiar cousin. It takes beautifully to sautéing or braising. Feel free to substitute broccoli in this recipe if you prefer. Cut a

2-pound head of broccoli into small florets, then peel the stems and cut in 1/2-inch pieces.

1. In a large, deep skillet, heat oil over medium-high heat. Add garlic and pepper flakes; sauté 30 seconds.
2. Add broccoli rabe, water, lemon juice and lemon zest; mix well. Cover skillet and cook over medium heat 8 minutes or until broccoli rabe is crisp-tender.
3. Season to taste with salt and freshly ground black pepper.
4. Transfer to a serving dish and sprinkle with Parmesan.

Browned Pumpkin with Maple and Sage

Servings: 8 | Prep: 10 m | Style: Italian | Cook: 15 m

Ingredients

- 1 lb Pumpkin
- 1/4 cup chopped Shallots
- 1 tbsp Unsalted Butter Stick
- 1/4 cup Bouillon Vegetable Broth
- 1/16 cup Sugar Free Syrup
- 1/4 tsp Sage (Ground)

Directions

Use fresh sage for this recipe if possible. You will need 7-8 leaves.

1. Heat butter in a medium skillet over medium-high heat. Cube pumpkin into 3/4-inch chunks.
2. Add pumpkin and shallots to pan and season with salt and freshly ground black pepper. Saute until pumpkin is lightly browned and the shallots are translucent; 5-6 minutes.
3. Turn heat to low, add 1/4 cup vegetable broth, and simmer covered for 8-10 minutes until pumpkin is tender.
4. Add maple syrup and sage. Tossing to combine. Serve immediately. Serving size is about 1/4 cup.

Brussels Sprouts with Bacon and Parmesan

*Servings: 10 | **Prep:** 10 m | **Style:** American | **Cook:** 20 m*

Ingredients

- 6 medium slice (yield after cooking) Bacon
- 2 lbs Brussels Sprouts
- 1/2 tsp Salt
- 1/4 tsp Black Pepper
- 1/2 cup Heavy Cream
- 1/2 cup Parmesan Cheese (Grated)

Directions

1. Wash, trim and cut Brussels sprouts in half.
2. Heat a medium skillet over medium-high heat. Brown bacon, transferring to a paper towel when done and set aside to cool. Once cool, cut or break into bite sized pieces. Set aside and remove all but 1-2 Tbsp bacon grease from the pan.
3. Add Brussels sprouts, salt and pepper to the pan. Sauté over medium-high heat, stirring occasionally until lightly golden and cooked through; about 15 minutes.
4. Add cream and Parmesan cheese. Stir to heat through another 1 minute. Transfer to a serving platter and sprinkle bacon over the top. Serve immediately.

Brussels Sprouts with Lemon and Parmesan

*Servings: 8 | **Prep:** 5 m | **Style:** American | **Cook:** 15 m*

Ingredients

- 1 tbsp Olive Oil
- 1 lb Brussels Sprouts
- 1 tbsp Fresh Lemon Juice
- 1 oz Parmesan Cheese (Hard)

Directions

1. Heat oil in a large skillet over medium-high heat. Add Brussels sprouts, season with salt and freshly ground black pepper, and saute until browned; about 5-8 minutes.
2. Add 1/3 cup water and 1 tsp lemon zest (optional). Continue to cook until the water has cooked off and the sprouts are tender; about 5 minutes.
3. Toss with 1 tbsp lemon juice, place in a serving bowl and top with shaved Parmesan.

Buffalo Chicken Salad

Servings: 2 | Style: American | Cook: 45 m

Ingredients

- 1/2 fruit (2-1/8" dia) Lemon
- 1 medium (4-1/8" long) Young Green Onions
- 1 head Cos or Romaine Lettuce
- 2 stalk medium (7-1/2" - 8" long) Celery
- 1 medium (approx 2-3/4" long, 2-1/2" dia) Red Sweet Pepper
- 1 medium Tomato
- 1 large Egg
- 5 1/3 tbsps Apple Cider Vinegar
- 1/8 tsp Celery Salt
- 1/8 tsp Red or Cayenne Pepper
- 2 thigh, bone removeds Chicken Thigh Meat and Skin (Broilers or Fryers)
- 1/4 cup Real Mayonnaise
- 2 tbsps Sour Cream
- 2/3 oz Blue Cheese
- 1/8 tsp Garlic Powder
- 1/3 tsp Salt
- 1/4 tsp Black Pepper

Directions

1. Preheat oven to 450ºF. Juice the lemon into a large bowl discarding any seeds. Finely chop the green onions and add to the bowl; set aside. To the

bowl with the lemon juice and green onions, add the mayonnaise, sour cream, blue cheese and garlic powder and stir to combine.

2. Cut the romaine lettuce into 1-inch pieces and place into the large bowl with the dressing. Cut the celery into ½-inch pieces on a bias and add to the romaine. Remove the stem, pith and seeds from the red bell pepper and discard. Cut the bell pepper into ¼-inch thin strips. Cut the tomato into 1" inch diced pieces and add to the bowl. Set in the refrigerator until step 5.
3. Using a fork, beat the egg in another medium bowl. Add the apple cider vinegar, ¼ cup canola oil, ¼ teaspoon of black pepper, ⅓ teaspoon of salt, the celery salt and cayenne pepper and stir until well combined.
4. Pat the chicken thighs with paper towels and add to the marinade, then place on a sheet pan lined with foil. Bake for 18 to 20 minutes, turning the thighs and brushing with the marinade several times, until cooked through and crisp. Cut the chicken thighs into ½-inch diced pieces and set aside for step 6.
5. Remove the salad from the refrigerator and toss to combine.
6. Divide the salad between to plates and place the chicken in the center. Enjoy!

Buffalo Hot Wing Cauliflower

*Servings: 4 | **Prep**: 10 m | **Style**: American | **Cook**: 45 m*

Ingredients

- 1 head large (6-7" dia) Cauliflower
- 2 tbsps Light Olive Oil
- 4 tbsps Red Hot Buffalo Wing Sauce
- 3 tsps Sriracha Hot Chili Sauce
- 2 tbsps Unsalted Butter Stick
- 1 1/2 oz Blue or Roquefort Cheese

Directions

1. Preheat oven to 375°F.
2. Cut cauliflower into smaller florets and sprinkle with 1 tablespoon olive oil. Roast on a baking sheet for 35-40 minutes or until tender.
3. While cauliflower is roasting, put hot wing sauce and siracha into a small sauce pan and heat until boiling. Lower heat and simmer for 10 minutes. Add butter, stir until melted and allow to cool to room temperature. Heat a large sauté pan with remaining oil. Add the cauliflower and sauté until

heated through, add the hot sauce and continue to cook for 1 minute, tossing continuously until fully coated. Serve immediately with blue cheese sprinkled on top.

Butternut Squash and Escarole Gratin

Servings: 8 | Prep: 30 m | Style: French | Cook: 60 m

Ingredients

- 3 tbsps Unsalted Butter Stick
- 16 oz Escarole
- 2 1/2 lbs Butternut Winter Squash
- 1/2 tsp Salt
- 1/4 tsp Black Pepper
- 3 leeks Leeks
- 1 fl oz Water
- 1 cup Heavy Cream
- 1/2 cup Chicken Broth, Bouillon or Consomme
- 2 tsps Thick-It-Up
- 1 cup shredded Gruyere Cheese
- 2 tbsps Parmesan Cheese (Grated)

Directions

1. Butter a 6- to 8-cup baking dish. Set oven rack in upper third of oven and heat oven to 400F.
2. Bring 3 inches of water to boil in a large saucepan. Add escarole and cook, stirring, until tender, 3 to 5 minutes. Drain in a colander and rinse under cold running water. Gently squeeze to remove as much moisture as possible.
3. Melt 1 tablespoon of the butter in a medium nonstick skillet over medium-high heat. Add half of the squash and season with 1/4 teaspoon of the salt and 1/8 teaspoon of the pepper; cook, turning occasionally, until lightly browned and nearly tender, about 8 minutes. Transfer to baking dish. Repeat and reserve.
4. Melt remaining tablespoon butter in skillet over medium-low heat. Add leeks and season with remaining 1/4 teaspoon salt; cook, stirring, 3 minutes. Add water, cover and cook, stirring occasionally, until tender, about 3 minutes. Stir in escarole and cook until heated through; spoon over squash in baking dish.

5. Top with reserved squash.
6. Wipe out skillet. Combine cream, broth and thickener in skillet, whisking until blended. Cook over medium heat, stirring, until thickened, about 2 minutes. Remove from heat and stir in Gruyre until melted.
7. Pour sauce over vegetables, spreading evenly. Sprinkle Parmesan on top and bake until bubbly and golden brown on top, about 30 minutes. Let stand 10 minutes before serving.

Cajun Blackened Salmon with Cucumber Relish

Servings: 2 | Style: French | Cook: 45 m

Ingredients

- 1/2 cucumber (8-1/4") Cucumber (with Peel)
- 1 lime yield Lime Juice
- 1/4 oz Dill
- 1/4 oz Thyme
- 1 individual packet Sucralose Based Sweetener (Sugar Substitute)
- 12 oz Cauliflower
- 1/2 tsp Basil (Dried)
- 1 tbsp Paprika
- 1/2 tsp Oregano
- 1/4 tsp Red or Cayenne Pepper
- 12 oz boneless Salmon
- 2 tbsps Olive Oil
- 3/4 tsp Salt

Directions

1. Place 4 cups of water in a medium saucepot over medium-high heat and bring to a boil. Cut the cucumber into ¼-inch dice pieces and place in a medium bowl. Squeeze the lime directly into the bowl with the cucumber; set aside. Remove the dill and thyme leaves from the stems and finely chop the leaves; set aside separately.
2. To make the relish, add the splenda, dill, 1 tablespoon of olive oil and a pinch of salt and pepper to the cucumber. Toss well to combine. To create the blackening rub, combine the dried basil, paprika, dried oregano, cayenne, fresh thyme, and ½ teaspoon of salt in a small bowl and stir. Set aside for step 4.

3. Add the cauliflower florets, cover, and reduce the heat to medium-low. Let the cauliflower cook for 10 minutes or until tender. Drain a colander and return to the saucepot. Cover and keep warm for step 5.
4. Pat dry the salmon with paper towels. Brush each piece of salmon with 2 teaspoons of olive oil and then coat evenly with the blackening rub. Heat a large sauté pan with 1 tablespoon of olive oil over medium-high heat. When the oil is hot, add the salmon and cook for 2 to 3 minutes until blackened. Turn the fish over and cook for 4 to 5 more minutes and the fish flakes easily with a fork.
5. Mash the cauliflower and add 1 tablespoon of olive oil, mashing until the oil is incorporated. Season with ¼ teaspoon each of salt and pepper.
6. Spoon equal amounts of the mashed cauliflower onto two plates. Place a salmon fillet on top, and then garnish with the cucumber relish. Enjoy!

Cali Mac and Cheese

Servings: 6 | Prep: 15 m | Style: French | Cook: 20 m

Ingredients

- 1 head large (6-7" dia) Cauliflower
- 1 cup Heavy Cream
- 2 oz Cream Cheese
- 1 1/2 tsps Mustard
- 1 1/2 cups shredded Cheddar Cheese
- 1 clove Garlic
- 1 tsp Salt
- 1/4 tsp White Pepper
- 1/4 tsp Original Pepper Sauce

Directions

1. Preheat oven to 375°F and prepare a baking dish with olive oil spray. Heat a large pot of water to boiling and add 1/2 tsp salt. Remove stem and leaves from cauliflower. Cut into small bite sized pieces and place in the boiling water; cook until crisp-tender; about 5 minutes. Drain well then pat between paper towels to remove all moisture.
2. In a medium sauce pan bring the cream to a simmer, whisk in the cream cheese and powdered mustard until smooth. Add the shredded Cheddar, minced garlic, 1/2 tsp salt, white pepper and pepper sauce (Tabasco®, to taste) whisking until the cheese melts; about 1-2 minutes. Remove from

the heat and stir in the cauliflower. Pour into the baking dish and top with remaining 1/2 cup of cheese. Bake for 15 minutes until browned and bubbly.

Candied-Ginger Sweet Potatoes

Servings: 6 | *Prep:* 20 m | *Style:* French | *Cook:* 40 m

Ingredients

- 1/2 cup Sugar Free Maple Flavored Syrup
- 3 tsps Ginger
- 3 tbsps Unsalted Butter Stick
- 4 medium (2" dia x 5" long, raw) Baked Sweetpotato (Peel Eaten)

Directions

1. Heat oven to 450°F. Butter an 8-by 10-inch baking dish.
2. Cook potatoes in boiling salted water until almost tender, 8-10 minutes. Drain.
3. Combine syrup and ginger in a small saucepan. Cook over low heat until syrup is warm and the flavors have blended, about 3 minutes.
4. Arrange potatoes in a single layer in baking dish. Pour syrup mixture over potatoes. Dot with butter. Cover with aluminum foil and bake until potatoes are very soft, about 40 minutes

Cauliflower and Onion Mash with Cheddar

Servings: 1 | *Prep:* 5 m | *Style:* American | *Cook:* 8 m

Ingredients

- 1/2 cup Cauliflower
- 1 tsp Extra Virgin Olive Oil
- 3 tbsps chopped Onions
- 1/4 cup shredded Cheddar Cheese

Directions

1. Steam cauliflower in a steamer basket over boiling water until tender, about 3 4 minutes. Mash with a fork.
2. Meanwhile, heat a nonstick skillet with 1 teaspoon virgin olive oil over medium-high heat. Add onions and sauté until tender.
3. Add onions to mashed cauliflower and top with cheese.

Cauliflower Risotto

Servings: 4 | Prep: 10 m | Style: American | Cook: 15 m

Ingredients

- 2 cups Cauliflower
- 1 tbsp Extra Virgin Olive Oil
- 1 tbsp chopped Shallots
- 1/2 cup Bouillon Vegetable Broth
- 2 tbsps Heavy Cream
- 2 tbsps Parsley
- 1/2 cup Parmesan Cheese (Grated)

Directions

1. Pulse cauliflower florets in a food processor until they are the size of grains of rice.
2. In a skillet over medium heat cook shallots in the olive oil until tender.
3. Add cauliflower and toss to coat; add vegetable stock and cook until tender, about 10 minutes.
4. Add cream, chopped parsley and cheese.
5. Season with salt and freshly ground black pepper to taste.

Cauliflower Shepherd's Pie

Servings: 6 | Prep: 15 m | Style: American | Cook: 60 m

Ingredients

- 1 head large (6-7" dia) Cauliflower
- 2 tbsps Unsalted Butter Stick
- 1/4 cup Cream Cheese
- 1 cup shredded Cheddar Cheese
- 1 tbsp Olive Oil
- 1 large Onion
- 2 cloves Garlic
- 1 carrot (7-1/2") Carrots
- 3 stalk large (11"-12" long) Celery
- 1 1/2 lbs Ground Beef (90% Lean / 10% Fat)
- 1/2 tbsp Cornstarch
- 2 tbsps Tomato Paste
- 6 tsps The Original Worcestershire Sauce
- 1/2 cup Beef Broth, Bouillon or Consomme
- 3 tsps Thyme
- 2/3 tbsp Parsley

Directions

1. Preheat the oven to 375°F.
2. MAKE THE TOPPING: In a large pot steam cauliflower for 15 minutes or until tender. Drain and return to warm pot. Add butter & cream cheese. Puree with immersion blender until smooth. You can use a potato masher but it will be lumpy. Taste and season with salt and pepper. Stir in 1/2 cup shredded cheese and set aside (reserve remaining 1/2 cup for later).
3. MAKE THE FILLING: Heat oil in a large skillet over medium heat. Add the onion, garlic, carrot and celery and saute for 5 minutes stirring occasionally. Add the ground meat and cook for 5 minutes. Sprinkle cornstarch over the meat mixture, stir and cook for a minute. Add the next 5 ingredients (tomato paste through parsley; note that you will need 2 tbsp of the Worcestershire sauce) and stir to combine. Bring to a boil, reduce heat to low, cover and simmer for about 10 minutes stirring occasionally.
4. ASSEMBLE: Place meat mixture in the bottom of an 11 X 7 inch baking dish. Spoon and gently spread cauliflower mixture evenly over the top with rubber spatula. The meat mixture should be completely covered. Finish by gently swirling the cauliflower with the spatula so you have some nice peaks.
5. COOK: Place the baking dish on a rimmed baking sheet and bake for 20 minutes. Top with remaining cheddar cheese and bake an additional 5-10 minutes or until the cheese melts and the top is lightly browned.

Cauliflower with Indian Spices

Servings: 6 | *Prep:* 8 m | *Style:* Indian | *Cook:* 15 m

Ingredients

- 2 tbsps Unsalted Butter Stick
- 1 tsp Cumin
- 1/2 tsp Coriander Seed
- 1/2 tsp Ginger (Ground)
- 1 medium whole (2-3/5" dia) Red Tomato
- 1 head large (6-7" dia) Cauliflower
- 1/2 cup Chicken Broth, Bouillon or Consomme
- 1 1/2 tsps Salt
- 1/2 tsp Black Pepper
- 1/2 oz Cilantro (Coriander)

Directions

1. To make this a vegetarian dish, simply use vegetable broth instead of chicken broth.
2. In a large skillet, melt butter over medium heat. Add cumin, coriander and ginger. Cook spices until fragrant, about 1 minute.
3. Add tomato and cauliflower to skillet. Raise heat to high, add broth, salt and pepper and bring to a boil. Cover, turn heat down to low and simmer until cauliflower is tender but still very firm, about 7 minutes.
4. Remove lid and continue cooking until broth has evaporated and cauliflower is very tender, about 5 more minutes. Sprinkle with chopped cilantro before serving.

Cauliflower-Cheddar Mash

Servings: 1 | *Prep:* 5 m | *Style:* American | *Cook:* 8 m

Ingredients

- 1 cup Cauliflower
- 1/4 cup shredded Cheddar Cheese

Directions

1. Steam cauliflower in a steamer basket over boiling water in a medium covered sauce pot until tender, about 5 minutes.
2. Remove to a bowl and mash with a fork. Top with Cheddar cheese and season to taste with salt and freshly ground pepper.

Cauliflower-Sour Cream Mash

Servings: 6 | Prep: 10 m | Style: American | Cook: 10 m

Ingredients

- 8 cups Cauliflower
- 2 tbsps Sour Cream (Cultured)
- 2 tbsps Heavy Cream
- 1 1/2 tbsps Unsalted Butter Stick
- 1 tsp Salt

Directions

1. Add a cup of water to a large pot and insert a steamer basket. Place cauliflower florets in the basket and bring water to a boil over high heat. Cover tightly, cook until tender, 10 12 minutes, and drain.
2. Purée cauliflower in a food processor, adding florets in batches.
3. Add sour cream, heavy cream, butter and salt; process until smooth and well combined.
4. Reheat gently, if necessary, before serving.

Celery Siciliano

Servings: 6 | Prep: 12 m | Style: Italian | Cook: 15 m

Ingredients

- 2 tbsps Extra Virgin Olive Oil
- 1/4 medium (2-1/2" dia) Onions
- 1 1/2 lbs Celery
- 1 tbsp Thick-It-Up
- 1 cup Bouillon Vegetable Broth
- 2 plums Red Tomatoes
- 6 Green Olives
- 2 tbsps Parsley

Directions

1. Heat oil in a large skillet over medium heat. Add celery and white onion; cook 5 minutes, until onion is softened. Sprinkle with thickener, salt and pepper and mix well. Sauté 2 minutes. Stir in broth; heat to boiling.
2. Cover and simmer 10-15 minutes, until celery is tender.Uncover and stir in tomatoes and olives. Simmer 3 minutes, until liquid thickens. Season to taste with salt and pepper. Sprinkle with parsley.

Chard and Cheese Casserole

Servings: 6 | Prep: 20 m | Style: American | Cook: 55 m

Ingredients

- 2 tbsps Extra Virgin Olive Oil
- 3/4 lb Swiss Chard
- 1 medium (approx 2-3/4" long, 2-1/2" dia) Sweet Red Peppers
- 1 small Onion
- 1/2 tsp Salt
- 1/4 tsp Black Pepper
- 1 1/2 cups shredded Muenster Cheese
- 1/2 cup Parmesan Cheese (Grated)

Directions

1. Heat oven to 350°F. Grease a 9- by 13-inch baking dish.

2. Heat 1 tablespoon oil in a large Dutch oven or heavy pot over high heat. Add chard and cook 3 -4 minutes, until wilted. Drain in colander; press with the back of a spoon to extract excess liquid and discard.
3. Heat remaining tablespoon of oil in a large skillet over medium heat. Sauté
4. bell pepper and white onion 8 minutes, until softened. Mix in chard; toss to coat. Season with salt and pepper. Mix in Muenster cheese.
5. Spoon into prepared baking dish. Evenly sprinkle Parmesan cheese over top. Cover with aluminum foil; bake 30 minutes.
6. Uncover and cook 10 minutes more, until cheese is brown and bubbly.

Chicken Braised in Sauerkraut

Servings: 6 | Prep: 25 m | Style: American | Cook: 35 m

Ingredients

- 4 thick slice packed 12/lbs Bacon (Cured)
- 40 oz, with bone (yield after cooking, bone removed) Chicken Thigh (Skin Eaten)
- 3/4 tsp Salt
- 1/4 tsp Black Pepper
- 1 small Red Onion
- 3 cups Sauerkraut (Solid and Liquids, Canned)
- 1 cup Chicken Broth, Bouillon or Consomme
- 1 tsp Dijon Mustard
- 1 tsp crumbled Bay Leaf
- 1 tsp Sucralose Based Sweetener (Sugar Substitute)

Directions

This recipe requires Juniper berries as an ingredient. You will need 3/4 teaspoon for 6 servings. If you cannot find them, leave them out of the recipe.

1. In a large, deep skillet over medium-high heat, cook bacon until crisp. Transfer to a bowl with a slotted spoon.
2. Sprinkle chicken with teaspoon salt and pepper. Brown in two batches in bacon drippings, 8 minutes per batch. Transfer chicken to bowl as it browns.
3. Cook onion in drippings 4-5 minutes, until softened. Add bacon, sauerkraut, chicken broth, mustard, juniper berries, bay leaf, sugar substitute, and remaining salt and mix well. Arrange chicken on top. Bring

to a simmer, cover, and cook on low 35 minutes, until chicken is cooked through.Transfer chicken to a platter. Discard bay leaf.
4. Increase heat to high and boil off most of the cooking liquid. Serve chicken with sauerkraut on the side.

Chicken Cauliflower Mac and Cheese

Servings: 2 | Prep: m | Style: American | Cook: 45 m

Ingredients

- 1 clove Garlic
- 12 oz Cauliflower
- 1/3 cup Heavy Cream
- 1 oz Cream Cheese
- 1/2 tsp Dry Mustard
- 1/2 cup Classic Cheddar Jack Cheese
- 1/8 tsp Original Pepper Sauce
- 3 oz Roasted Red Peppers
- 12 oz raw Chicken Breast
- 1 tsp Olive Oil
- 1/2 tsp Salt
- 1/2 tsp Black Pepper

Directions

1. Preheat oven to 375ºF. Spray a baking dish with non-stick spray. Finely chop the garlic and set aside. Bring a large sauce pot with 4 cups of water and ½ teaspoon salt to a boil over high heat.
2. Cut the cauliflower into bite-sized pieces and add to the water when it begins to boil. Cook for 5 minutes, or until crisp-tender. Drain in a colander and lay on paper towels to dry.
3. Pour the whipping cream into a medium sauce pot over medium-high heat. When the cream begins to simmer, whisk in the cream cheese and the powdered mustard until smooth. Add half of the shredded Cheddar cheese, garlic, ¼ teaspoon of salt and ¼ teaspoon of pepper and the Tabasco sauce, whisking until the cheese melts, about 1 to 2 minutes.
4. Remove the cheese sauce from the heat and stir in the cauliflower, making sure the cauliflower is well coated. Pour into the baking dish and top with the roasted red peppers and the remaining cheddar cheese. Place in the oven and bake for 15 minutes, until browned and bubbly.

5. While the Cali mac and cheese is baking, pat dry the chicken breasts with paper towels. Season the chicken with ¼ teaspoon each of salt and pepper. Heat 1 teaspoon of olive oil in a medium sauté pan over medium-high heat. -- When the pan is hot, add the chicken and sauté for 4 minutes on each side until cooked through.
6. Place a chicken breast on two plates. Scoop the Cali mac and cheese next to the chicken and enjoy!

Chicken Curry

Servings: 26 | Prep: 8 m | Style: Indian | Cook: 20 m

Ingredients

- 3 tbsps Unsalted Butter Stick
- 32 oz boneless, cooked Chicken Breast
- 1 tsp Cumin
- 1/2 tsp Coriander Leaf (Dried)
- 1/2 tsp Ginger (Ground)
- 1/4 tsp Crushed Red Pepper Flakes
- 2 tsps Garlic
- 1/2 cup Chicken Broth, Bouillon or Consomme
- 1/3 cup Heavy Cream
- 1/16 cup Cilantro (Coriander)

Directions

1. Heat butter in a heavy skillet over medium-high heat until the foam from the butter subsides. Add chicken strips and cook in batches until browned, 5 minutes per batch.
2. Add cumin, coriander, ginger, red-pepper flakes (if using) and garlic and cook, stirring occasionally, 2 minutes. Add chicken stock and bring to a boil. Reduce heat to medium-low; simmer, stirring occasionally, 5 minutes.
3. Slowly add heavy cream and simmer (do not let mixture come to a boil) until heated through, 3 minutes.Transfer chicken and sauce to a serving plate. Garnish with cilantro.
4. Place a chicken breast on two plates. Scoop the Cali mac and cheese next to the chicken and enjoy!

Chicken Legs with Spicy Avocado-Tomatillo Salsa

*Servings: 4 | **Prep:** 15 m | **Style:** Mexican | **Cook:** 20 m*

Ingredients

- 1 California Avocado
- 1 cup chopped or diced Tomatillos
- 10 sprigs Cilantro
- 10 cloves Garlic
- 4 tbsps Red Wine Vinegar
- 1 cup (8 fl oz) Water
- 4 peppers Serrano Pepper
- 1 small Red Onion
- 1 1/2 lbs Chicken Leg Meat and Skin (Broilers or Fryers)
- 1/2 tsp Salt
- 1/2 tsp Black Pepper
- 3 tbsps Olive Oil

Directions

1. Place the avocado, tomatillos, cilantro, roasted garlic, vinegar, water and chiles in a blender; purée just until smooth. Transfer to a bowl and fold in onion and salt. Set aside.
2. Heat oven to 350°F.
3. Sprinkle the chicken with salt and pepper. Heat the oil in a large ovenproof sauté pan or skillet over medium-high heat. Add the chicken legs with skin side down and sear for 1 2 minutes until golden-brown. Flip the chicken, transfer skillet to the oven and bake uncovered for 15-20 minutes until just done. (Juices will run clear.)
4. Place one chicken leg on each plate and spoon one-quarter of the salsa around each plate and on the chicken. Garnish each with a sprig of cilantro.

*To roast garlic, toss the cloves in just enough olive oil to coat and place in a square of aluminum foil with about 1/8 cup of water. Fold and crimp foil pouch to close and place in a preheated 350°F oven for about 40 minutes. **Wear rubber gloves when handling chile peppers and be careful not to rub your eyes.

Chicken Paprikash

Servings: 6 | Prep: 10 m | Style: Middle Eastern | Cook: 45 m

Ingredients

- 2 tbsps Unsalted Butter Stick
- 2 medium (4-1/8" long) Scallions or Spring Onions
- 1 tsp Garlic
- 3/4 tsp Crushed Red Pepper Flakes
- 1 1/2 tbsps Paprika
- 32 oz Chicken Breast Meat and Skin (Broilers or Fryers)
- 2 cups Mushroom Pieces and Stems
- 3/4 cup Tap Water
- 3/4 tsp Salt
- 1 Bay Leaf
- 1/2 cup Sour Cream (Cultured)
- 1 tsp Thick-It-Up

Directions

1. Melt butter in a large skillet or Dutch oven set over high heat. Add chopped scallions and minced garlic; sauté until softened, about 2 minutes. Stir in red pepper flakes and 1 Tablespoon paprika; sauté until fragrant, about 30 seconds.
2. Add chicken pieces, skin side down, and sear 3 minutes. Add mushrooms, water, salt, and bay leaf; bring to a boil. Reduce heat to low, cover, and simmer until chicken is cooked through, about 45 minutes; turn chicken halfway through.
3. Transfer chicken to a plate. Spoon off fat from sauce and discard. Remove and discard bay leaf. Increase heat to high and boil liquid until reduced to about 1 cup, 5 minutes.
4. Remove from heat and gradually stir in sour cream, thickener, and remaining 1/2 Tablespoon paprika. Reduce heat to medium-low and bring sauce to a simmer, stirring constantly. Return chicken to pot and simmer until heated through.

Chicken Picatta with Capers and Tomoatoes

Servings: 2 | Style: Italian | Cook: 45 m

Ingredients

- 1 medium (4-1/8" long) Young Green Onions
- 1 clove Garlic
- 18 oz Asparagus
- 2 italian Tomatoes
- 1 cube Chicken Stock Cubes (Dry, Dehydrated)
- 2 medium Chicken Thighs
- 1 tbsp drained Capers
- 1 tbsp Olive Oil
- 3/4 tsp Salt
- 3/4 tsp Black Pepper

Directions

1. Cut the green onion into ¼-inch pieces; set aside. Finely chop the garlic clove; set aside. Trim asparagus by snapping the thicker bottom ends where they break naturally; set aside. Cut the tomato into ¼-inch diced pieces; set aside. Add the chicken stock concentrate to 1 cup of water in a small bowl; stir and set aside.
2. Pat dry the chicken thighs with paper towels. Season with ¼ teaspoon each of salt and pepper. Heat 1 tablespoon of olive oil in a large sauté pan over medium-high heat. When the oil is hot, add the chicken and cook for 3 to 5 minutes per side, until cooked through. Transfer the chicken to a plate, cover with foil and keep warm
3. Keeping the heat at medium-high, add 1 tablespoon of olive oil. When hot, add the green onions and garlic to the pan and reduce the heat to medium. Cook for about 30 seconds until garlic is fragrant.
4. Add the tomatoes, 2 tablespoons of the chicken stock, capers and ¼ teaspoon each of salt and pepper. Cook, stirring occasionally until slightly thickened, about 5 minutes.
5. Meanwhile, heat 2 teaspoons of olive oil in a medium sauté pan over medium-high heat. When hot, add the asparagus and ¼ teaspoon each of salt and pepper and sauté for 3 minutes. Return the chicken to the pan with the tomato mixture and coat the chicken in the sauce. Heat until warmed through.
6. Divide the asparagus evenly between two plates. Place the chicken next to the asparagus, spoon the sauce over the chicken and enjoy!

Chicken Stuffed with Apple, Almond and Cheese

Servings: 4 | Prep: 10 m | Style: American | Cook: 15 m

Ingredients

- 1/4 cup sliced Almonds
- 8 tbsps Garlic & Fine Herbs Gournay Cheese
- 1/3 cup quartered or chopped Apple
- 3 tbsps Parsley
- 1/2 tsp Garlic
- 1/4 tsp Salt
- 1/4 tsp Black Pepper
- 28 oz raw Chicken Breast
- 1 tbsp Light Olive Oil

Directions

1. Toast almonds in a dry skillet turning once for 2-3 minutes or in a 350°F oven on a sheet pan. Set aside to cool.
2. In a small bowl thoroughly mix the cheese (Boursin brand can be found in most supermarkets), chopped unpeeled apples, chopped parsley, almonds, garlic, 1/2 teaspoon salt and 1/4 teaspoon pepper in a small bowl.
3. Slice the chicken breasts lengthwise creating a pocket for the stuffing; generously salt and pepper on the inside and outside of each breast. Divide the stuffing and fill each breast and secure with a tooth pick(s) on the open end.
4. Heat the skillet over medium high heat with oil. Cook the chicken breasts for about 6 minutes each side until the juices run clear and they are no longer pink in the center. Increase time if the breasts are thick. Serve immediately.

Chimichurri Steak and Cauliflower Mash

Servings: 2 | Style: Mexican | Cook: 45 m

Ingredients

- 1/4 oz Cilantro
- 1/4 oz Parsley
- 1 oz Shallots
- 1 fruit (2-1/8" dia) Lemon
- 4 tbsps Olive Oil

- 2/3 tbsp Red Wine Vinegar
- 1/4 tsp Crushed Red Pepper Flakes
- 1 clove Garlic
- 12 oz Cauliflower
- 1 tbsp Sour Cream
- 1 1/2 tsps Unsalted Butter Stick
- 16 oz boneless (yield after cooking) Steak
- 1/2 tsp Salt
- 1/2 tsp Black Pepper

Directions

1. Remove the leaves from the cilantro and parsley stems and discard stems. Place the leaves in the bowl of a food processor. Chop the shallot and add to the herbs. Zest half of the lemon directly into the processor. Juice the lemon into a small bowl, discard the seeds and add the juice to the herbs along with the red wine vinegar, red chili flakes, garlic cloves and ½ teaspoon each of salt and pepper.
2. Pulse until all the ingredients are well combined, but not over processed. Pour into a medium bowl and stir in 4 tablespoons of olive oil; hold. Wash and rinse the food processor for use in step 4.
3. Add 2 cups of water to a medium sauce pot and insert a steam basket. Place the cauliflower florets in the steamer basket and bring the water to a boil over high heat. Cover and cook until tender, 10 to 12 minutes and drain in a colander.
4. Puree the cauliflower in the food processor, adding the florets in small batches. Add the sour cream, butter and ⅓ teaspoon of salt and process until smooth and well combined. Keep warm and hold for plating.
5. Pat dry the steaks with paper towels and season with ¼ teaspoon each of salt and pepper. Heat a large non-stick sauté pan over medium-high heat and when the pan is hot, add the steak and sear on one side for 3 to 4 minutes on each side. Remove the steak and place on a cutting board to rest for 5 to 10 minutes. Slice into ¼-inch pieces against the grain.
6. Divide the cauliflower mash between two plates. Arrange the steak slices next to the cauliflower and drizzle the chimichurri over the steak. Enjoy!

Creamy Spinach and Parmesan Puff

Servings: 8 | Prep: 10 m | Style: American | Cook: 30 m

Ingredients

- 2 large Eggs (Whole)
- 1 cup Heavy Cream
- 1/4 tsp Nutmeg (Ground)
- 1 lb Spinach
- 4 oz Parmesan Cheese (Shredded)

Directions

Use either fresh or frozen chopped spinach for this recipe. For the frozen: thaw first and squeeze out any excess moisture. For fresh: chop it and then place into a microwave safe bowl. Heat for 1 minute intervals until it is cooked, drain and cool to room temperature.

1. Prepare a 1-quart souffle dish with a small amount of oil.
2. In a small bowl, whisk together the eggs, cream and nutmeg. Add the spinach and cheese (leaving 1/4 cup for the top) mixing to combine.
3. Pour into the prepared dish, top with reserved cheese and bake at 350°F for 30 minutes until puffed and golden on top. Serve immediately.

Crispy Buttermilk Fried Chicken

Servings: 8 | Prep: 20 m | Style: American | Cook: 50 m

Ingredients

- 1 1/2 cups Buttermilk (Reduced Fat, Cultured)
- 1 tbsp Fresh Lemon Juice
- 48 oz Chicken Leg
- 1 cup Whole Grain Soy Flour
- 1 tsp Salt
- 1/2 tsp Black Pepper
- 1/2 cup Canola Vegetable Oil

Directions

1. In a large bowl, mix buttermilk and lemon juice. Add chicken, cover and refrigerate for at least 3 hours (can marinate overnight).
2. Preheat oven to 350°F.

3. Drain chicken and pat dry with paper towels. Combine soy flour, salt and pepper in a plastic bag. In two batches, add chicken and shake to coat. Place chicken on wire rack and let dry 15 minutes.
4. Heat 1/2 cup oil in a large skillet over medium heat, and fry chicken in batches 4 to 5 minutes per side, until golden brown.
5. Place chicken on baking sheet and bake 25 to 30 minutes minutes, until chicken is cooked through.

Easy and Festive Chicken Casserole

Servings: 6 | *Prep:* 20 m | *Style:* American | *Cook:* 40 m

Ingredients

- 1 cup (8 fl oz) Chicken Stock
- 1 cup Heavy Cream
- 3 cups cooked, diced Rotisserie Chicken
- 4 cups chopped Broccoli
- 1 cup chopped Sweet Red Peppers
- 1 tbsp Parsley
- 1/2 tsp Tarragon
- 3 tbsps Sherry Cooking Wine
- 1/2 tsp Black Pepper
- 4 oz Parmesan Cheese (Shredded)

Directions

1. Preheat oven to 350°F.
2. In a medium pot reduce the chicken stock and heavy cream to about 1 cup over medium-high heat; 20 minutes.
3. Shred rostisserie chicken (you will need 1 chicken for this recipe) and place in a 3 quart casserole dish with the broccoli and chopped red peppers.
4. Add parsley, tarragon, cooking sherry and black pepper and half of the cheese to the cream mixture. Pour this over the chicken and vegetables in the casserole dish. Top with remaining Parmesan cheese and bake for 30 minutes covered with foil. Remove the foil and bake an additional 10 minutes until golden on top.

Eggplant Stacks

Servings: 4 | Prep: 70 m | Style: American | Cook: 10 m

Ingredients

- 1/2 tsp Black Pepper
- 1 medium whole (2-3/5" dia) Red Tomato
- 4 slice (1 oz) Whole Milk Mozzarella Cheese
- 6 1/2 tbsps Extra Virgin Olive Oil
- 3 tbsps Red Wine Vinegar
- 1/2 tsp Garlic
- 1 tsp leaf Oregano
- 1 tsp Salt
- 1 peeled (yield from 1-1/4 lb) Eggplant
- 16 tbsps Basil
- 1/4 cup Parmesan Cheese (Grated)
- 1/4 cup Dried Pine Nuts
- 1/3 tbsp Balsamic Vinegar

Directions

1. Combine 1 1/2 tablespoons olive oil, red wine vinegar, minced glove of garlic, oregano, 1/2 teaspoon salt and 1/2 teaspoon pepper in a large bowl. Add eggplant, toss well, and let stand 1 hour; turning eggplant occasionally. Optional: brush eggplant with olive oil and grill for 2-3 minutes per side; allow to cool and set aside.
2. In a food processor pulse the basil, Parmesan, 1/2 tablespoon olive oil and pine nuts until a smooth paste forms. Transfer to bowl and cover entire surface with plastic wrap.
3. Combine 1/4 cup oil (4 Tbsp), balsamic vinegar, 1/2 teaspoon salt and a pinch (1/8 tsp) of black pepper in a pie plate; add sliced tomato and turn to coat.
4. To assemble stack: Arrange 4 eggplant slices, spread 1/2 tablespoon pesto over the top. Top with 1 tomato slice then with 1 mozzarella slice. Add another layer of eggplant, pesto, tomato and cheese. Drizzle any extra tomato juices around each stack.

Ginger, Almond and Garlic Broccoli

Servings: 6 | Prep: 10 m | Style: Asian | Cook: 10 m

Ingredients

- 2 tbsps Canola Vegetable Oil
- 1/2 cup, slivered Almonds
- 1 tbsp Ginger
- 1 tsp Garlic
- 4 cup flowerets Broccoli Flower Clusters
- 1/2 cup Chicken Broth, Bouillon or Consomme
- 2 tbsps Tamari Soybean Sauce
- 1 tbsp Sodium and Sugar Free Rice Vinegar
- 1/2 tsp Sesame Oil

Directions

1. In a large heavy skillet, heat oil over high heat. Add almonds and cook until browned, about 1-2 minutes. Add ginger and garlic and cook until aromatic, another 30 seconds.
2. Add broccoli to skillet and sauté until browned in spots, about 3 minutes. Stir in chicken broth, soy sauce and vinegar. Bring to a boil, and cook until liquid has almost evaporated and broccoli is crisp-tender, about 5 more minutes. Drizzle in sesame oil and serve.

Greek Hamburger with Feta and Roasted Zucchini Salad

Servings: 2 | Style: Mediterranean / Greek | Cook: 45 m

Ingredients

- 1 large Young Green Onion
- 1 oz Baby Spinach
- 1/4 oz Dill
- 1 italian Tomato
- 1 fruit (2-1/8" dia) Lemon
- 1 medium Zucchini
- 8 oz Ground Beef (85% Lean / 15% Fat)
- 1 oz Feta Cheese
- 1/4 tsp Oregano

- 4 oz Butterhead Lettuce (Includes Boston and Bibb Types)
- 2 tbsps Olive Oil
- 1/2 tsp Salt
- 1/2 tsp Black Pepper

Directions

1. Finely chop the green onion and place in a large bowl. Roughly chop the baby spinach and add to the bowl with the green onion. Remove enough dill leaves from their stems to yield 1 teaspoon of roughly chopped dill and add to the bowl.
2. Slice the tomato into ¼-inch sliced rounds; set aside. Zest the lemon into a small bowl. Juice the lemon into the same bowl, discarding any seeds; set aside. Cut the zucchini into ¼-diced pieces; set aside.
3. Pat dry the ground beef with paper towels and add to the bowl with the spinach mixture. Add the crumbled feta cheese, ¼ teaspoon each of salt and pepper and the dried oregano. Mix until all ingredients are well combined.
4. Form the ground beef mixture into two patties. Heat a large sauté pan over medium-high heat and when hot, add the burger patties and cook for 5 to 6 minutes per side until cooked through.
5. While the burgers are cooking, heat 2 tablespoons of olive oil in a medium sauté pan over medium-high heat. Add the zucchini and sauté for 1 to 2 minutes to soften and get slightly browned. Season with the lemon zest and juice and ¼ teaspoon each of salt and pepper. Stir to combine.
6. Place the burgers between two slices of bibb lettuce and top with the sliced tomatoes. Place a burger on each plate and arrange the sautéed zucchini next to the burgers. Enjoy!

Greek-Style Chicken Thighs

*Servings: 2 | **Prep:** 15 m | **Style:** Mediterranean / Greek | **Cook:** 30 m*

Ingredients

- 1 fruit (2-1/8" dia) Lemon
- 12 oz boneless (yield after cooking) Chicken Thigh (Skin Eaten)
- 3 cloves Garlic
- 2 tsps Extra Virgin Olive Oil
- 1/3 tsp Salt
- 1/3 tsp Black Pepper

- 1 tbsp Peppermint (Mint)
- 1 tsp leaf Oregano
- 4 olives Pitted Kalamata Olives
- 1 medium Zucchini
- 4 oz Brown Mushrooms (Crimini Italian)
- 1 tbsp Olive Oil

Directions

1. Arrange rack in center of oven. Heat oven to 350°F. Layer lemon slices on the bottom of a 13x9 baking dish; set aside. Gently run your fingers between chicken thigh and the skin to loosen skin. Slice 2/3rd of the lemon and juice the remaining. Line a pan prepared with oil spray with the lemon slices. Set aside.
2. Press 2 garlic cloves through a garlic press. Lift the skin from 1 breast and rub garlic between skin and breast. Repeat process with remaining chicken and garlic. Drizzle olive oil and lemon juice over chicken breasts. Sprinkle with salt and pepper and rub into skin. Place chicken breasts over the lemon slices in prepared pan.
3. Combine mint and oregano in a small bowl; evenly sprinkle over chicken breasts. Sprinkle olives over chicken and bake for 45 minutes, until juices run clear when chicken is pricked with a fork. Remove from oven and sprinkle with 4 oz of feta cheese (this is optional and adds .77g NC per serving). Bake 5 minutes more. Serve with pan juices.

Green and Yellow Squash Kebabs

*Servings: 8 | **Prep:** 25 m | **Style:** American | **Cook:** 10 m*

Ingredients

- 2 medium Zucchinis
- 1/4 cup Parsley
- 2 tbsps Extra Virgin Olive Oil
- 3 tbsps Real Mayonnaise
- 1 tsp Garlic
- 1/2 cup Cilantro (Coriander)
- 1 tbsp Fresh Lime Juice
- 2 medium Summer Squashes

Directions

1. Soak eight 12-inch bamboo skewers in warm water for 20 minutes before threading them with squash. Or use metal skewers.
2. In a small bowl, combine 1/2 cup chopped cilantro, 1/4 cup chopped parsley, oil, mayonnaise, lime juice and garlic and mix well. Let stand for 15 minutes to allow flavors to blend.
3. Preheat grill to medium-high.
4. Alternating colors, thread 6 pieces of squash on each of 8 skewers. Brush half the mayonnaise mixture over the vegetables. Cover and grill 4 to 5 minutes, turn, brush with remaining mayonnaise mixture and grill 4 to 5 minutes more, until lightly charred.

Green Bean Casserole Topped with Crispy Onions

Servings: 12 | Prep: 15 m | Style: American | Cook: 40 m

Ingredients

- 24 oz Green Snap Beans
- 1 1/2 lbs Brown Mushrooms (Crimini Italian)
- 6 tbsps Unsalted Butter Stick
- 1 tsp Garlic
- 1 medium (2-1/2" dia) Onions
- 1 tsp Salt
- 2 tsps Thyme
- 1/8 tsp Nutmeg (Ground)
- 1/8 tsp Red or Cayenne Pepper
- 1/2 tsp Black Pepper
- 1/2 cup Sour Cream (Cultured)
- 3/4 tsp Thick-It-Up
- 1/2 cup Heavy Cream
- 1/2 cup Parmesan Cheese (Grated)
- 1/4 cup Whole Grain Soy Flour
- 1/4 cup Canola Vegetable Oil
- 1 cup Chicken Broth, Bouillon or Consomme

Directions

1. Thaw green beans completely (or use fresh, ends trimmed).

2. In a large sauté pan heat butter until bubbly. Add mushrooms, garlic and salt. Cook mushrooms until nicely browned; about 10 minutes. Combine with the green beans in a 2-quart casserole dish.
3. To the pan, add the thyme, cayenne, nutmeg, black pepper and chicken broth. Sprinkle the Thick-It-Up over the top and whisk over medium heat for 1-2 minutes until thickened. Whisk in the sour cream and heavy cream and continue to cook an additional 3 minutes until thoroughly combined and thickened. Poor evenly over the green beans and mushrooms. Top with Parmesan cheese and bake for 20 minutes until bubbly throughout.
4. While the casserole is cooking, cut the onion into thin slices and separate into rings. Coat evenly with soy flour and fry in oil in small batches for 1-3 minutes until golden and crispy. Drain away excess oil on a paper towel and continue until all onion rings are fried. Top casserole with onion rings and serve immediately.

Green Beans Almondine

*Servings: 8 | **Prep:** 10 m | **Style:** American | **Cook:** 10 m*

Ingredients

- 2 lbs Green Snap Beans
- 4 tbsps Unsalted Butter Stick
- 1 1/2 oz Almonds

Directions

1. Place beans in a steamer basket steamer fitted over a pot of boiling water and cook until crisp-tender, about 7 9 minutes.
2. In a large skillet over medium heat melt butter with almonds. Cook 1-2 minutes until butter is browned and almonds are fragrant.
3. Add green beans to skillet and toss to coat. Season to taste with salt and freshly ground black pepper.

Grilled Bell Peppers and Onions

*Servings: 4 | **Prep:** 15 m | **Style:** American | **Cook:** 10 m*

Ingredients

- 2 medium (approx 2-3/4" long, 2-1/2" dia) Green Sweet Pepper
- 2 small Onions
- 3 tbsps Extra Virgin Olive Oil
- 1 tbsp Balsamic Vinegar
- 1/8 tsp Black Pepper
- 1/8 tsp Salt
- 1 oz Black Olives
- 1 tbsp drained Capers

Directions

1. Heat grill to medium.
2. Grill vegetables 4 5 minutes per side until peppers are blistered and White onions are nicely browned. Remove from grill; cool 5 minutes. Rub skin off peppers.
3. In a medium bowl mix olive oil, vinegar, black pepper, salt, diced olives and capers.
4. Cut peppers into 1/2-inch strips and onions into 1/2-inch pieces. Add vegetables to bowl.Toss gently to combine ingredients. Adjust seasonings if necessary.

Grilled Chicken with Asparagus and Tomato Salad

Servings: 1 | Prep: 10 m | Style: American | Cook: 15 m

Ingredients

- 6 oz raw Chicken Breast
- 1 cup Asparagus
- 5 Cherry Tomatoes
- 5 leaves Basil
- 1 tbsp Olive Oil
- 2/3 tbsp Balsamic Vinegar

Directions

1. Preheat a grill. Season the chicken breast with salt and freshly ground black pepper. Grill until the juices run clear and the inside is no longer pink. About 7 minutes per side. Place lightly oiled asparagus on the grill during the last 5 minutes of cooking the chicken.
2. While the chicken cooks, cut the cherry tomatoes in half and arrange on a serving plate topped with minced basil leaves, olive oil and balsamic vinegar. Season with salt and freshly ground black pepper. Once cooked sliced the chicken and serve with the asparagus and tomato salad.

Grilled Chicken with Cali Mac and Cheese

Servings: 6 | Prep: 10 m | Style: American | Cook: 20 m

Ingredients

- 32 oz raw Chicken Breast
- 6 servings Cali Mac and Cheese

Directions

Use the Atkins recipe to make Cali Mac and Cheese to serve with the grilled chicken.

1. Prepare the Cali Mac and Cheese.
2. Heat a charcoal or gas grill to medium or heat a grill pan. Season chicken with salt and freshly ground black pepper or add any sugar-free rub to the chicken.
3. Grill chicken, turning occasionally, until it is no longer pink in the center and the juices run clear; about 7 minutes.
4. Serve with the Cali Mac and Cheese.

Grilled Pineapple

Servings: 8 | Prep: 10 m | Style: American | Cook: 12 m

Ingredients

- 8 slice (3-1/2" dia x 3/4" thick) Pineapple
- 4 tbsps Unsalted Butter Stick
- 1 tsp Cinnamon

Directions

1. Preheat grill to medium. In a small bowl, mix butter with ground cinnamon. Brush pineapple rings with mixture.
2. Grill rings until soft and nicely browned, about 3 to 4 minutes per side.

Herbed Mahi Mahi Fish en Papillote

Servings: 2 | **Prep:** m | **Style:** American | **Cook:** 35 m

Ingredients

- 5 Cherry Tomatoes
- 1 medium Zucchini
- 1/4 oz Parsley
- 1 fruit (2-1/8" dia) Lemon
- 1 oz Shallots
- 2 tbsps Unsalted Butter Stick
- 12 oz boneless Mahi Mahi
- 1/4 tsp Salt
- 1/4 tsp Black Pepper

Directions

1. Preheat oven to 475°F. Rub 1 pat of butter over each piece of parchment paper. Cut the cherry tomatoes in half; set aside. Cut the zucchini into ½-inch rounds and set aside.
2. Remove the parsley leaves from the stems and discard. Roughly chop the parsley leaves; set aside. Cut the lemon into ¼-inch slices; set aside. Finely chop the shallots; set aside.
3. Melt the remaining butter in a medium sauté pan over medium-high heat. Add the shallots and ¼ teaspoon each of salt and pepper and sauté for 3 minutes until caramelized. Turn off the heat and set aside.

4. Pat dry the mahi-mahi fillets with paper towels. Place the fillets in the center of each piece of parchment paper. Cover each fillet with shallots then top with the tomatoes and zucchini. Lay the slices of lemon over the top. Bring the edges of the parchment paper to the center and fold tightly
5. Bake until the fish is just cooked through, about 10 minutes
6. To serve, carefully cut open each packet, (Use caution as steam will escape). Gently transfer each portion to a plate, spooning any of the remaining veggies and sauce over the fish. Garnish with parsley. Enjoy!

Italian Chicken Cacciatore

Servings: 2 | *Style:* Italian | *Cook:* 45 m

Ingredients

- 1/4 medium (2-1/2" dia) Onions
- 1 clove Garlic
- 1/4 oz Rosemary
- 1/4 oz Parsley
- 1/2 lemon yield Lemon Juice
- 3 Cherry Tomatoes
- 12 oz raw Chicken Breast
- 1 tbsp White Cooking Wine
- 1/4 tsp Crushed Red Pepper Flakes
- 7 1/4 oz Stewed Tomatoes
- 4 oz Arugula (Rocket)
- 2 tbsps Olive Oil
- 1/2 tsp Salt
- 1/2 tsp Black Pepper

Directions

1. Peel the onion and cut in half. Cut 1/4 of the onion into ¼-inch dice; set aside. Finely chop the garlic clove; set aside. Remove the rosemary needles from the stems. Roughly chop the rosemary; set aside. Remove the stems from the parsley leaves and discard stems. Rough chop the parsley leaves and set aside for garnish.
2. Juice only HALF of the lemon into a large bowl; discard seeds. Add 2 tablespoons of olive oil and ¼ teaspoon each of salt and pepper. Mix to combine. Cut the cherry tomatoes in half; add to large bowl with the vinaigrette.

3. Pat dry the chicken breasts with paper towels. Season with ¼ teaspoon each of salt and pepper. Heat 3 tablespoons of olive oil in a large non-stick sauté pan over medium-high heat. Add the chicken and sauté about 4 minutes per side. Transfer the chicken to a plate and set aside for next step.
4. Add the onion, garlic and rosemary to the sauté pan and over medium-high heat, cook for 4 minutes, stirring, until the onion has softened. Add the white cooking wine and bring to a boil, scraping the bottom of the pan to loosen any browned bits. Add red chili flakes and a pinch of salt. Return the chicken and any accumulated juices to the pan.
5. Cook until almost all of the wine has evaporated, about 2 minutes. Add tomatoes. Cover, reduce the heat to low and simmer for 10 minutes until the chicken is cooked through. Remove from heat and set aside. Add the arugula to the lemon vinaigrette and toss to combine.
6. In the center of two plates, place the chicken cacciatore. Place the arugula salad in two bowls and enjoy!

Italian Sausage and Cauliflower Sauté

Servings: 2 | Style: Italian | Cook: 35 m

Ingredients

- 1/4 oz Basil
- 6 oz Turkey Sausage
- 12 oz Cauliflower
- 7 1/4 oz Stewed Tomatoes
- 1/4 tsp Crushed Red Pepper Flakes
- 1/2 tsp Oregano
- 2 tbsps Parmesan Cheese (Grated)
- 1 tbsp Olive Oil
- 1/4 tsp Salt
- 1/4 tsp Black Pepper

Directions

1. Remove the basil leaves from the stems and discard stems. Roughly chop the leaves and hold.
2. Remove the sausage from its casing and break into pieces. Heat a medium non-stick sauté pan over medium heat. When hot, add the sausage and cook until browned and cooked through, about 5 to 7 minutes.

3. Cut the cauliflower into bite sized pieces and place in a large non-stick sauté pan over medium-high heat. Add 1 tablespoon olive oil and sauté until the cauliflower just begins to brown, about 2 minutes. Add 1 tablespoon of water and cook until the water evaporates and the cauliflower is crisp-tender, about 3 minutes.
4. Once the cauliflower is crisp-tender, add the sausage and stir. Add the stewed tomatoes, basil, red chili flakes, dried oregano and ¼ teaspoon each of salt and pepper. Cook, stirring occasionally until everything is well incorporated and heated through.
5. Top the cauliflower and sausage mixture with the Parmesan cheese, cover and cook for 2 minutes, or until the cheese has melted.
6. Divide the sausage and cauliflower sauté evenly between two plates. Enjoy!

Kale with Pears and Onions

Servings: 2 | Prep: 15 m | Style: American | Cook: 30 m

Ingredients

- 1 medium (2-1/2" dia) Onions
- 3 tbsps Extra Virgin Olive Oil
- 1 medium (approx 2-1/2 per lb) Pears
- 1/4 tsp Curry Powder
- 1/8 tsp Nutmeg (Ground)
- 1/2 tsp Salt
- 1/4 tsp Black Pepper
- 1 lb Kale

Directions

1. Cook kale in a large pot of boiling, lightly salted water until bright green and wilted, about 3 minutes. Drain, cool 10 minutes, and squeeze out excess liquid, coarsely chop.
2. Heat oil in a large nonstick skillet over medium-high heat. Add onion and cook, stirring occasionally, until lightly golden, about 6 to 7 minutes.
3. Stir in pear and cook until crisp-tender, 2 to 3 minutes.
4. Add curry and nutmeg and cook until fragrant, about 30 seconds.
5. Add kale and salt and pepper and cook, stirring frequently, until tender, about 3 to 4 minutes. Serve warm.

Layered Turnips with Cheese and Bacon

*Servings: 12 | **Prep:** 20 m | **Style**: American | **Cook:** 70 m*

Ingredients

- 2 tbsps Unsalted Butter Stick
- 8 oz cooked Bacon
- 1 tbsp Organic High Fiber Coconut Flour
- 3/4 tsp Thyme
- 1/2 tsp Salt
- 1/2 tsp Black Pepper
- 32 oz, raw, yields Turnip
- 1 cup shredded Gruyere Cheese

Directions

1. Preheat oven to 425°F. Prepare a 9-inch glass pie pan by greasing with butter (about 1/2 Tbsp; use remaining to grease pan in step 4). Set aside. A metal pan can be used; turn oven down to 400°F.
2. Cook bacon in a pan over medium-high heat until crisp, drain on paper towels, allow to cool, then chop. Place in a small bowl and add cheese, coconut flour, thyme, salt, and pepper. Set aside.
3. Thinly slice turnips into rounds using a mandoline. Arrange slices beginning in the center and working out to the edges so that they overlap slightly. Sprinkle 1/4 of the bacon mixture and drizzle with the remaining 11/2 tablespoons butter. Repeat three times with remaining turnips and bacon mixture ending with a layer of turnips.
4. Lightly butter the bottom of another pie pan, fill pan with pie weights and set it on top of the final layer of turnips. Bake on a sheet pan (to catch any drippings) for 55 minutes or until the edges turn golden brown. Remove top pie pan and continue to cook another 10-12 minutes until the top is browned. Serve immediately by loosening the edges and flipping onto a serving platter. Cut into 12 equal pie-wedge servings.

Lemon Chicken and Shrimp Kabobs

Servings: 2 | *Prep:* 20 m | *Style:* American | *Cook:* 40 m

Ingredients

- 1 fruit (2-1/8" dia) Lemon
- 1 1/2 tbsps Lemon Peel
- 2 cloves Garlic
- 1/2 medium (2-1/2" dia) Onions
- 6 oz Brown Mushrooms (Crimini Italian)
- 8 oz raw Chicken Breast
- 8 medium Shrimps
- 3 1/2 Cherry Tomatoes
- 1/4 tsp Crushed Red Pepper Flakes
- 2 tbsps Olive Oil
- 1/4 tsp Salt

Directions

You will need wooden or metal skewers for this recipe. You will also need 2 lemons. The marinade is not fully eaten so the recipe ingredients only show 1 lemon. You will need both for the marinade.

1. Preheat oven to 375ºF. Soak the wooden skewers in warm water for 30 minutes. Zest the lemons into a medium bowl. Juice both lemons into the bowl, discarding any seeds. Finely chop the garlic and add to the bowl.
2. Peel and cut the red onion in half. Cut only HALF of the onion into 1-inch chunks; set aside. Remove the stems from the mushroom caps and discard. Set the caps aside. To the lemon and lemon zest, stir in ½ cup of olive oil, ¼ teaspoon of salt, 1 teaspoon of pepper and the red chili flakes; set aside ¼ cup of the marinade for step 4.
3. Pat dry the chicken breast with paper towels and cut into 2-inch pieces; set aside. Pat dry the shrimp and set aside. Place the chicken and the shrimp in the zip lock bag. Pour in the larger portion of the marinade and seal the bag tightly, pressing out any air. Refrigerate for 20 minutes.
4. Thread the chicken, shrimp, onion, mushrooms, and cherry tomatoes alternately onto the skewers, dividing all the ingredients equally. Discard the marinade in the bag, and lightly brush the skewers with the reserved ¼ cup of marinade.
5. Place the skewers on a sheet pan lined with foil and place in the oven and bake for 12 to 14 minutes until chicken is cooked through and vegetables are tender.
6. Serve the skewers on two plates, or remove the ingredients from the skewers and divide all of the ingredients evenly. Enjoy!

Lemon-Thyme Halibut with Sautéed Green Beans

Servings: 4 | *Prep:* 10 m | *Style:* American | *Cook:* 15 m

Ingredients

- 2 tbsps Olive Oil
- 1 fl oz Lemon Juice
- 1 clove Garlic
- 1 tsp leaf Dried Thyme Leaves
- 1 1/4 lbs Atlantic and Pacific Halibut
- 16 oz Green String Beans
- 2 tsps Lemon Peel
- 4 tbsps Butter

Directions

1. For fish: Sprinkle fish with salt, pepper then make a paste with 1 Tbsp lemon juice, minced garlic and thyme. Heat 1 Tbsp oil in a large nonstick skillet over medium-high heat.
2. Cook fish until just cooked through, about 4 minutes per side. Transfer to a plate, add remaining lemon juice, and cover to keep warm.
3. Sauté green beans in the same skillet with the remaining 1 Tbsp oil and 2 tsp lemon zest. Season with salt and freshly ground black pepper and cook until tender-crisp; about 5 minutes. Serve with the halibut topped with 1 Tbsp butter.

Maple Mustard Glazed Salmon and Asparagus

Servings: 2 | *Style:* American | *Cook:* 35 m

Ingredients

- 12 oz Asparagus
- 1 clove Garlic
- 1/8 cup Sugar Free Syrup

- 1/2 oz Dijon Mustard
- 12 oz boneless Salmon
- 1 oz Shallots
- 1 tbsp Vegetable Oil
- 1/4 tsp Salt

Directions

1. Preheat oven to broil. Prepare the sheet pan by lining it with foil and lightly coating it with 1 teaspoon of canola oil; hold.
2. Trim asparagus by snapping the thicker bottom ends where they break naturally; set aside. Finely chop the garlic clove; set aside.
3. In a small sauce pot over medium heat, combine the sugar-free maple syrup, ¼ cup of water, the Dijon mustard and garlic. Add a pinch of salt and bring to a simmer until liquid is reduced by about half. When the glaze has reduced, remove from heat and let cool.
4. Pat dry the salmon fillets with paper towels. Place the salmon on one half of the sheet pan and place the asparagus and shallots on the other half. Sprinkle the asparagus and shallots with 1 tablespoon canola oil and sprinkle with ¼ teaspoon of salt. Roast for 5 minutes.
5. Remove from oven and brush the salmon fillets with the maple-mustard glaze and broil until just cooked through, about 4 more minutes.
6. Divide the asparagus between two plates. Place the salmon next to the asparagus and enjoy!

Mashed Autumn Vegetables with Bacon and Scallions

*Servings: 8 | **Prep:** 12 m | **Style:** American | **Cook:** 20 m*

Ingredients

- 1 1/2 lbs Turnips
- 16 oz, raw, yields Baked Sweetpotato (Peel Eaten)
- 4 medium slice (yield after cooking) Bacon
- 1 tbsp Unsalted Butter Stick
- 1/8 tsp Cinnamon
- 1/8 tsp Salt
- 1/4 tsp Black Pepper
- 2 small (3" long) Scallions or Spring Onions

Directions

1. Put turnips and sweet potatoes in a large saucepan fitted with steamer basket with just enough water to clear the bottom of the basket. Cover and bring to a boil over high heat. Reduce heat to medium-low and steam vegetables until very tender, 10 12 minutes.
2. Meanwhile, cook bacon in a medium skillet over medium heat until crisp. Drain on paper towels and coarsely crumble. Reserve drippings.
3. Drain vegetables and return to saucepan. Beat with an electric mixer or mash with a potato masher until fairly smooth. Add butter and bacon drippings. Stir in cinnamon, salt and pepper.
4. Spoon into a serving dish and top with scallions and bacon.

Mediterranean Swordfish Steaks

Servings: 4 | Prep: 35 m | Style: American | Cook: 10 m

Ingredients

- 1/4 cup Extra Virgin Olive Oil
- 1 fl oz Fresh Lemon Juice
- 1 tsp leaf Oregano
- 1/2 tsp Lemon Peel
- 1/2 tsp Rosemary (Dried)
- 1/2 tsp Salt
- 1/2 tsp Black Pepper
- 1 1/2 lbs Swordfish

Directions

1. Zest the lemon and then juice it reserving 2 tablespoons juice. Mix olive oil, lemon juice, oregano, lemon zest, rosemary, salt and pepper in a resealable plastic bag. Add swordfish steaks; toss to coat. Marinate at room temperature 30 minutes, turning occasionally.
2. Prepare a medium grill. Remove steaks from the marinade (discard marinade) and cook about 5 minutes per side for medium doneness.

Mixed Greens Cooked with Tomatoes and Ginger

*Servings: 6 | **Prep:** 10 m | **Style:** American | **Cook:** 15 m*

Ingredients

- 1/2 tsp Garlic
- 2 medium whole (2-3/5" dia) Red Tomatoes
- 3 tsps Ginger
- 32 1/16 cups Spring Mix Salad
- 1 small Onion
- 1/8 tsp Salt
- 1/8 tsp Black Pepper
- 3 tbsps Unsalted Butter Stick

Directions

1. For the mixed greens you can use 2 pounds total of the following: arugula, chard, collard, dandelion, mustard, sorrel and turnips. For collard, mustard and turnip greens, you need to blanch them after chopping for the best flavor.
2. In a large saucepan over medium heat, melt butter. Add onion; cook 5 minutes, until softened. Add garlic and cook 1 minute more.
3. Add tomatoes and ginger and cook 5 minutes, stirring occasionally. Stir in greens. Mix well, cover and cook 5 minutes, until wilted. Season with salt and pepper to taste.

Pork Tenderloin Medallions with Mustard Sauce

*Servings: 2 | **Style:** American | **Cook:** 45 m*

Ingredients

- 1 clove Garlic
- 1/4 oz Dill
- 12 oz Green String Beans
- 1 cube Chicken Stock Cubes (Dry, Dehydrated)
- 14 oz Pork Loin (Tenderloin)
- 1 tbsp Unsalted Butter Stick
- 1/4 cup Sour Cream
- 2 tsps Olive Oil

- 4 tsps Country Dijon Mustard
- 1/2 tsp Salt
- 1/2 tsp Black Pepper

Directions

1. Finely chop the garlic clove; set aside. Remove the dill leaves from the stems and roughly chop the leaves; set aside. Remove the ends from the green beans and discard the ends; set the beans aside. Combine the chicken stock concentrate and ¾ cup water in a small bowl; set aside. Pat dry the pork tenderloin with paper towels. Cut the pork into ½-inch slices.
2. Heat the butter in a large sauté pan over medium-high heat until foam subsides. Add the pork medallions and sauté until browned, about 1 minute per side. Transfer the pork to a plate and cover with foil to keep warm.
3. Add the garlic to the pan and sauté until fragrant, about 10 seconds. Stir in the chicken stock, scraping up any browned bits from the bottom of the pan. Reduce the heat to medium and simmer for 2 to 3 minutes to reduce slightly.
4. Remove the pan from heat and mix in the sour cream, Dijon, dill and ¼ teaspoon each of salt and pepper. Return the pork to the pan along with any juices that have accumulated and reheat over medium heat for 2 to 3 minutes. Cover and keep warm for plating.
5. Heat 2 teaspoons of olive oil a medium sauté pan over high heat. When the oil is hot, add the green beans, season with ¼ teaspoon each of salt and pepper and cook until they are slightly charred, about 5 minutes.
6. Divide the green beans between two plates. Arrange the pork medallions next to the green beans and spoon the sauce over the pork. Enjoy!

Red Snapper with Tomatoes and Olives

Servings: 2 | Style: American | Cook: 35 m

Ingredients

- 12 olives Pitted Kalamata Olives
- 3 1/2 Cherry Tomatoes
- 1 clove Garlic
- 1/2 medium (2-1/2" dia) Onions
- 2/3 tbsp drained Capers
- 2 tbsps Red Cooking Wine

- 1/8 tsp Crushed Red Pepper Flakes
- 1 1/2 tsps Unsalted Butter Stick
- 12 oz Snapper (Fish) (Mixed Species)
- 1/4 tsp Salt
- 1 tbsp Olive Oil
- 1/4 tsp Black Pepper

Directions

1. Cut the Kalamata olives in half lengthwise; set aside. Cut the cherry tomatoes in half; set aside. Finely chop the garlic cloves; set aside. Peel the onion cut only HALF of the onion into ¼-inch diced pieces; set aside.
2. Heat 1 tablespoon olive oil in a large sauté pan over medium-high heat. When the oil is hot, add the onion and the olives. Cook, stirring occasionally, 3 minutes, or until the onion is translucent.
3. Add the tomatoes, capers, garlic, red cooking wine and the red chili flakes. Bring the mixture to a boil and reduce the heat to medium. Cover and simmer for 5 minutes.
4. Meanwhile, pat dry the red snapper with paper towels. Season each fillet with ¼ teaspoon each of salt and pepper. Heat another large sauté pan with the butter over medium-high heat. Add the fillets and cook for 2 minutes on each side until lightly browned.
5. Transfer the fish to the tomato mixture, cover again and cook for 3 to 4 minutes, just until the fish is cooked through.
6. Place a red snapper fillet on each of two plates. Spoon the tomato mixture over the fish and enjoy.

Red, White and Blue Coleslaw

Servings: 12 | Prep: 75 m | Style: American

Ingredients

- 3/4 tbsp Real Mayonnaise
- 1/4 cup Sour Cream (Cultured)
- 1 cup crumbled Blue or Roquefort Cheese
- 1 1/3 tbsps Red Wine Vinegar
- 1/2 tsp Garlic
- 1 1/2 tsps Salt
- 1/4 tsp Sucralose Based Sweetener (Sugar Substitute)
- 1/2 cup chopped Cabbage

- 1/2 head medium (about 5" dia) Red Cabbage

Directions

1. Combine mayonnaise, sour cream, blue cheese, vinegar, garlic, salt, and sugar substitute in a large bowl. Add green and red cabbage and toss well.
2. Cover and chill at least 1 hour before serving. (Can be made ahead. Store in an airtight container and refrigerate up to 24 hours.)

Roasted Asparagus and Red Peppers with Dijon and Thyme

Servings: 4 | Prep: 5 m | Style: American | Cook: 15 m

Ingredients

- 16 spear medium (5-1/4" to 7" long) Asparagus
- 2 tbsps Unsalted Butter Stick
- 2 tbsps chopped Shallots
- 6 tsps Dijon Mustard
- 1 fl oz Fresh Lemon Juice
- 2 tbsps Extra Virgin Olive Oil
- 3 tsps Thyme
- 2 tsps Lemon Peel
- 1 large (2-1/4 per lb, approx 3-3/4" long, 3" dia) Sweet Red Peppers

Directions

1. Heat oven to 425°F. Cut the bell pepper in half, remove seeds and then slice into 1/2-inch thick strips. Place pepper strips and asparagus on a rimmed sheet pan covered with aluminum foil; set aside.
2. Sauté shallot in butter in a small saucepan over medium heat until translucent, about 3 minutes. Transfer to a small bowl; add mustard, lemon juice, oil, thyme and lemon zest; whisk the dressing together.
3. Brush asparagus and red peppers with the dressing; set remainder aside. Roast vegetables in oven for 10-15 minutes, until asparagus is tender.
4. Drizzle with remaining sauce, season with salt and black pepper to taste, and serve right away.

Roasted Brussels Sprouts and Onions with Siracha Cream

*Servings: 10 | **Prep:** 5 m | **Style:** American | **Cook:** 20 m*

Ingredients

- 1 lb Brussels Sprouts
- 1 medium Red Onion
- 2 tbsps Olive Oil
- 1/4 cup Real Mayonnaise
- 1 tsp Sriracha Hot Chili Sauce

Directions

1. Preheat oven to 425°F. Trim Brussels sprouts. Cut onion into 1/4-inch wedges.
2. Place sprouts and onions on a sheet pan. Toss with olive oil and season with salt and freshly ground black pepper. Cook for 15-20 minutes until sprouts are tender and onions are translucent. Place into a serving bowl.
3. In a small bowl, stir the mayonnaise and siracha until incorporated. Place sauce in mircrowave for 30 seconds, stir in 1/2-1 tsp water to thin it then drizzle it over the Brussels sprouts and onions. Serve immediately. 1 serving is about 3 whole sprouts with some onion pieces.

Rosemary Turkey Burger Over Baby Kale Salad

*Servings: 4 | **Prep:** 10 m | **Style:** American | **Cook:** 10 m*

Ingredients

- 20 oz Ground Turkey
- 2 tbsps Heavy Cream
- 2 tbsps Rosemary
- 1 tbsp Black Pepper
- 1 tsp Salt
- 2 cups chopped Kale
- 6 cups shredded Cos or Romaine Lettuce
- 4 oz Feta Cheese

- 4 oz hulled (142 seeds) Dried Pumpkin and Squash Seed Kernels
- 1 lemon yield Lemon Juice
- 1 clove Garlic
- 1/2 cup Real Mayonnaise
- 1/2 cup Olive Oil
- 1/4 cup (8 fl oz) Water

Directions

1. Preheat a medium non-stick skillet with a small amount of oil. Combine the turkey and cream and form into 4 equal patties. Combine the rosemary, pepper and salt in a small bowl then sprinkle all side of the burgers. Press seasonings into the patty then pan fry until cooked through. They also taste great grilled.
2. Prepare salad and dressing while meat is cooking. For the salad: combine the kale (pull it off of the rib and slice it thin or chop it), Romaine lettuce (slice it thin), feta and pepitas. Plate equally on four plates and set aside to make the dressing. For the dressing: place the lemon juice and 1 tsp of lemon zest, garlic, mayonnaise, olive oil and water in a blender. Blend until smooth then season to taste with salt and freshly ground black pepper. Drizzle onto the four salads then serve the burger on top.

Rosemary-Roasted Sweet Potatoes

Servings: 12 | Prep: 10 m | Style: American | Cook: 30 m

Ingredients

- 2 lbs Sweet Potato
- 2 tbsps Canola Vegetable Oil
- 1 tbsp Rosemary
- 1/2 tsp Cumin
- 1 tsp Salt
- 1/8 tsp Red or Cayenne Pepper

Directions

1. Heat oven to 425ºF. Place oven racks in the upper third and lower third of oven. Lightly oil 2 rimmed baking sheets. Cut potatoes 1/4-1/2 inch spears.

2. Combine potato spears, oil, rosemary, ground cumin, salt and cayenne in a large bowl; toss well to coat. Arrange potatoes in a single layer on baking sheets.
3. Roast potatoes, rotating pans and tossing potatoes every 10 minutes, until lightly golden and tender, about 30 minutes.

Sausage and Peppers

Servings: 8 | Style: Italian

Ingredients

- 12 link (4 oz, raw, yield after cooking) Italian Sausage
- 20 medium (approx 2-3/4" long, 2-1/2" dia) Bell Peppers
- 2 large Onions
- 1 clove Garlic
- 1/4 cup Canola Vegetable Oil

Directions

1. Preheat oven to 400°F. In a roasting pan, place all 24 links of sausage in pan with 1/4 cup water and 2 tbsp vegetable oil and cover with aluminum foil. Cook for 30 minutes. Remove foil, turn sausages over and recover. Cook another 25 minutes.
2. While the sausage is cooking, cut up the peppers and onions into 3-4" squares and place in a large frying pan with 2 tbsp vegetable oil over medium-high heat. Add the garlic clove (thinly sliced), salt & pepper (to taste) and stir occasionally making sure they don't stick to the pan. Cook until onions and peppers are softened; up to 45 minutes.
3. When the sausage is done, remove foil, drain water and cook for another 12-15 minutes uncovered (to get brown) then flip them and do the same. When finished, leave out to cool.
4. When the peppers and onions are done, remove from heat and drain all juice from the pan.
5. After 20 minutes, cut all the sausage into pieces and add to the frying pan. Cook, stirring occasionally, on low heat for about another 20 minutes. Serve immediately. Leftovers freeze very well!

Sautéed Green and Yellow Squash with Fresh Mint

Servings: 4 | Prep: 10 m | Style: American | Cook: 5 m

Ingredients

- 2 tbsps Extra Virgin Olive Oil
- 1/2 tsp Garlic
- 2 1/2 oz Peppermint (Mint)
- 3 medium Zucchinis
- 1/8 tsp Crushed Red Pepper Flakes
- 1 small Red Onion
- 1 fl oz Fresh Lemon Juice

Directions

1. Cook garlic and onion with olive oil in a skillet over medium-low heat till softened.
2. Increase heat to medium-high and add zucchini, onion and red pepper flakes. Use salt and pepper to taste. Cook an additional 5 minutes.
3. Drizzle with lemon juice and add mint.

Sautéed Okra

Servings: 1 | Prep: 5 m | Style: American | Cook: 5 m

Ingredients

- 1 cup Okra
- 1 tbsp Extra Virgin Olive Oil

Directions

1. Add oil to a skillet over medium-high heat. Add okra and sauté until tender, about 5 7 minutes.
2. Season to taste with salt and freshly ground black pepper.

Scrambled Eggs with Turkey Sausage Topped with Smoked Gouda

Servings: 1 | Prep: 5 m | Style: American | Cook: 10 m

Ingredients

- 2 large Eggs
- 1 tbsp Heavy Cream
- 2 oz Turkey Sausage
- 1 oz Smoked Gouda

Directions

1. Heat a nonstick skillet over medium-high heat with a small amount of oil. Whisk the eggs with the heavy cream and set aside.
2. Cook the turkey sausage in the skillet breaking it up into bite sized pieces with a spatula until it is cooked through, about 5 minutes. Pour the egg mixture over the top and continue to cook while stirring with the spatula until the eggs are set.
3. Place the egg and sausage on a serving plate, season with salt and freshly ground black pepper and then sprinkle the Gouda over the top allowing it to melt. Enjoy immediately.

Seared Lemon Chicken

Servings: 4 | Style: American | Cook: 15 m

Ingredients

- 32 oz raw Chicken Breast
- 1 oz Lemon Juice
- 1 clove Garlic
- 1 tsp Salt
- 1/2 tsp Black Pepper
- 1/4 cup Olive Oil

Directions

1. Use the zest from 2 whole lemons and the juice from one for this recipe to impart the most lemon flavor.
2. Combine all ingredients in a zip top plastic bag and marinate 3-12 hours (overnight is best).
3. Pan sear over medium high heat until browned and the juices run clear.

Sesame Broccoli, Red Pepper and Spinach

Servings: 6 | Prep: 10 m | Style: American | Cook: 10 m

Ingredients

- 1 tbsp Dried Whole Sesame Seeds
- 1 tsp Canola Vegetable Oil
- 3 cup flowerets Broccoli Flower Clusters
- 1 medium (approx 2-3/4" long, 2-1/2" dia) Red Sweet Pepper
- 1 clove Garlic
- 10 oz Baby Spinach
- 1 Jalapeno Pepper
- 1 tbsp Tamari Soybean Sauce
- 2/3 tbsp Toasted Sesame Oil

Directions

1. Toast sesame seeds in a large nonstick skillet over medium heat, stirring until golden brown and fragrant. Transfer to a small bowl.
2. Heat oil over medium heat in same skillet until hot. Add chopped broccoli and red pepper; cook until broccoli is crisp-tender, about 5 minutes. Add garlic, spinach, jalapeño, soy sauce, and sesame oil; mix well.
3. Cover and cook until spinach is wilted, about 2 minutes. Sprinkle with toasted sesame seeds.

Shanghai Bok Choy with Oyster Sauce

*Servings: 6 | **Prep:** 5 m | **Style:** American | **Cook:** 10 m*

Ingredients

- 23 oz Chinese Cabbage (Bok-Choy, Pak-Choi)
- 1 cup Chicken Broth, Bouillon or Consomme
- 3 tbsps Oyster Sauce
- 1 tsp Thick-It-Up

Directions

1. Cook bok choy in a large pan of lightly salted boiling water 5 minutes, until tender but still firm. Drain well.
2. In a small saucepan, bring broth and oyster sauce to a simmer. Stir in thickener; cook 2 minutes.
3. Add chili oil to taste; pour over bok choy. Toss gently to coat.

Slow Roasted Chicken with Cauliflower Bake

*Servings: 4 | **Prep:** 10 m | **Style:** American | **Cook:** 10 m*

Ingredients

- 32 oz with bone and skins Chicken Breast
- 3 cloves Garlic
- 1 tsp Thyme
- 2 tbsps Olive Oil
- 1 head medium (5-6" dia) Cauliflower
- 1 cup Tomato Sauce
- 1 cup shredded Mozzarella Cheese (Whole Milk)
- 1/4 tsp Crushed Red Pepper Flakes

Directions

1. Preheat oven to 300°F. Prepare a sheet pan with aluminum foil. Set aside.
2. Mince 1 clove of garlic and fresh thyme then blend together with olive oil, salt and freshly ground black pepper to make a paste. Coat the chicken

breasts with the paste then roast for one hour on the sheet pan. Allow to cook then remove the bone and slice.

3. While the chicken cooks, cut the cauliflower into pieces and boil or steam until tender; drain well and set aside.
4. Combine the tomato sauce, 2 minced garlic cloves, mozzarella cheese, chili pepper flakes, the chicken slices and the cauliflower to a baking dish. Bake for 40 minutes uncovered until hot and bubbly.

Slow Roasted Lemon-Rosemary Chicken with Asparagus

Servings: 4 | Prep: 5 m | Style: American | Cook: 60 m

Ingredients

- 24 oz with bone and skins Chicken Breast
- 2 cloves Garlic
- 1 tsp Rosemary
- 2 tbsps Olive Oil
- 32 spear large (7-1/4" to 8-1/2") Asparagus

Directions

1. Preheat oven to 300°F. Prepare a sheet pan with aluminum foil. Set aside.
2. Mince 1 clove of garlic and fresh minced rosemary then blend together with 1 Tbsp olive oil, salt and freshly ground black pepper to make a paste. Coat the chicken breasts with the paste then roast for one hour on the sheet pan.
3. While the chicken cooks, prepare the asparagus by cutting off the hard/root end. Toss with the remaining 1 Tbsp olive oil and minced remaining clove of garlic, season with salt and freshly ground black pepper. During the last 15 minutes the chicken cooks add the asparagus to the same pan and continue to bake until the chicken is no longer pink in the center and the juices run clear. Remove the bone from the chicken before serving.

Southwestern Cornbread

Servings: 12 | Prep: 15 m | Style: American | Cook: 25 m

Ingredients

- 1/3 cup Heavy Cream
- 8 oz Whole Grain Soy Flour
- 1/3 cup Canola Vegetable Oil
- 1/2 cup Tap Water
- 1 tsp Baking Powder (Straight Phosphate, Double Acting)
- 1/8 cup White Bolted Self-Rising Cornmeal (Enriched)
- 2 large Eggs (Whole)
- 1/2 small Red Onion
- 1/2 cup Cilantro (Coriander)

Directions

1. Heat oven to 350°F. Grease an 8-inch square baking pan; set aside.
2. Combine soy flour, corn meal, baking powder, cilantro, onion and 1 tsp lime zest (optional) together in a large bowl.
3. Whisk in the water, oil, heavy cream and eggs; mix with a wooden spoon until smooth. Pour into prepared pan.
4. Bake until bread is set and a toothpick inserted in center comes out clean, about 25 minutes. Cool in pan on a wire rack. Cut into 12 squares.
5. Serve warm or at room temperature.

Spaghetti Squash Surprise

Servings: 8 | Style: American

Ingredients

- 1 squash yield Cooked Spaghetti Squash
- 3 tbsps Unsalted Butter Stick
- 2/3 cup sliced Onions
- 1 tsp Crushed Red Pepper Flakes
- 1/4 tsp Garlic Salt
- 1/3 cup Sour Cream
- 1 cup shredded Cheddar Cheese

Directions

1. You will need 1 medium whole spaghetti squash for this recipe.
2. Cut the spaghetti squash in half and remove seeds. Place in covered dish with ¼ inch of water. Microwave 10-12 min. Set aside to cool.
3. In a medium-sized skillet over medium heat melt the butter and add the onions, red pepper flakes, garlic salt and black pepper (to taste). Cook until the onions are browned and softened.
4. Using a fork, scrape the insides of the squash and transfer to a small bowl. Mix the squash, cooked onions, sour cream, and half the cheese together until fully combined. Transfer the mixture to a buttered baking dish and top with the remaining cheese. Bake at 375°F for 20-25 minutes. (Broil for the last minute to brown the top, if desired). You can also place the mixture back into the spaghetti squash shells and bake it!

Spicy Collards and Okra

Servings: *8* | **Prep:** *20 m* | **Style:** *American* | **Cook:** *30 m*

Ingredients

- 2 lbs Collards
- 3 tbsps Light Olive Oil
- 2 tsps Garlic
- 1/2 tsp Crushed Red Pepper Flakes
- 1/4 lb Okra
- 1 1/2 cups Chicken Broth, Bouillon or Consomme
- 1/2 tsp Salt

Directions

1. Bring a large stockpot filled two-thirds with water to a boil; add collards and cook 2 minutes. Drain.
2. Heat oil in 12 skillet over medium heat. Add garlic and pepper; cook 1 minute, until garlic is golden. Add okra and cook 4 to 5 minutes more. Add broth and collards to skillet and bring to a simmer.
3. Cook 20 minutes, turning collards occasionally, until tender. Stir in salt.

Spicy Shrimp Diablo

*Servings: 2 | **Style:** Mexican | **Cook:** 45 m*

Ingredients

- 2 oz Brown Mushrooms (Crimini Italian)
- 1/2 medium (2-1/2" dia) Onions
- 1 stalk medium (7-1/2" - 8" long) Celery
- 1/2 medium (approx 2-3/4" long, 2-1/2" dia) Bell Peppers
- 1/2 Jalapeno Peppers
- 1/4 oz Thyme
- 1/4 oz Basil
- 1/2 fruit (2-1/8" dia) Lemon
- 1 clove Garlic
- 1 tbsp Unsalted Butter Stick
- 1/2 cup Diced Canned Tomatoes
- 12 large Shrimps
- 1/4 cup Heavy Cream
- 2 oz Baby Spinach
- 1/2 tsp Salt
- 1/2 tsp Black Pepper

Directions

1. Remove the stems from the mushrooms and discard. Cut the mushrooms into ¼-inch slices; set aside. Peel the onion and cut into¼-diced pieces; set aside. Cut the celery into ¼-inch diced pieces; set aside.
2. Remove the stems, pith and seeds from the green bell pepper and the jalapeño. Cut each pepper into ¼-inch diced pieces and set each aside separately.
3. Remove the thyme and basil leaves from the stems and discard the stems. Finely chop the thyme leaves; set aside. Rough chop the leaves and set aside. Juice the lemon into a small bowl, discarding any seeds; set aside. Cut the garlic cloves into slices; set aside. Pat dry the shrimp with paper towels and set aside for step 5.
4. Melt the butter in a large sauté pan over medium-high heat. Add the onion, celery, and green bell pepper. Sauté until soft, about 4 minutes. Add the garlic and sauté until fragrant, about 30 seconds. Add only HALF can of diced tomatoes, the mushrooms and ¼ cup of water. Reduce the heat to medium and simmer until the sauce thickens slightly, about 5 minutes.

5. Add ¼ cup of whipping cream, the shrimp, lemon juice and only HALF of the jalapeño, to the pan and cover. Simmer until the shrimp turn pink, about 4 minutes. Stir in the basil, thyme, baby spinach and ¼ teaspoon each of salt and pepper.
6. Divide the shrimp Diablo between two bowls and enjoy.

Spinach with Pine Nuts and Garlic

*Servings: 4 | **Prep:** 5 m | **Style:** Other | **Cook:** 5 m*

Ingredients

- 1/4 cup Dried Pine Nuts
- 3 tbsps Extra Virgin Olive Oil
- 1 tsp Garlic
- 18 cups Baby Spinach
- 1/4 tsp Salt
- 1/4 tsp Black Pepper

Directions

1. Gently toast nuts in a dry sauté pan until they start to brown. Set aside.
2. In a very large pan, heat olive oil and garlic over medium heat until garlic sizzles and starts to turn golden (do not allow garlic to brown).
3. Add pine nuts and one third of the spinach; sauté until spinach wilts. Add remaining spinach in batches, seasoning with salt and pepper as it cooks.
4. Serve with lemon wedges (if desired, add 1g NC per wedge per serving added).

Spinach, Swiss Chard and Cheese Bake

*Servings: 8 | **Prep:** 10 m | **Style:** American | **Cook:** 40 m*

Ingredients

- 3 10 oz packages Frozen Chopped Spinach

- 20 oz Swiss Chard
- 3 large Eggs (Whole)
- 1 cup Sour Cream (Cultured)
- 1/8 tsp Nutmeg (Ground)
- 1/2 tsp Salt
- 1/4 tsp Black Pepper
- 6 oz Cheddar Cheese

Directions

1. If you can't find frozen Swiss chard, replace it with additional frozen spinach.
2. Defrost spinach and Swiss chard; pour off excess water and squeeze dry.
3. Preheat oven to 350°F.
4. In a large bowl, mix spinach, chard, eggs, sour cream and nutmeg; season well with salt and pepper.
5. Transfer to a shallow buttered baking dish. Using a spatula, even out the mixture; top with cheese.
6. Bake 40 minutes until bubbly and browned on top. Serve immediately or at room temperature.

Steak au Poivre

Servings: 2 | Prep: 10 m | Style: French | Cook: 10 m

Ingredients

- 2 tsps Whole Black Peppercorns
- 14 oz Beef Top Sirloin (Lean Only, Trimmed to 1/8" Fat, Choice Grade)
- 2 tbsps Light Olive Oil
- 6 oz Mushrooms
- 1 oz Shallots
- 1/2 cup Heavy Cream
- 1 tbsp Unsweetened Ketchup
- 1/2 fl oz (no ice) Brandy
- 1 tbsp Parsley

Directions

Green peppercorns are used instead of black peppercorns in this recipe. Purchase them brined in a jar for the best flavor and consistency. You will need 2 tablespoons drained from the brine.

1. Spread peppercorns on a work surface and press onto both sides of the steaks in an even layer.
2. Heat oil in a large, heavy skillet over medium-high heat until very hot. Cook steaks 5 minutes per side for medium-rare. Remove steaks from the skillet and keep warm.
3. To the same skillet add the mushrooms and shallots. Cook over medium-high heat 3-5 minutes and season with salt and freshly ground black pepper. Add cream, ketchup, brandy, and up to 1/2 tsp additional salt to skillet. Bring to a boil, stirring, loosening any browned bits from bottom of skillet.
4. Lower heat and simmer the sauce for 2 minutes until slightly thickened. Pour sauce over steaks, sprinkle with fresh minced parsley and serve immediately.

Steamed Brussels Sprouts with Browned Butter and Lemon Zest

Servings: 2 | Prep: 10 m | Style: Other | Cook: 15 m

Ingredients

- 1/4 lb Brussels Sprouts
- 1/4 cup Unsalted Butter Stick
- 1/2 tsp Salt
- 1 fruit without seed Lemons (with Peel)

Directions

1. In a medium cooking pot with a tight-fitting lid, set a steamer basket over 1 1/2 water. Add Brussels sprouts, and steam over high heat until tender, about 10 minutes.
2. Melt butter in a large skillet over medium-high heat. Add salt and cook, watching carefully, until butter sizzles, browns slightly, and gives off a nutty aroma.
3. Zest the entire lemon (about 1 tablespoon) then squeeze juice from lemon halves into the pan and add the zest.
4. Stir in Brussels sprouts; cook, shaking pan occasionally, until warmed through.

Swiss Chard with Garlic Butter

*Servings: 8 | **Prep**: 15 m | **Style**: Other | **Cook**: 15 m*

Ingredients

- 2 lbs Swiss Chard
- 2 tbsps Unsalted Butter Stick
- 1 tbsp Light Olive Oil
- 2 tsps Garlic
- 1/2 tsp Salt
- 1/4 tsp Black Pepper

Directions

1. Cut chard stems crosswise into 1/2-inch pieces. Cut leaves in half lengthwise, stack them and cut crosswise into 2-inch pieces.
2. Heat butter and olive oil in a large saucepan over medium heat. Add garlic and cook, stirring, until just fragrant, about 30 seconds. Add chard stems; cover and cook, stirring occasionally, until crisp-tender, about 4 minutes.
3. Add chard leaves in batches, tossing to coat; season with salt and pepper. Cover and cook, stirring once, until stems are tender and leaves are wilted, 4 to 5 minutes.

Tabbouleh Salad

*Servings: 6 | **Prep**: 25 m | **Style**: American | **Cook**: m*

Ingredients

- 1/2 cup, dry, yield Bulgur
- 1 cup Tap Water
- 2 plums Red Tomatoes
- 3/4 cup Parsley
- 1 cucumber (8-1/4") Cucumber (with Peel)
- 8 tbsps Peppermint (Mint)

- 1/4 cup Extra Virgin Olive Oil
- 3 large Scallions or Spring Onions
- 1/4 cup Fresh Lemon Juice
- 1 tsp Salt
- 1/2 tsp Black Pepper

Directions

1. Combine bulgur and water in a large heatproof bowl; cover tightly with plastic wrap and let stand until water is absorbed, about 15 minutes.
2. Line a sieve with cheesecloth or a dish towel, place bulgur in it, and press firmly with your hands to remove any excess water.
3. Add tomatoes, cucumber, parsley, mint, lemon juice, oil, scallions, salt, and pepper; toss gently to combine. Serve cold or at room temperature.

Texas Barbecued Beef Brisket

*Servings: 8 | **Prep:** 390 m | **Style:** American | **Cook:** 180 m*

Ingredients

- 2 tbsps Extra Virgin Olive Oil
- 2 tbsps Black Pepper
- 1 tbsp Chili Powder
- 1/2 tsp Cumin
- 1 tbsp Yellow Mustard Seed
- 3 cloves Garlic
- 1/2 tsp Coriander Leaf (Dried)
- 2 tsps Paprika
- 1 tsp Dry Mustard
- 8 oz Beef Brisket (Flat Half, Lean Only, Trimmed to Trimmed to 1/8" Fat, Cooked, Braised)
- 4 1/2 oz Light Beer
- 1 serving Chili-Barbecue Sauce

Directions

Use the Atkins recipe to make Chili-Barbecue Sauce for this recipe.

1. In a small bowl, combine the olive oil, pepper, chili powder, cumin, 1 tablespoon mustard seeds (or coarse grained prepared mustard), garlic (minced), coriander, paprika and 1 teaspoon dry mustard. Mix well to form a thick paste.
2. Place brisket in a shallow dish. Rub paste on both sides of brisket. Cover with plastic wrap, and marinate in the refrigerator for at least 6 hours or overnight.
3. Heat grill to medium-high, following manufacturers instructions for indirect cooking (stacking coals on both sides of grill, if using charcoal).
4. Place brisket, fat side up, on a wire rack in a large disposable aluminum baking pan. Place in center of grill. Cover, and cook until tender and an instant-read meat thermometer inserted in center registers 180°F, 2 1/2 to 3 hours.
5. Turn brisket every 1/2 hour, and baste with 3 tablespoons low-carb beer every 45 minutes. Remove from grill, tent with aluminum foil, and let stand for 15 minutes before cutting.
6. Thinly slice brisket across the grain. Serve with 1/4 cup Chili-Barbecue Sauce per serving.

Alternate directions for the oven:

1. Season the brisket as directed in the instructions. The longer it is marinated the better – so overnight works great too.
2. Once seasoned, wrap in tin foil with the fat side up. Seal at the top as tightly as possible. Place on a roasting pan or something to catch any juices that may seep out. You will need these for step 3.
3. Cook at 300°F for 45 minutes per pound. Once done remove any excess fat (if you prefer not to eat it) and then slice the meat against the grain and place the pieces in a baking dish (helpful to line with tinfoil for easy cleaning). Pour about ½ cup of the drippings from the pan over the top along with the Chili-Barbecue sauce. Bake for another hour; cover the top with tinfoil. Once baked, turn oven to lowest setting to keep warm until ready to serve.

Thai Basil Chicken Stir Fry

Servings: 2 | Style: Asian | Cook: 45 m

Ingredients

- 1 medium (4-1/8" long) Young Green Onions
- 1/4 oz Basil
- 1 clove Garlic

- 12 oz raw Chicken Breast
- 1/2 tbsp Fish Sauce
- 1 tbsp Organic Tamari
- 1 tsp Sucralose Based Sweetener (Sugar Substitute)
- 1/4 tsp Crushed Red Pepper Flakes
- 1 medium (approx 2-3/4" long, 2-1/2" dia) Bell Peppers
- 6 oz Broccoli
- 2 1/3 tbsps Vegetable Oil

Directions

1. Preheat oven to 400º. Cut the green onion into ¼-inch pieces on a bias; set aside. Remove the basil leaves from the stems and roughly chop the basil; set aside. Finely chop the garlic; set aside. Remove the stem, pith and seeds from the red bell pepper and discard. Cut the bell pepper into ½-inch pieces; set aside.
2. Pat dry the chicken breasts with paper towels and cut into ¼-inch strips. In a medium bowl, combine the fish sauce, tamari sauce, 2 tablespoons of water and 1 teaspoon of Splenda; stir to combine. Remove HALF of the marinade from the bowl and reserve for step 5. Add the chicken to the medium bowl and cover with plastic wrap. Let the chicken marinate in the refrigerator for ready to use.
3. Heat 2 tablespoons of peanut oil/ canola oil in a large non-stick sauté pan over medium-high heat. When the oil is hot (but not smoking) add the green onions and stir-fry for 30 seconds, until softened. Add the garlic and red chili flakes and stir-fry for 10 more seconds.
4. Remove the chicken from the marinade and discard marinade. Add to the onion mixture and stir-fry until the chicken is almost cooked through, about 3 minutes. Remove from heat and place on a plate. Coat the same pan with 1 teaspoon of peanut oil/ canola oil; set over medium-high heat. When hot, add the red bell peppers and broccoli. Cook, stirring occasionally, until broccoli is crisp-tender about 5 to 7 minutes.
5. Meanwhile, bring the marinade to a boil in a small saucepot over high heat. Boil for 1 minute, then reduce the heat to low and simmer for 2 more minutes. Set aside Return the chicken mixture to the pan with the vegetables and gently fold in the marinade. Remove from heat and stir in HALF of the basil.
6. Divide the stir-fry between two bowls, garnish with the remaining basil and enjoy!

Turkey and Roasted Zucchini Lasagna

Servings: 6 | Prep: 30 m | Style: Italian | Cook: 75 m

Ingredients

- 6 medium Zucchinis
- 8 oz Turkey Sausage
- 8 oz Ground Turkey
- 1 small Onion
- 6 cloves Garlic
- 3 cups Crushed Tomatoes
- 16 tbsps Mascarpone Cheese
- 10 leaves Basil
- 1 large Egg (Whole)
- 1 cup shredded Mozzarella Cheese (Whole Milk)

Directions

This dish is best served the following day to allow the flavors to blend and the lasagna to settle.

1. Preheat an oven to 350°F. Prepare a square baking pan with aluminum foil and spray with oil; set aside.
2. Slice the zucchini thin (with a knife or mandoline). Spray with a little oil then roast on a sheet pan in the oven for 15-20 minutes until browned but not crispy. When done set aside to cool.
3. Sauté the meats with chopped onion and 4 minced garlic cloves in a large skillet until browned. Add the crushed tomatoes and cook for additional 40 minutes on low and let cool.
4. Puree the mascarpone, basil leaves, 2 cloves of garlic, a dash of salt and egg in a food processor until smooth; set aside.
5. Layer the zucchini, meat sauce then mascarpone two times. Top with cheese and bake for one hour covered with aluminum foil. Remove the foil and bake an additional 15 minutes. Serve immediately or allow it to fully cool and then place in the refrigerator overnight and pull out and slice into 6 servings.

Turkey Meatloaf with Cauliflower Mash

Servings: 4 | Prep: 15 m | Style: American | Cook: 60 m

Ingredients

- 2 tbsps Olive Oil
- 1/2 cup chopped Onions
- 1/2 cup chopped Green Peppers
- 2 cloves Garlic
- 2 stalk medium (7-1/2" - 8" long) Celery
- 1 tsp ground Thyme (Dried)
- 1 tsp Salt
- 1/2 tsp Black Pepper
- 1/2 cup Tomato Sauce
- 12 oz Ground Turkey
- 8 oz Turkey Sausage
- 1 large Egg (Whole)
- 3 cups Cauliflower

Directions

- Preheat oven to 325°F. Use a loaf pan with a meatloaf insert or prepare a sheet pan with aluminum foil. Set aside.
- Heat a non-stick skillet with oil over medium high heat. Mince the onion and garlic, chop the green pepper and the celery then sauté them with the thyme; seasoning with salt and freshly ground black pepper until softened. Set aside to cool slightly.
- Mix together the cooled vegetable mixture with the tomato sauce, ground turkey, turkey sausage and egg until thoroughly combined.
- Bake for 1 hour or until the juices run clear and it is cooked through.
- While it is baking, make the cauliflower mash by boiling the cauliflower for 10 minutes (or until very soft) in salted water. Mash with a fork and season with salt and freshly ground black pepper. Keep warm until ready to serve with the meatloaf.

Chapter 5: Snacks Recipes

***

Atkins Garlic Toast Crisps

Servings: 20 | *Prep:* 10 m | *Style:* American | *Cook:* 60 m

Ingredients

- 1/4 cup Extra Virgin Olive Oil
- 1 oz Garlic
- 2 cups Whole Grain Soy Flour
- 3 tsps Baking Powder (Straight Phosphate, Double Acting)
- 2 large Eggs (Whole)
- 1/2 tsp Salt
- 1/2 can or bottle (16 fl oz) Club Soda
- 6 servings All Purpose Low-Carb Baking Mix

Directions

Use the Atkins recipe to make All Purpose Low-Carb Baking Mix for this recipe. Have these crispy crackers with olive tapenade or guacamole.

1. Heat oven to 350°F. Lightly coat an 8-inch by 4-inch loaf pan with olive oil spray.
2. Place olive oil and garlic in a small microwave-safe cup and microwave on high until garlic turns golden, about 1 minute. (Or cook in a small saucepan over medium-high heat, for 4 to 5 minutes, stirring occasionally.) Set aside.
3. In a large mixing bowl, combine baking mix (2 cups), baking powder and salt and blend well. Add club soda, eggs and 1 tablespoon of the garlic oil. Mix by hand or with an electric mixer until just combined.
4. Transfer dough to prepared pan, smooth top and bake 45 minutes, until a tester inserted into the center comes out clean.
5. Transfer loaf to a wire rack to cool for 20 minutes. Meanwhile, increase oven temperature to 400°F.
6. When loaf has cooled, using a serrated knife, cut loaf into 20 thin slices. Place them on an ungreased baking sheet and brush with the remaining garlic oil, turning to coat both sides.
7. Bake until golden and crisp, about 14 minutes.

Atkins Peanut Butter Granola Bar Parfait with Yogurt and Strawberries

*Servings: 1 | **Prep:** 5 m | **Style:** American*

Ingredients

- 1/2 cup Greek Yogurt - Plain (Container)
- 1 serving Atkins Meal Peanut Butter Granola Bar
- 5 large (1-3/8" dia) Strawberries

Directions

1. In a parfait glass, layer the granola bar (chopped) with the yogurt and strawberries.

Avocado Salsa

*Servings: 4 | **Prep:** 10 m | **Style:** Mexican*

Ingredients

- 1 small whole (2-2/5" dia) Red Tomato
- 1/8 cup Cilantro (Coriander)
- 1 small Red Onion
- 1/2 Jalapeno Peppers
- 1 California Avocado
- 2 tbsps Fresh Lime Juice
- 1/8 tsp Salt
- 1/8 tsp Black Pepper

Directions

Wear rubber gloves when handling chile peppers and be careful not to touch your eyes. Remove the seeds to keep the "fire" under control. Serve with simple chicken, fish or shellfish dishes or as a dip.

1. Chop the tomato and cilantro, set aside. Finely dice the onion and jalapeno.
2. Remove the avocado from the skin, chop it and place it in a serving bowl. Add the onion, jalapeño and lime juice to the avocado and gently combine; do not mash.
3. Fold in tomato and chopped cilantro and season with salt and pepper.
4. Cover and refrigerate until ready to serve.

Bagna Cauda

Servings: 8 | Prep: 5 m | Style: Italian | Cook: 5 m

Ingredients

- 1/2 cup Extra Virgin Olive Oil
- 1/4 cup Unsalted Butter Stick
- 3 tsps Garlic
- 8 anchovies Anchovy (Drained Solids In Oil, Canned)

Directions

1. In a small saucepan, heat olive oil and butter over medium heat.
2. Add garlic and anchovies. Cook gently for 5 minutes, until garlic is fragrant (but not brown).
3. Add pepper to taste. Transfer to a hot pot or heated dish and serve with vegetables.

Baked Brie with Sun-Dried Tomatoes and Pine Nuts

Servings: 6 | Prep: 5 m | Style: American | Cook: 10 m

Ingredients

- 8 oz Brie Cheese
- 1 tbsp chopped Sun-Dried Tomato
- 1 tbsp Parsley

- 1/2 oz Dried Pine Nuts

Directions

1. Heat oven to 450°F.
2. With a sharp knife, trim white rind off top of cheese. Place cheese in a pie plate.
3. Mix chopped sun-dried tomatoes and parsley, spread evenly over surface of cheese, sprinkle with pine nuts and bake 10 minutes until heated through.

Baked Eggplant Puree

Servings: 8 | Prep: 15 m | Style: Other | Cook: 40 m

Ingredients

- 1 lb Eggplant
- 3/4 cup Extra Virgin Olive Oil
- 2 tsps Garlic
- 1 tbsp Parsley
- 1/8 tsp Salt
- 1/8 tsp Black Pepper

Directions

1. Preheat oven to 425°F.
2. Cut the eggplant on all sides with deep slashes and place in a baking pan. Roast until soft, 30 to 40 minutes. Set aside until cool enough to handle, about 15 minutes.
3. Peel eggplant and coarsely chop (or briefly pulse in a food processor or blender)and place in a medium bowl. Mix in oil, garlic and parsley. Salt and pepper to taste.

Black Olives with Cheddar

Servings: 1 | Prep: 5 m | Style: American

Ingredients

- 7 greek olives Black Olives
- 1 slice (1 oz) Cheddar Cheese

Directions

1. Dice the cheese and place into hole in the olive.
2. Pop into your mouth and enjoy!

Blackberry-Peach Compote

Servings: *12* | **Prep:** *10 m* | **Style:** *American* | **Cook:** *20 m*

Ingredients

- 4 fl ozs Sauvignon Blanc Wine
- 2 tbsps Xylitol
- 1 tsp Ginger
- 1 tsp Cinnamon
- 3 medium (2-1/2" dia) (approx 4 per lb) Peaches
- 6 oz Blackberries
- 1/2 tsp Thick-It-Up

Directions

This sauce is delicious over lemon ice cream or pancakes.

1. Combine the wine, granular sugar substitute, ginger, ground cinnamon and peaches in a medium sauce pan. Bring to a boil then reduce heat to low and simmer for about 15 minutes until very tender. Add the blackberries and Thick-It-Up; continue to simmer for another 5 minutes.
2. Take off heat and cool to room temperature or serve warm. Maybe be refrigerated for up to 1 week. Makes 3 cups; 1 serving = 1/4 cup.

Blue Cheese Dip

Servings: 16 | *Prep:* 10 m | *Style:* American

Ingredients

- 1 tbsp Red Wine Vinegar
- 1 1/2 tsps Thyme
- 1 cup Sour Cream (Cultured)
- 2/3 cup Real Mayonnaise
- 4 oz Blue or Roquefort Cheese

Directions

1. Whisk together the vinegar, thyme, sour cream and mayonnaise.
2. Add the blue cheese and season with salt and freshly ground black pepper.
3. Serve immediately with assorted fresh vegetables. Can be made 2 days ahead, cover and keep refrigerated.

Blue-Cheese Ghosts

Servings: 8 | *Prep:* 10 m | *Style:* American

Ingredients

- 8 oz Cream Cheese
- 2 oz Blue or Roquefort Cheese
- 1/4 cup Sour Cream (Cultured)
- 1/4 tsp Black Pepper
- 1 Black Olives

Directions

1. Line two 1-cup molds with plastic wrap.
2. Mix cream cheese and blue cheese in a bowl until blended. Stir in sour cream and pepper. Divide between molds, cover with plastic wrap, and refrigerate for at least 2 hours.

3. Unmold ghosts onto plates, then carefully remove plastic wrap.
4. Cut olive into thin slices, and place on ghosts faces for eyes, or finely chop and sprinkle over molds.
5. Serve with fresh blanched vegetables such as broccoli, asparagus, celery (do not blanch), bell pepper slices and cherry tomatoes.

Buffalo Chicken Egg Salad

Servings: 8 | Prep: 20 m | Style: American | Cook: 10 m

Ingredients

- 6 large Boiled Eggs
- 6 oz boneless, cooked Chicken Thigh
- 3 tbsps Real Mayonnaise
- 1 1/2 tbsps Red Hot Buffalo Wing Sauce
- 1/4 cup crumbled Blue or Roquefort Cheese
- 8 stalk medium (7-1/2" - 8" long) Celery

Directions

Be sure to use a Buffalo hot sauce that has only a few ingredients including red pepper, vinegar and salt; 0g NC per serving.

1. Hard boil the eggs: cover 6 eggs with water, bring to a boil, remove from heat and allow to sit for 10 minutes. Immediately plunge eggs into an ice water bath, allow to cool then peel and dice. Reserve in a medium bowl.
2. While eggs are cooking cook chicken over medium heat in a skillet or on the grill until the juices run clear and the meat is no longer pink in the center. Cool and dice; add to the eggs in the bowl.
3. To the bowl with the diced eggs and chicken add the mayonnaise, Buffalo hot sauce and blue cheese. Mix to combine and blend flavors. Add salt and pepper to taste. Serve with celery stalks for dipping or carefully fill celery stalks. Drizzle with additional Buffalo hot sauce as a garnish or if more heat is desired.

Caesar Salad Dressing

Servings: 4 | Prep: 5 m | Style: Mediterranean / Greek | Cook: m

Ingredients

- 1/4 cup Real Mayonnaise
- 3 tbsps Parmesan Cheese (Grated)
- 1 tbsp Anchovy Paste
- 1 tbsp Fresh Lemon Juice
- 1 tsp Garlic
- 2 tsps Extra Virgin Olive Oil
- 1 tsp Worcestershire Sauce
- 1 tsp Dijon Mustard
- 1/2 tsp Black Pepper
- 1/4 tsp Tabasco Sauce

Directions

This is the classic dressing for a Caesar salad made with Romaine, but it enlivens any salad greens. For a real treat, make this dressing with homemade mayonnaise. See the Atkins recipe: Mayonnaise. Each serving is 2 Tbsp.

1. Combine mayonnaise, cheese, anchovies (or 2 Tbsp paste), lemon juice, garlic, olive oil, Worcestershire sauce, mustard, pepper and hot sauce in a small bowl.
2. Use immediately or refrigerate in an airtight container for up to 2 days.

Caprese Salad

Servings: *1 |* **Prep:** *10 m |* **Style:** *Italian*

Ingredients

- 5 Cherry Tomatoes
- 2 oz Fresh Mozzarella
- 1 tbsp Extra Virgin Olive Oil
- 1 tbsp Basil

Directions

1. Slice tomatoes and mozzarella.
2. Drizzle with olive oil.
3. Julienne the fresh chopped basil leaves and sprinkle on top. Serve immediately.

Carrot-Nut Muffins

Servings: 12 | Prep: 10 m | Style: Other | Cook: 25 m

Ingredients

- 1 cup Whole Grain Soy Flour
- 1 cup Blanched Almond Flour
- 1 1/4 cups Sucralose Based Sweetener (Sugar Substitute)
- 2 tsps Cinnamon
- 1/2 tsp Salt
- 1/2 tsp Baking Powder (Straight Phosphate, Double Acting)
- 1 cup Canola Vegetable Oil
- 4 large Eggs (Whole)
- 1 cup grated Carrots
- 2 tsps Vanilla Extract
- 1/3 second spray Original Canola Cooking Spray

Directions

1. Preheat oven to 350°F. Grease one 12-cup muffin tin; set aside.
2. In a large bowl whisk together soy flour, ground almonds, 1 1/2 cups sugar substitute, cinnamon, salt and baking powder.
3. In a medium bowl, whisk vegetable oil, eggs, carrot, and vanilla extract. Pour carrot mixture into soy mixture. Mix until just combined. Divide batter in muffin tins.
4. Bake 20-25 minutes until golden brown, and a cake tester inserted in centers comes out clean. Cool on wire rack

Cattle Ranch Beef Spread

*Servings: 12 | **Prep:** 60 m | **Style:** American*

Ingredients

- 3 oz Beef Jerky
- 8 oz Cream Cheese
- 1/2 cup Sour Cream (Cultured)
- 2 medium (4-1/8" long) Scallions or Spring Onions
- 1/8 cup chopped Green Sweet Pepper
- 1/2 tbsp Worcestershire Sauce

Directions

1. Mix beef, cream cheese, sour cream, green onions, green pepper and Worcestershire sauce. Add black pepper to taste.
2. Let stand 1 hour for flavors to blend. Serving size is 2 Tbsp.
3. Serving suggetion: Serve 1-2 tablespoons in the cavity of a celery stalk (don't forget to add in the extra Net Carbs; 1 stalk celery = 1g NC)

Cauliflower Fritters

*Servings: 12 | **Prep:** 15 m | **Style:** American | **Cook:** 10 m*

Ingredients

- 1/2 head medium (5-6" dia) Cauliflower
- 1/3 cup Total 2% Greek Yogurt
- 1/2 tsp Baking Powder (Sodium Aluminum Sulfate, Double Acting)
- 1/4 tsp Salt
- 1/4 tsp White Pepper
- 1/4 tsp Cumin
- 1/4 tsp Coriander Seed
- 1/8 tsp Nutmeg (Ground)
- 3 large Egg Whites
- 1 tbsp Olive Oil
- 2 tbsps Organic High Fiber Coconut Flour

Directions

1. Boil salted water in a medium pot. Add cauliflower and cook 3 minutes. Drain water and dry on a kitchen towel until cool enough to touch then puree in a food processor until finely chopped.
2. Add the yogurt to the food processor along with the coconut flour, baking powder, salt, pepper, cumin, coriander and nutmeg. Process 1-2 times until combined.
3. Add the egg whites to the bowl of a stand mixer or use a handheld mixer to whip the egg whites (and 1/8 tsp lemon juice or cider vinegar) to stiff peaks. Fold egg whites into cauliflower mixture in 3 additions.
4. Place a non-stick skillet over medium-high heat and heat the oil until it shimmers. Drop cauliflower mixture by tablespoonfuls onto the skillet; space about 1 inch apart for best results. Cook for 1-2 minutes on each side until puffed and golden. Serve warm or cold. 1 serving is 1 fritter. Makes 12 fritters.

Cheddar and Scallion Pie Squares

Servings: 24 | *Prep*: 45 m | *Style*: American | *Cook*: 47 m

Ingredients

- 4 oz Vital Wheat Gluten
- 1/4 cup dry Whole Grain Soy Flour
- 1 large Egg Yolk
- 3/4 tsp Salt
- 1/2 cup Unsalted Butter Stick
- 8 large Eggs (Whole)
- 1/2 tsp Tap Water
- 3/4 cup Heavy Cream
- 1/4 tsp Black Pepper
- 1/4 tsp Tabasco Sauce
- 3 cups shredded Cheddar Cheese
- 1 cup shredded Fontina Cheese
- 6 medium (4-1/8" long) Scallions or Spring Onions
- 1/2 cup 100% Stone Ground Whole Wheat Pastry Flour

Directions

1. FOR CRUST: Combine pastry flour, gluten, soy flour, 1/4 teasponn salt, and butter in a food processor. Pulse until mixture is the texture of coarse meal. Add egg yolk and water; continue pulsing until dough begins to come together. Turn onto a sheet of wide plastic wrap, form into a square and cover with another sheet of plastic. Flatten to a 40-inch by 8-inch rectangle. Freeze for 10 minutes.
2. Roll dough between the plastic wrap to an 8 ½- by 12 1/2-inch rectangle (to facilitate rolling, occasionally remove plastic and dust each side with ½ teaspoon of wheat gluten). Remove top sheet of plastic. Invert pastry into a 9-inch by 13-inch buttered baking pan. Press to fill bottom of pan. Remove the remaining plastic. Freeze dough for 10 minutes.
3. Heat oven to 375ºF. Line the dough with foil and a layer of dried beans or pie weights. Bake 10 minutes. Remove beans and foil. Bake until golden brown, an additional 5 to 6 minutes. Cool on a wire rack 10 minutes. (May be made up to 1 day in advance)
4. FOR FILLING: Heat oven to 350ºF. Combine eggs, cream, 1/2 teaspoon salt, pepper, and hot pepper sauce in a bowl; mix well. Stir in cheddar cheese, fontina cheese, and scallions. Pour mixture into baked crust and smooth with spatula.
5. Bake until filling is set and lightly browned, about 35 minutes. Remove from oven. Cool 5 minutes, then cut into 24 squares. Serve warm or at room temperature.
6. Makes 24 squares. Nutritional information is for 1 square.

Cheese Straws

Servings: 13 | ***Prep:*** *150 m* | ***Style****: American* | ***Cook:*** *12 m*

Ingredients

- 6 tbsps Unsalted Butter Stick
- 1/2 tsp Garlic Powder
- 3/4 cup shredded Cheddar Cheese
- 1/4 cup Parmesan Cheese (Grated)
- 2 large Eggs (Whole)
- 1/8 tsp Garlic Salt
- 3 servings All Purpose Low-Carb Baking Mix

Directions

Use the Atkins recipe to make All Purpose Low-Carb Baking Mix for this recipe. You will need 1 cup = 3 servings (1/3 cup each).

1. Preheat oven to 375°F.
2. Place baking mix, butter, and garlic powder in a food processor. Process until mixture resembles coarse crumbs. Add cheeses and eggs. Pulse just until dough comes together.
3. Transfer dough onto a large piece of plastic wrap. Lightly form into a flat round.Place second piece of wrap over dough. Press or roll dough to a 6 x 12 rectangle, about 1/2 thick. Refrigerate until very firm, at least 2 hours (or overnight).
4. Place dough horizontally on countertop. Remove top sheet of plastic from dough. Sprinkle with garlic salt; gently press into dough. With a sharp knife cut dough into forty 6-inch long strips.Transfer strips to an ungreased baking sheet. Bake 12-15 minutes, until lightly browned. Slide straws onto a cooling rack. When cool, store in an airtight container. 3 sticks equals one serving.

Chile Roasted Macadamia Nuts

Servings: 6 | Prep: 5 m | Style: Other | Cook: 20 m

Ingredients

- 2 cup whole or halveds Macadamia Nuts
- 1 tsp Canola Vegetable Oil
- 1 1/2 tsps Chili Powder
- 1 tsp Salt

Directions

1. Heat oven to 300°F.
2. Toss nuts with oil, spread on a sheet pan and bake 25 minutes, until golden.
3. Transfer to a bowl; toss nuts with chili powder and salt.

Chipotle Chicken Bites with Creamy Blue Cheese Dip

Servings: 4 | Style: American

Ingredients

- 1 /4 cup Organic High Fiber Coconut Flour
- 2 tbsps Chili Powder
- 1/2 tsp Garlic Powder
- 1/2 tsp Onion Powder
- 1 dash Salt
- 2 tbsps Olive Oil
- 32 oz raw Chicken Breast
- 1/2 cup Sour Cream
- 1/4 cup Real Mayonnaise
- 1/4 fl oz Lemon Juice
- 1 tsp Dill (Dried)
- 1/3 tbsp Chives (Freeze Dried)
- 1/2 tsp Garlic Powder
- 1/2 tsp Black Pepper
- 1/4 cup crumbled, not packed Blue Cheese

Directions

For this recipe use chipotle powder in place of the chili powder.

1. Preheat oven to 400°F.
2. Combine first 5 ingredients (coconut flour through salt) in medium mixing bowl. Cut chicken breast into cubes and toss to coat with the coconut flour mixture.
3. Heat oil over medium heat in a large cast iron or oven proof skillet. Add the chicken cubes and brown for 4 minutes, turn over and place skillet in preheated oven. Bake for 5 minutes or until cooked through.
4. Skewer and serve with Creamy Blue Cheese Dipping Sauce.

For the Creamy Blue Cheese Dipping Sauce:

1. Whisk the sour cream, mayonnaise, lemon juice, dill, chives, garlic powder, and black pepper together until fluffy.
2. Stir in blue cheese.

Chocolate Ganache Macarons

*Servings: 20 | **Prep:** 15 m | **Style:** French | **Cook:** 40 m*

Ingredients

- 3 large Egg Whites
- 1 tsp Fresh Lemon Juice
- 3/4 cup Almond Meal Flour
- 2 tbsps Xylitol
- 6 oz Sugar Free Chocolate Chips
- 2 tbsps Heavy Cream

Directions

This recipe is suitable for all phases except for the first two weeks of Induction due to the nuts. Please measure the granulated xylitol first for this recipe and then powder in a blender before use.

1. Preheat oven to 250°F. Prepare a silicon baking mat or parchement paper on a baking sheet. Drawing 1-inch circles on the backside of the parchment can be helpful. Set aside.
2. Using a stand mixer with the whip attachment, whip the egg whites, lemon juice, a pinch of salt and 1 tablespoon of the xylitol until stiff peaks form.
3. Sift together the remaining 1 tablespoon xylitol and almond flour. Add to the egg whites and gently fold in to fully incorporate. Using a piping bag or simply cut the end of a large zippered plastic bag, fill with the meringue and pipe onto the baking sheet making 1-inch rounds. Tap the tops with a slightly wet finger if tips remain. Bake for 35-45 minutes. If they begin to brown, decrease temperature by 25 degrees and bake a little longer. Remove from oven and allow to cool down. Once cooled remove with a spatula and set on a fresh piece of parchment paper.
4. Make Filling: melt chocolate in the microwave at 30 second intervals. Add heavy cream and using a handheld blender; whip until thick. Using a small piping bag, pipe chocolate onto the flat side of 1 macaron then top with the another on the flat side sandwiching together. Sprinkle with a little cocoa powder as a garnish if desired. 1 Macaron = 1 serving.

Chocolate-Cinnamon Smoothie

Servings: 1 | Style: American

Ingredients

- 1 cup Coconut Milk Unsweetened
- 1/2 oz Chocolate Whey Protein
- 1/4 tsp Cinnamon
- 3 ice cubes (3/4 fl oz) Water
- 1 tsp Cocoa Powder (Unsweetened)
- 1/2 packet Sweetener (Splenda Packets, Sucralose)

Directions

1. Combine all ingredients in a blender and blend until smooth. This recipe can also be heated after blending (omit the ice). Do not allow it to boil; may be heated in the microwave at 30 second intervals until warm but not hot. Makes a terrific late night slightly sweet snack.

Cranberry-Ginger Loaf

Servings: 20 | Prep: 5 m | Style: American | Cook: 30 m

Ingredients

- 1/3 second spray Original Canola Cooking Spray
- 1 1/4 cups Whole Grain Soy Flour
- 3 tsps Baking Powder (Straight Phosphate, Double Acting)
- 1/2 cup shelled (50 halves) English Walnuts
- 1/4 tsp Salt
- 2 large Egg Whites
- 1/2 cup Unsalted Butter Stick
- 2/3 cup Sucralose Based Sweetener (Sugar Substitute)
- 2 tbsps Sour Cream (Cultured)
- 1 tbsp Ginger
- 1 tsp Vanilla Extract
- 1 cup whole Cranberries
- 2 large Eggs (Whole)

Directions

1. Preheat over to 350°F. Toast walnuts in an even layer on a cookie sheet for 8 minutes. Cool, place walnuts in food processor until finely ground.
2. Grease a 9x5x3 inch loaf pan with oil spray.
3. In a large bowl, combine soy flour, baking soda, walnuts and salt. In a medium bowl, with an electric mixer on medium, beat butter and sugar substitute until fluffy, about 3 minutes. Add eggs, sour cream, ginger and vanilla and beat until well-combined, about 1 minutes. Fold in cranberries. Fold in bake mix mixture. Set aside.
4. In another medium bowl, beat whites until stiff, but not dry, peaks form. Gently fold whites into batter until just combined. Spoon batter into prepared pan and bake 40 to 45 minutes until a toothpick inserted in the center comes out clean.
5. Cool in pan on wire rack for 10 minutes before removing. Cook loaf on wire rack for at least 30 minutes before slicing.

Creamy Crab Dip

Servings: 6 | Prep: 10 m | Style: American

Ingredients

- 1/4 cup Real Mayonnaise
- 2 medium (4-1/8" long) Scallions or Spring Onions
- 1/4 cup Sour Cream (Cultured)
- 1 tsp Old Bay Seasoning
- 6 oz Blue Crab (Canned)
- 1 tsp Fresh Lemon Juice
- 1/2 small (5 per pound) Red Sweet Pepper
- 1/8 tsp Salt
- 1/8 tsp Black Pepper

Directions

1. In a medium bowl, mix mayonnaise, sour cream, seasoning and lemon juice until smooth.
2. Add crab, chopped green onions and pepper; stir until ingredients are well combined.
3. Season to taste with salt and pepper. Serve with vegetables for dipping.

Creamy Italian Dressing

Servings*: 10 | ****Prep:*** *15 m | ****Style:*** *American*

Ingredients

- 1/2 cup Real Mayonnaise
- 5 1/3 tbsps White Wine Vinegar
- 6 tsps Xylitol
- 1/4 cup Parmesan Cheese (Grated)
- 1/2 tsp Garlic
- 2 tsps Italian Seasoning
- 1/4 tsp Crushed Red Pepper Flakes
- 1/4 tsp Salt
- 1/4 tsp Black Pepper
- 2 tbsps Parsley

Directions

If you don't have Italian seasoning on hand, use a combination of basil, oregano and parsley instead. Xylitol crystals are available in natural foods stores and the baking department of most well-stocked supermarkets. Each serving is 2 Tbsp.

1. Whisk mayonnaise, vinegar and 2 tablespoons xylitol in a medium bowl. Stir in Parmesan, garlic, Italian seasoning, pepper flakes, salt, pepper and parsley until well blended. Let stand for 5 minutes.
2. Use immediately or refrigerate in an airtight container for up to 3 days. Stir before using.

Creamy Sun-Dried Tomato and Goat Cheese Dip

Servings*: 16 | ****Prep:*** *10 m | ****Style:*** *American*

Ingredients

- 4 oz Cream Cheese
- 4 oz Goat Cheese (Soft)
- 1/3 cup Sour Cream (Cultured)

- 3/4 cup Sun-Dried Tomatoes
- 3 oz Roasted Bell Peppers
- 1/4 cup chopped Onions
- 2 Jalapeno Peppers
- 1/2 tsp Garlic
- 1/8 cup Cilantro (Coriander)

Directions

1. Blend the softened cream cheese, goat cheese and sour cream until thoroughly incorporated. Add the diced sun-dried tomatoes, red peppers, yellow onion, jalapenos, garlic and cilantro; blend to combine.
2. Season with salt and freshly ground black pepper. Refrigerate for 8 hours or up to 1 day and serve with fresh vegetables. Will keep refrigerated in an airtight container for up to 1 week. Makes 2 cups; serving size is about 2 tablespoons per person.

Crockpot Reuben Dip

Servings: 8 | **Prep:** 10 m | **Style:** American | **Cook:** 10 m

Ingredients

- 4 oz Cream Cheese
- 1/2 cup Sour Cream (Cultured)
- 1/3 tbsp Horseradish Sauce
- 3 tsps Original Stone Ground Mustard
- 2 tbsps Unsweetened Ketchup
- 4 oz Corned Beef Brisket (Cured)
- 1/2 cup shredded Swiss Cheese
- 1/2 cup Sauerkraut (Solid and Liquids, Canned)

Directions

1. Shred swiss cheese. Drain sauerkraut.
2. In a small saucepan blend the softened cream cheese, sour cream, mustard, horseradish and unsweetened ketchup until combined. Add the corned beef, siwss cheese and sauerkraut. Mix to distribute all ingredients.
3. Cook over medium heat until the cheese melts and it is warmed through. Place into a 2-cup capacity small crockpot to stay warm about 10 minutes

before serving. Alternatively it may be placed in an oven proof bowl and heated at 350°F for 30 minutes. Serve immediately. Serve with celery stalks or other vegetables.

Crunchy Almond Pretzels

Servings: 6 | Prep: 10 m | Style: American | Cook: 30 m

Ingredients

- 1 1/2 tsps Bakers Yeast (Active Dry)
- 2 tbsps Tap Water
- 1 1/2 cups Blanched Almond Flour
- 1/8 tsp Salt
- 3/4 tsp Baking Powder (Straight Phosphate, Double Acting)
- 1/4 tsp Guar Gum
- 1/4 tsp Crushed Red Pepper Flakes
- 1/4 tsp Black Pepper
- 1/4 tsp White Pepper
- 1 large Egg (Whole)
- 1/4 tsp Baking Soda
- 1 large Egg White
- 1 tsp Coarse Kosher Salt

Directions

1. Preheat oven to 350°F. Combine the yeast with 1 tablespoon warm water in a small bowl. Set aside and allow to foam.
2. In a medium bowl combine the almond flour, baking powder, 1/8 tsp salt, guar gum, crushed red pepper, black pepper, white pepper and a pinch of stevia (optional) Mix to combine.
3. Whisk the whole egg into the yeast and water mixture then blend into the flour mixture with a fork until thoroughly combined forming a stiff dough; divide into 6 portions. Use a small amount of oil on your hands, pick up a portion of pretzel dough and begin to roll into a 10-inch snake. Form pretzel shapes or into a round for each piece of dough. The dough may crack or break; use a little water and your fingers to press it back into shape.
4. Set each finished pretzel onto a piece of greased parchment paper. Whisk together the egg white, 1 tablespoon of water and 1/4 teaspoon baking soda. Brush egg wash over pretzels then sprinkle coarse salt over the tops.

Bake for 30 minutes rotating pan halfway through. Allow to cool for 20 minutes before eating with your favorite mustard or party dip.

Cucumber Guacamole

*Servings: 4 | **Prep**: 10 m | **Style**: Mexican*

Ingredients

- 1/4 cucumber (8-1/4") Cucumber (with Peel)
- 1 Jalapeno Pepper
- 1/16 cup chopped Red Onions
- 1/2 tsp Garlic
- 1/4 cup Cilantro (Coriander)
- 1 California Avocado
- 1 tbsp Fresh Lime Juice
- 1/2 tsp Chili Powder

Directions

1. Dice the cucumber into 1/4-inch pieces, remove the seeds and gills from the jalepno and finley dice, finely dice the red onion, mince the garlic and chop the cilantro; set all aside.
2. Mash the avocado in a bowl with a fork. Add the lime juice, chili powder, and salt and freshly ground black pepper to taste.
3. Add the cucumber, jalpeno, onion, garlic and cilantro. Mix to combine and adjust seasonings to your taste.

Cucumber, Onion and Tomato Salad with Creamy Feta Dressing

*Servings: 4 | **Prep**: 105 m | **Style**: Mediterranean / Greek*

Ingredients

- 3 cup slices Cucumber (with Peel)
- 1/4 medium Red Onion

- 1 large whole (3" dia) Red Tomato
- 2 oz Pitted Kalamata Olives
- 1/4 cup crumbled Feta Cheese
- 4 tbsps Peppermint (Mint)
- 6 tbsps Extra Virgin Olive Oil
- 2 tbsps White Wine Vinegar
- 1 tsp Sucralose Based Sweetener (Sugar Substitute)

Directions
1. Combine the cucumbers, onions, tomatoes and olives in a large bowl. Set aside.
2. Combine the feta cheese, mint, olive oil, vinegar and sugar substitute in a blender and blend until thoroughly combined. If the dressing is too thick add a little water till desired consistency. Season dressing with salt and freshly ground black pepper.
3. Arrange salad on 4 serving plates and pour dressing on top. Serve immediately

Cucumbers and Hummus

Servings: 1 | Prep: 5 m | Style: American

Ingredients
- 1 cup slice Cucumber (with Peel)
- 4 tbsps Organic Hummus Classic

Directions
1. Slice cucumber and dip slices in hummus.

French Dressing

Servings: 10 | Prep: 10 m | Style: American

Ingredients

- 1/2 cup Canola Vegetable Oil
- 1/4 cup Vinegar (Cider)
- 1/2 tsp Salt
- 1/4 tsp Garlic Powder
- 1 tbsp Xylitol
- 1/2 cup Unsweetened Ketchup
- 1/8 tsp Red or Cayenne Pepper

Directions

Despite its name, this is a classic American salad dressing. Its sweet-tart flavor is ideal with crisp pieces of iceberg lettuce and wedges of sweet ripe tomatoes. If you don't have garlic powder, crush one garlic clove with the flat side of a chef's knife and add it to the dressing; remove and discard the garlic before serving or storing. Light olive oil may also be substituted for the canola oil. Each serving is 2 Tbsp.

1. Whisk together ketchup, oil, vinegar, salt, garlic powder, xylitol and cayenne pepper in a medium bowl.
2. Use immediately or refrigerate in an airtight container for up to 3 days.

Garlic Ranch Dressing

Servings: 10 | Prep: 20 m | Style: American

Ingredients

- 3/4 cup Real Mayonnaise
- 1/2 cup Buttermilk (Reduced Fat, Cultured)
- 3/4 tsp Onion Powder
- 2 tbsps Parsley
- 1/2 tsp Garlic
- 1 tsp Dijon Mustard
- 1/8 tsp Salt
- 1/8 tsp Black Pepper
- 1 tsp Fresh Lemon Juice

Directions

1. Combine all ingredients in a blender; puree until smooth. Season to taste with salt and freshly ground black pepper. Makes: 10 servings, 2 tablespoons per serving.

Garlicky White Bean Dip

Servings: *8* | ***Prep:*** *5 m* | ***Style:*** *American*

Ingredients

- 1 tbsp Extra Virgin Olive Oil
- 2 cloves Garlic
- 1 tsp Rosemary
- 2 cups Cannellini Beans
- 1/2 tsp Salt
- 1/8 tsp Black Pepper

Directions

1. Heat oil in a small skillet over medium heat. Add garlic (minced) and rosemary; sauté until aromatic, about 1 minute. Add beans, salt, and pepper; cook to heat through, about 3 minutes.
2. Transfer mixture to a food processor; puree with reserved beans. Serve, or refrigerate in an airtight container for up to 3 days.

Ginger, Soy and Sesame Dipping Sauce

Servings: *10* | ***Prep:*** *5 m* | ***Style:*** *American*

Ingredients

- 4 tbsps Tamari Soybean Sauce
- 1/4 cup Chicken Broth, Bouillon or Consomme
- 2 tbsps Sesame Oil
- 2 tbsps Sodium and Sugar Free Rice Vinegar

- 2 tsps Sucralose Based Sweetener (Sugar Substitute)
- 1 tsp Ginger
- 1/2 tsp Garlic

Directions

1. In a small bowl, whisk together soy sauce, chicken broth, sesame oil, vinegar, sugar substitute, ginger, and garlic cloves.

Goblin Eyes

Servings: 6 | Prep: 120 m | Style: American | Cook: 20 m

Ingredients

- 6 large Eggs (Whole)
- 1/4 cup Real Mayonnaise
- 1/2 tsp Wasabi Paste in Tubes
- 2 Black Olives
- 1/2 tsp Pimento (Canned)

Directions

1. Bring the eggs covered with 1 inch of water to a boil over medium-high heat. Once the water boils, take it off the heat and begin timing the eggs for 12 minutes. After 12 minutes, transfer the eggs to a bowl with cold water. Allow the eggs to cool until they are easy to handle.
2. Crack each egg all over but do not peel. Place in a 1 quart resealable plastic bag along with 1 cup of cold water, 1 teaspoon each of vinegar, red and blue food coloring or color of your choice. Seal bag and place in the refrigerator for 1-2 hours or overnight.
3. Remove the eggs from the dye and discard the dye and bag. Carefully peel eggs and cut each in half. Remove the yolks placing them in a small bowl and place each egg half on a serving platter. Mash the yolks with mayonnaise, wasabi paste (if using; alternate choices include 1 teaspoon of dry mustard or hot pepper sauce) and a few drops of green food coloring. Place this mixture in a piping bag or use a small sandwich bag with the corner clipped off. Pipe the mixture into the egg halves, top with a slice of olive and a piece of pimento (can also use chopped red bell pepper or tomato).

Green Goddess Dressing

Servings: 68 | Prep: 10 m | Style: American | Cook: 20 m

Ingredients

- 1/2 cup Real Mayonnaise
- 1/2 cup Sour Cream (Cultured)
- 1 tbsp White Wine Vinegar
- 1/4 cup Parsley
- 2 tbsps Chives
- 1 tbsp Tarragon
- 1/8 tsp Salt
- 1/8 tsp Black Pepper

Directions

1. The classic dressing can also be used as a sauce for fish and shellfish. For extra tang, add 1 tablespoon of anchovy paste.
2. Pulse mayonnaise, sour cream, vinegar, parsley, chopped chives, tarragon and optional anchovy paste, along with 2 tablespoons of water in a food processor or blender until smooth.
3. Add salt and freshly ground black pepper to taste. Use immediately or refrigerate for up to 1 day.

Guacamole

Servings: 8 | Prep: 105 m | Style: Mexican

Ingredients

- 3 large Scallions or Spring Onions
- 1 Jalapeno Pepper
- 1 medium whole (2-3/5" dia) Red Tomato
- 2 California Avocados
- 1/2 fl oz Fresh Lime Juice

- 1/8 cup Cilantro (Coriander)
- 1/8 tsp Salt

Directions

1. Dice the onions, pepper and tomato and place them in a medium bowl.
2. Slice avocados in half lengthwise, remove pits and scoop pulp into bowl with a spoon then mash with a fork.
3. Add the diced onions, pepper, and tomato mixing to combine and then mix in lime juice and cilantro. Add salt to taste.

Jerk Chicken Wings and Drummettes

*Servings: 8 | **Prep:** 10 m | **Style:** Other | **Cook:** 40 m*

Ingredients

- 40 oz, with bone cooked (yield after bone removed) Chicken Wing
- 2 tbsps Canola Vegetable Oil
- 1/2 tsp Cinnamon
- 1 tbsp Xylitol
- 1/2 packet Stevia
- 2 tsps Salt
- 3/4 tsp Black Pepper
- 1/2 tsp Ginger (Ground)
- 1/2 tsp Nutmeg (Ground)
- 1/2 tsp Garlic Powder
- 1 tsp ground Thyme (Dried)
- 1/2 tsp Onion Powder
- 1/2 tsp Paprika
- 1 tsp Allspice Ground
- 1/2 tsp Red or Cayenne Pepper

Directions

1. Preheat oven to 400°F. Combine all spice ingredients and set aside.
2. Place wings and drummettes in a gallon sized zip top bag with the oil, shake to distribute the oil over all pieces. Add the combined spices and shake to evenly coat.

3. Place chicken on a sheet pan and put into the oven for 30-40 minutes until cooked through and fragrant. Serve immediately with Sweet Ginger Chili Sauce (see Atkins recipe) if desired. Each 1 1/2 Tbsp serving of sauce = 1.7g NC additional.

Kale Chips

Servings: 6 | Prep: 5 m | Style: American | Cook: 30 m

Ingredients

- 7 oz Kale
- 1 tbsp Extra Virgin Olive Oil
- 1/8 dash Salt

Directions

Note: Purchase at least 13oz of kale (a large bunch). Once the stems are removed you will have about 7oz of leaves.

1. Preheat oven to 250°F and prepare two sheet pans with parchment paper.
2. Remove the leaves from the stems of the kale stalk by cutting away with kitchen shears or tearing. Tear leaves into bite sized pieces (it will shrink so pieces should be about 3-inches long otherwise you will end up with tiny pieces) then wash and thoroughly dry on a towel or in a salad spinner. Discard the stems.
3. Toss kale with olive oil by hand in a bowl then arrange equally spaced on the baking sheets and season with sea salt to your taste.
4. Place pan in the oven and set a timer for 30 minutes. After 20 minutes check to see if pieces are dried and crispy, if not continue to check at 5 minute intervals. Store in an airtight container up to 1 week.

Yummy flavors to try:

1. Cheesy: add 2 Tbsp finely grated Parmesan cheese along with the salt just before baking. Add 0.1g NC to the net carb count per serving.
2. Truffle: add flavored salts such as truffle salt. Or a drop or two of truffle oil can be added to the olive oil. This will not change the net carb count.
3. Chipotle: add a pinch of ground chipotle with the salt. This will not change the net carb count.

4. Wasabi: add 1/8 tsp ground wasabi powder with the salt. This will not change the net carb count.

King Crab Dip

*Servings: 8 | **Prep**: 60 m | **Style**: American*

Ingredients

- 2 oz Cream Cheese
- 2/3 tbsp Real Mayonnaise
- 2 tsps Fresh Lemon Juice
- 1/2 tsp Garlic Powder
- 3/4 cup Blue Crab (Canned)
- 2 medium (4-1/8" long) Scallions or Spring Onions
- 1/2 cup chopped Sweet Red Peppers
- 1 oz, raw, yield Green Sweet Pepper
- 3 tsps fresh Dill

Directions

1. Mix cream cheese, 2 tsp mayonnaise, lemon juice and garlic powder until smooth. Mix in crab meat, peppers, green onion and dill.
2. Add Tabasco to taste. Refrigerate 1 hour for flavors to blend.

Lemon Zest Tuna Salad

*Servings: 1 | **Prep**: 5 m | **Style**: American*

Ingredients

- 6 oz Tuna in Water (Canned)
- 1 oz Lemon Juice
- 3 tbsps Real Mayonnaise
- 2 cups Arugula (Rocket)
- 1/2 cup slice Cucumber (with Peel)
- 1 tbsp Olive Oil

Directions

Be sure to zest the full lemon before juicing.

1. Combine the tuna, 1 1/2 Tbsp lemon juice, zest, and mayonnaise in a small bowl. Season with salt and freshly ground black pepper.
2. Serve over arugula and slice cucumber seasoned with 1 Tbsp olive oil and 1/2 Tbsp lemon juice.

Low-Carb Grilled Cheese with Tomato

Servings: 1 | Style: American

Ingredients

- 1/4 cup shredded Cheddar Cheese
- 2 medium slice (1/4" thick) Tomatoes
- 1 tsp Unsalted Butter Stick
- 1 serving Low-Carb Bread

Directions

Use the Atkins recipe to make Atkins Cloud Bread.

1. Preheat a non-stick skillet over medium-high heat. Add the butter and allow it to melt.
2. Slice 1 piece of Atkins Cloud Bread into two thinner slices and place them into the skillet. Brown one side and then flip over and brown the other side; add the cheese to the top of one slice of bread while they brown on the other side.
3. Place two slices of tomato onto the melted cheese, season with salt and freshly ground black pepper, and then place the other piece of bread on top.

Mixed Fruit Salad

Servings: 1 | Prep: 10 m | Style: Other

Ingredients

- 1/4 small (2-1/2" dia) (approx 4 per lb) Apples
- 1/4 medium (7" to 7-7/8" long) Bananas
- 1/2 fruit Kiwi Fruit
- 1/4 cup Raspberries

Directions

1. Combine apples, banana, kiwi and raspberries in a bowl and serve.

Mushrooms Stuffed with Sausage and Mozzarella

Servings: 24 | Prep: 35 m | Style: Italian | Cook: 10 m

Ingredients

- 24 whole Mushroom Pieces and Stems
- 2 tbsps Extra Virgin Olive Oil
- 6 oz Pork Italian Sausage
- 3 large Scallions or Spring Onions
- 1 tsp Garlic
- 1/4 tsp Italian Seasoning
- 1/2 cup shredded Whole Milk Mozzarella Cheese
- 1/4 cup Parmesan Cheese (Grated)

Directions

Although this recipe calls for pork sausage, you could also substitute turkey sausage or even vegetarian "sausage" made from soy. Also feel free to use more garlic if you wish.

1. Preheat oven to 400°F.
2. Remove stems from mushrooms; finely chop enough stems to equal 1/2 cup and reserve. Place mushroom caps in a bowl and toss with 1 tablespoon oil.
3. Arrange caps cavity side up on a shallow baking pan and set aside.

4. Heat remaining oil in a medium skillet over high heat. Add sausage, green onion, garlic (minced), Italian seasoning and reserved chopped mushroom stems. Sauté, breaking up sausage into smaller pieces, for about 5 minutes, until cooked through and nicely browned.
5. Remove from heat; add both cheeses and stir just until cheese melts.
6. Stuff mushroom caps with sausage mixture and bake 10 15 minutes, until mushrooms are tender and cheese is slightly golden.

Olive Tapenade

Servings: 24 | *Prep:* 15 m | *Style:* Italian

Ingredients

- 1 cup whole Black Olives
- 8 cups whole Green Olives
- 2 tsps Fresh Lemon Juice
- 1/2 tsp Garlic
- 1/16 tsp Crushed Red Pepper Flakes
- 1/4 cup Extra Virgin Olive Oil

Directions

1. Pulse black and green olives, garlic, lemon juice, red pepper flakes, and oil in a food processor until finely chopped.
2. Transfer to a bowl and serve, or refrigerate in an airtight container for up to 1 week.

Parsley Butter

Servings: 4 | *Prep:* 120 m | *Style:* American

Ingredients

- 6 tbsps Salted Butter Stick
- 2 tbsps chopped Shallots

- 2 tbsps Parsley
- 2 tsps Fresh Lemon Juice
- 1/4 tsp Salt
- 1/8 tsp Black Pepper

Directions

1. Top vegetables or grilled meats and poultry with this seasoned butter or use it to cook eggs. Substitute a minced clove of garlic and a little onion if shallots aren't available. Feel free to substitute chopped fresh cilantro for the parsley, lime juice for the lemon juice and a pinch of cayenne pepper for the pepper. Each serving is 2 Tbsp.
2. Combine butter, shallot, parsley, lemon juice, salt and pepper in a medium bowl; blend well to distribute ingredients thoroughly.
3. Spoon seasoned butter onto waxed paper; roll paper around butter to form a log. Twist ends to secure butter; roll gently across counter to form an even cylinder.
4. Refrigerate until chilled, at least 2 hours and up to 1 week. Slice into small pats and use as desired.

Peachy Prosciutto Bites

*Servings: 2 | **Prep:** 10 m | **Style:** American*

Ingredients

- 1/2 medium (2-1/2" dia) (approx 4 per lb) Peaches
- 2 oz Cream Cheese
- 1 tsp Cinnamon
- 1/4 cup whole Almonds
- 6 leaves Basil
- 6 thin slices Prosciutto

Directions

1. The basil in this recipe adds a bit of complexity and balance when a pinch of pure stevia (optional) is added to the cream cheese mixture. Enjoy without the basil (or stevia) if you prefer.

2. Preheat oven to 350°F. Toast nuts in a single layer for 10 minutes. Cool and then coarsely chop. Set aside. Slice the peach into 6 wedges and set aside.
3. In a small bowl combine the softened cream cheese with 1 teaspoon ground cinnamon and a pinch of stevia (optional). Add the nuts, blend to combine.
4. Lay out a single slice of proscuitto, place 1 tablespoon cheese mixture on top of peach wedge and top with a basil leaf, place the wedge at one end of the proscuitto and roll-it-up. Repeat with remaining ingredients. 1 serving = 3 wrapped peach wedges.

Pico de Gallo

*Servings: 2 | **Prep**: 75 m | **Style**: Mexican*

Ingredients

- 1 fruit without skin and seed California Avocado
- 1 medium whole (2-3/5" dia) Red Tomato
- 3 medium (4-1/8" long) Scallions or Spring Onions
- 1 Jalapeno Pepper
- 1/8 cup Cilantro (Coriander)
- 1 tbsp Fresh Lemon Juice
- 1 tbsp Canola Vegetable Oil

Directions

1. In a small bowl, combine avocado, tomato, onions, jalapeno, cilantro, juice, and oil. Add salt and pepper to taste.
2. Refrigerate 1 hour for flavors to blend.

Pimento Cheese

*Servings: 8 | **Prep**: 10 m | **Style**: American*

Ingredients

- 4 oz Sharp Cheddar Cheese
- 4 oz Vintage White Extra Sharp Cheddar Cheese
- 1/3 cup Real Mayonnaise
- 2 oz Pimento (Canned)
- 1 tsp smoked Paprika
- 1/2 tsp Dijon Mustard
- 1/4 tsp Salt
- 1/8 tsp Red or Cayenne Pepper

Directions

1. Shred cheeses and set aside.
2. Combine mayonnaise, diced pimento, smoked paprika, Dijon mustard, salt, and cayenne pepper (to your taste) in a small bowl. Stir with a fork to blend flavors.
3. Add the cheeses to the mayonnaise mixture stirring to fully incorporate. Wrap and chill for 2-3 hours before serving for best flavor. May be kept tightly covered in the refrigerator for 1 week. Serve with celery sticks or other vegetables. Each serving is about 2 Tbsp.

Pina Colada

Servings: 2 | Prep: 5 m | Style: Other

Ingredients

- 2 oz Vanilla Whey Protein
- 1 oz Sugar Free French Vanilla Syrup
- 2 tsps Coconut Extract
- 1/4 cup diced Pineapple

Directions

1. Place the pineapple, syrup and coconut extract (add just enough to flavor it - start with 1 tsp and add more as desired) in a blender Blend until the pineapple is broken down.

2. Add the protein powder and 10-12 ice cubes, blend until very smooth, adding a small amount of water, and stirring with a wooden spoon if necessary.

Pumpkin Prosciutto Bites

*Servings: 9 | **Prep:** 15 m | **Style:** American | **Cook:** 33 m*

Ingredients

- 5 oz Pumpkin
- 1 tsp Extra Virgin Olive Oil
- 1/2 tsp Pumpkin Pie Spice
- 1 pinch Stevia
- 4 oz boneless Prosciutto
- 4 oz Cream Cheese
- 1/2 cup shredded Gruyere Cheese

Directions

1. Preheat oven to 425°F. Cut pumpkin into 18 1-inch cubes.
2. In a small bowl toss the pumpkin cubes with the oil, pumpkin pie spice, and a pinch of granular sugar substitute (stevia; use more if using sucralose or other sweetener - up to 1 teaspoon). Place on a piece of parchment and roast for 25-30 minutes until tender. Set aside to cool.
3. Combine softened cream cheese with Gruyere in a medium bowl mixing with a fork. Set aside.
4. Cut prosciutto slices in half (18 equal 3x3 squares). Place into a mini muffin tin pressing down into the tin, leave excess to overlap outside the well. Fill each prosciutto well with 1 1/3 teaspoons cheese mixture then place a piece of pumpkin in the center. Fold the excess prosciutto in towards the center and press together. Bake for 5-8 minutes until cheese is bubbly and prosciutto has cooked edges. 1 serving = 2 pieces.

Pumpkin-Nut Bake

*Servings: 10 | **Prep:** 15 m | **Style:** Other | **Cook:** 60 m*

Ingredients

- 2 cups Pumpkin (Without Salt, Canned)
- 1/4 tsp Allspice Ground
- 1/2 tsp Salt
- 1/2 cup Mascarpone
- 1/4 tsp Nutmeg (Ground)
- 12 large Eggs (Whole)
- 1/2 cup Sugar Free Maple Flavored Syrup
- 1/4 cup chopped Pecans

Directions

1. Heat oven to 350°F.
2. In an electric mixer on high speed, whip eggs 5 minutes until thick.
3. In a large bowl, whisk pumpkin purée until smooth; gradually whisk in eggs, nutmeg, allspice, salt, mascarpone and syrup. Pour in a buttered 9-inch x 13-inch baking pan.
4. Bake 45 minutes. Sprinkle chopped pecans evenly over top; bake 15 minutes more. Cool slightly before cutting.

Raita

*Servings: 8 | **Prep:** 75 m | **Style:** Other*

Ingredients

- 1 cucumber (8-1/4") Cucumber (with Peel)
- 1 1/2 cup (8 fl oz) Whole Milk Plain Yogurt
- 2 tbsps Peppermint (Mint)
- 1 oz Cilantro (Coriander)
- 1/2 tsp Salt
- 1/8 tsp Curry Powder

Directions

Cooling raita is a staple in Indian and Middle Eastern cuisines. It cools hot curries, but it's also great with mild dishes and spiced grilled meats and even as a dip. See

below for a variation. Please use fresh cilantro in this recipe for the best flavor.
Each serving is 1/4 cup.

1. Peel and grate the cucumber, squeeze out excess water and place into a
    medium bowl.
2. To the bowl add the yogurt, minced mint and cilantro, salt and curry
    powder. Cover and refrigerate for 1 hour to allow flavors to blend.

Ranch Dressing

Servings: 8 | Prep: 10 m | Style: American

Ingredients

*   3/4 cup Real Mayonnaise
*   1/2 cup Heavy Cream
*   2 tbsps Parsley
*   2 tbsps chopped Chives
*   2 tsps Fresh Lemon Juice
*   2 tsps Dijon Mustard
*   1/2 tsp Garlic
*   1 tsp fresh Dill
*   1/2 tsp Salt
*   1/4 tsp Black Pepper

Directions

1. An all-American favorite, this homemade version of the creamy garlic-and-
    herb dressing is smooth and satisfying without the added sugar. Each
    serving is just over 2 Tbsp.
2. Whisk mayonnaise, cream, parsley, chives, lemon juice, mustard, garlic,
    dill, salt and pepper in a small bowl.
3. Use immediately or refrigerate in an airtight container for up to 3 days.

Raspberry Sauce

Servings: 8 | Prep: 5 m | Style: French | Cook: 5 m

Ingredients

- 10 oz Unsweetened Frozen Raspberries
- 1 1/2 oz Sugar Free French Vanilla Syrup

Directions

1. In medium saucepan, cook frozen berries over medium heat 5 minutes until they begin to give off liquid and are defrosted.
2. Remove from heat, press through a strainer into a bowl to remove seeds.
3. Mix in vanilla syrup.

Remoulade

Servings: 8 | Prep: 25 m | Style: French

Ingredients

- 3/4 cup Real Mayonnaise
- 1 oz Pickles
- 1 tbsp drained Capers
- 1 large Hard-Boiled Egg
- 2 tsps Dijon Mustard
- 1 tsp Sucralose Based Sweetener (Sugar Substitute)
- 1 tbsp Parsley
- 1/2 tsp Tarragon

Directions

1. Each serving is 2 Tbsp.
2. Combine mayonnaise, capers, dill pickle, chopped egg, mustard, sugar substitute, parsley and tarragon in a small bowl until thoroughly combined.
3. Let stand 15 minutes for flavors to blend.

Rhubarb Muffins

Servings*: 10 | **Prep***: 10 m | ***Style****: American | **Cook***: 25 m*

Ingredients

- 1/3 cup Unsalted Butter Stick
- 1/3 cup Xylitol
- 3 large Eggs (Whole)
- 1/3 cup Coconut Milk Unsweetened
- 1 tsp Vanilla Extract
- 1/2 cup Organic High Fiber Coconut Flour
- 1 tsp Baking Powder (Straight Phosphate, Double Acting)
- 1/4 tsp Salt
- 1 1/2 tsps Cinnamon
- 1/3 tsp Nutmeg (Ground)
- 1 1/2 cups diced Rhubarb

Directions

1. Preheat oven to 350°F. Prepare 10 wells of a muffin tin with paper liners or spray with oil.
2. Whisk the melted butter, xylitol, eggs, coconut milk and vanilla until blended.
3. In a small bowl combine the coconut flour (reserve 1 tablespoon), baking powder, salt, ground cinnamon and nutmeg. Add mixture to the wet ingredients and blend until combined.
4. Toss the rhubarb with 1 tablespoon reserved coconut flour and then add it to the batter, mix to incorporate and divide into the muffin wells and bake for 25-30 minutes until golden brown and set. Allow to cool for 10 minutes in the pan and then place on a cooling rack for 15 minutes. Enjoy slightly warm or at room temperature.

Rhuberry Margarita

Servings*: 1 | **Prep***: 5 m | ***Style****: American*

Ingredients

- 1/2 tbsps Fresh Lime Juice
- 1 tsp Sweetener
- 1 fl oz (no ice) Tequila
- 4 ice cubes Tap Water
- 1 serving Strawberry Rhubarb Sauce
- 2 fl ozs Club Soda

Directions

Use the Atkins recipe to make Strawberry Rhubarb Sauce for this recipe. You will need 2 Tbsp for each serving. Truvia is the recommended sweetener (if using sucralose use 4 tsp and add 2g NC to the total).

1. Combine 2 tablespoons of Strawberry Rhubarb Sauce with the lime juice, sugar substitute and tequila in a blender. Pulse 2-3 times to puree the sauce.
2. Add 4 ice cubes to a glass, pour the tequila mixture over the top and add club soda or seltzer. Or make it frozen by putting all in a blender.

Roast Beef, Red Bell Pepper and Provolone Lettuce Wraps

Servings: 1 | Prep: 5 m | Style: American

Ingredients

- 2 leaves Cos or Romaine Lettuce
- 2 oz Provolone Cheese
- 1 tbsp Real Mayonnaise
- 1/8 tbsp Horseradish Sauce
- 4 oz boneless Roast Beef
- 1/4 medium (approx 2-3/4" long, 2-1/2" dia) Red Sweet Pepper

Directions

1. Remove bottom portion of lettuce leaves. Lay flat on a clean surface. Top each with a slice of cheese.

2. Combine the mayonnaise with horseradish adding garlic powder (optinal, to taste) and season with salt and freshly ground black pepper. Spread onto cheese slices. Then place a layer of roast beef.
3. Cut the red bell pepper into 1/4-inch thick strips and lay on one end of the roast beef, cheese and lettuce. Roll up, starting where you placed the pepper strips until fully rolled. Secure with a tooth pick, repeat for second roll-up and enjoy immediately.

Roasted Garlic-Basil Dressing

Servings: 5 | *Prep:* 5 m | *Style:* American | *Cook:* 45 m

Ingredients

- 10 cloves Garlic
- 17 tbsps Extra Virgin Olive Oil
- 5 1/4 tbsps Sodium and Sugar Free Rice Vinegar
- 10 leaves Basil
- 1 oz Parmesan Cheese (Grated)
- 1/2 tsp Salt
- 1 tsp Black Pepper
- 2 tbsps Xylitol

Directions

Roasted garlic emulsifies this creamy dressing, keeping it from separating into oil and vinegar. Roasting tames the garlic's pungency resulting in a paste that's actually sweet. If you have a ceramic garlic roaster, use it instead of aluminum foil. Each serving is 2 Tbsp.

Note: 17 tablespoons of olive oil is equivalent to 1 cup plus 1 tablespoon.

1. Preheat oven to 400°F. Trim the top 1/4 inch off the garlic bulb to expose the cloves. Place on a large square of aluminum foil, drizzle the top with one tablespoon of the olive oil and close tightly to form a packet. Bake until garlic is very soft, about 45 minutes. Remove from oven and let cool at room temperature for about 25 minutes.
2. Place vinegar, basil and grated Parmesan in food processor and pulse until very finely ground. Separate garlic into cloves. Squeeze roasted garlic out of skins into food processor and add olive oil, 2 Tbsp of xylitol, salt and

pepper. Process until smooth, 2 or 3 minutes. Refrigerate in a squeeze bottle or closed container for up to a week.

Samurai Crisps with Garlic Ginger Shrimp

Servings: 8 | Prep: 20 m | Style: American | Cook: 15 m

Ingredients

- 1 1/2 cups Parmesan Cheese (Grated)
- 2 tbsps Dried Whole Sesame Seeds
- 16 tbsps Chives & Onion Cream Cheese
- 6 tsps Sriracha Hot Chili Sauce
- 2 tbsps Sugar Free Orange Marmalade
- 2 tbsps Basil
- 2 tbsps Unsalted Butter Stick
- 2 cloves Garlic
- 3 tsps Ginger
- 24 medium Shrimps

Directions

1. Make the crisps. Preheat oven to 375°F. Line a baking sheet with parchment paper or aluminum foil then coat with cooking spray and set aside. Using a 2-inch cookie cutter or biscuit cutter as a mold, fill with 1 tablespoon of the grated Parmesan cheese and sprinkle with a portion of sesame seeds. Pat cheese down to flatten with fingers, remove cookie cutter and continue creating the rest of your cheese crisps. Bake for 8-10 minutes or until golden brown. While warm, remove crisps with spatula and place on a serving plate to cool.
2. While the crisps are baking, mix cream cheese, Sriracha (or hot pepper sauce) and marmalade in a small bowl with a rubber spatula. Transfer mixture to a decorating bag fitted with a star tip, or place cream cheese mixture into a heavy duty zipper sealed bag and snip off the corner to create your own decorating bag. Set aside.
3. In a skillet over medium high heat, add butter, shrimp, garlic and ginger. Cook until shrimp are opaque, about 4-5 minutes. When crisps are cool, pipe a heaping teaspoon of cream cheese mixture onto each crisp. Sprinkle with basil, and top each with a shrimp.

Sautéed Cocktail Meatballs

Servings: 4 | Prep: 20 m | Style: Mediterranean / Greek | Cook: 10 m

Ingredients

- 1/2 cup Blanched Almond Flour
- 1/2 lb Ground Beef (90% Lean / 10% Fat)
- 1/2 lb Ground Pork
- 1/4 tsp Cinnamon
- 1/4 cup Parmesan Cheese (Grated)
- 2 large Eggs (Whole)
- 1/4 cup sprig Dill
- 1/2 tsp Garlic
- 1 tbsp Peppermint (Mint)
- 1/2 tsp leaf Oregano
- 1/2 lb Ground Veal
- 1 tbsp Salt
- 1/2 tsp Black Pepper

Directions

This recipe is marked as a Phase 2 recipe in the cookbook. It is low enough in NC however to be considered Phase 1 unless you are in the first two weeks of Induction due to the nuts.

1. Combine almond meal, meat, cheese, eggs, dill, garlic, mint, oregano, cinnamon, salt, and pepper; mix gently with your hands.
2. Moisten your hands (this helps prevent mixture from sticking); shape mixture into 1-inch balls and set aside.
3. Place 2 tablespoons olive oil in a large nonstick skillet over medium-high heat. Add half the meatballs; cook, turning frequently, until browned on all sides and cooked through, about 8 minutes. Repeat with 2 more tablespoons olive oil and remaining meatballs. Serve with toothpicks or wooden skewers as an appetizer.

Savory Meatballs

Servings: 12 | Prep: 5 m | Style: Other | Cook: 15 m

Ingredients

- 1/3 second spray Original Canola Cooking Spray
- 16 oz Ground Beef (80% Lean / 20% Fat)
- 1/3 cup Whole Grain Soy Flour
- 1/2 cup Parmesan Cheese (Grated)
- 2 tbsps Parsley
- 2 tsps Italian Seasoning
- 2 tbsps Tap Water
- 1/2 tsp Black Pepper
- 1/2 tsp Salt

Directions

1. Preheat oven to 375°F. Lightly oil baking sheet.
2. In a large mixing bowl, combine sirloin, soy flour, cheese, parsley, seasoning, water, salt and pepper. Roll into 24 balls and place on baking sheet.
3. Bake 10 minutes.

Savory Popcorn and Nut Mix

Servings: 10 | **Prep:** 10 m | **Style:** Other | **Cook:** 15 m

Ingredients

- 12 oz Roasted Mixed Nuts with Peanuts
- 4 cups Air Popped Popcorn
- 3 tbsps Unsalted Butter Stick
- 2 tsps Thyme
- 1 tsp Coarse Kosher Salt
- 1/4 tsp Red or Cayenne Pepper
- 1/4 tsp Garlic Powder

Directions

1. Heat oven to 275°F.

2. On a large roasting pan, toss nuts and popcorn with butter. Sprinkle evenly with thyme. Combine kosher salt, cayenne pepper (to taste) and garlic powder; sprinkle over top and toss well.
3. Bake 15 minutes. Transfer to large sheet of wax paper and let cool.
4. Store in an airtight container.

Scotch Eggs

Servings: 4 | Prep: 20 m | Style: Other | Cook: 20 m

Ingredients

- 1 large Egg (Whole)
- 8 large Boiled Eggs
- 1 tsp Tap Water
- 2 /4 cups Organic High Fiber Coconut Flour
- 12 oz raw (yield after cooking) Turkey Breakfast Sausage

Directions

1. Prepare hard-boiled eggs. Cover 8 eggs in a heavy pan with 1-inch of cold water. Bring to a rolling boil, remove from the heat and allow eggs to cook for 10 minutes. Immediately drain off hot water and immerse eggs in an ice-water bath until cool enough to peel. Peel eggs and dry thoroughly on a paper towel.
2. Whisk 1 egg and water in a small bowl. In another shallow bowl place the coconut flour (season with salt and pepper if desired). Set both aside.
3. Prepare sausage by forming into 8 equal balls. Take each ball and flatten into an oblong disk. Wrap each egg into the sausage disk making sure to cover the entire surface evenly. Set each sausage covered egg on a plate.
4. Heat about 1-inch of oil in a large frying pan over medium-high heat. Roll each egg in the whisked egg, then the coconut flour until coated all over. When the oil is shimmering, place all 8 eggs (if they fit, allowing at least 1/2-inch in between) in the pan. Fry on one side until golden in color then using tongs flip to another side, continue until all sides are golden brown, about 8 minutes total. Drain on a paper towel and serve immediately.

Simple Baked Tofu

Servings: 1 | *Prep:* 5 m | *Style:* American | *Cook:* 30 m

Ingredients

- 6 oz Firm Silken Tofu
- 1 tsp Extra Virgin Olive Oil

Directions

1. Drain and pat tofu dry with a paper towel. Cut into 1/4 inch strips. Pour olive oil over tofu. Season with salt and pepper or other seasonings of choice.
2. Preheat oven to 375°
3. Bake on a greased flat pan for 15 minutes, turn over and bake an additional 15 minutes till golden brown and slightly crispy.

Smoked Salmon, Cucumber and Cream Cheese Roll-Ups

Servings: 1 | *Prep:* 5 m | *Style:* American

Ingredients

- 3 oz Smoked Chinook Salmon (Lox)
- 2 tbsps Cream Cheese
- 1/2 cucumber (8-1/4") Cucumber (with Peel)

Directions

1. Use a mandoline or a vegetable peeler to cut long thin strips of cucumber. You may have leftover strips to enjoy!
2. Spread cream cheese onto smoked salmon, place a strip of cucumber at one edge and roll up with the salmon and cream cheese. Pin in place with a tooth pick!

Smoked Salmon, Tomato and Cream Cheese

Servings: 1 | Prep: 10 m | Style: American

Ingredients

- 3 oz Smoked Chinook Salmon
- 1 medium whole (2-3/5" dia) Red Tomato
- 2 tbsps Cream Cheese

Directions

1. Cut smoked salmon into small chunks. Dice tomato. Mix cream cheese, diced tomato, and salmon chunks together. Season with salt and freshly ground black pepper. Serve in celery boats if desired. (Remember to add in 1g NC per stalk of celery.)
2. Alternate method: spread salmond with cream cheese then layer on top of tomato. Also great with a spinkle of fresh or dried dill weed.

Smoked Sausage Deviled Eggs

Servings: 4 | Prep: 8 m | Style: American

Ingredients

- 4 large Hard-Boiled Eggs
- 2 tbsps Real Mayonnaise
- 1/4 tsp Tabasco Sauce
- 3 tbsps chopped Scallions or Spring Onions
- 6 oz cooked Smoked Beef Sausage
- 1/4 serving Barbecue Sauce

Directions

Use the Atkins recipe to make Barbecue Sauce. Please note that the Barbecue Sauce recipe is a Phase 2 recipe but it can be used in this Phase 1 recipe because only a small amount is being used and the ingredients are Phase 1 acceptable (it is the high NC per serving of the sauce that makes it a Phase 2 sauce).

1. Cut hard-boiled eggs in half lengthwise; put yolks in a small mixing bowl; set whites aside.
2. Add mayonnaise to yolks and mash with a silicone spatula or fork until smooth.
3. Fold in Tabasco, scallions and 1 tsp barbecue sauce (or to taste) then season to taste with salt and freshly ground black pepper.
4. Fill each egg white half with the yolk mixture; top with sausage slices

Smoked Trout Mousse in Cucumber Cups

Servings: 12 | Prep: 60 m | Style: Other | Cook: 7 m

Ingredients

- 3 thick slice packed 12/lbs Bacon (Cured)
- 1/3 envelope (1 tbsp) Gelatin Powder (Unsweetened)
- 3 cucumber (8-1/4") Cucumber (with Peel)
- 1 tbsp chopped Onions
- 1/2 cup Tap Water
- 8 oz boneless Smoked Trout
- 3 tbsps chopped Chives
- 1/2 tsp Salt
- 1 tsp Worcestershire Sauce
- 1/4 tsp Tabasco Sauce
- 1/2 cup Heavy Cream
- 2 tsps Fresh Lemon Juice

Directions

1. Cook bacon, drain on paper towels, and cool. Crumble into small pieces.
2. Sprinkle gelatin over 1/4 cup cold water in a small bowl. Let stand until dissolved, about 2 minutes. Pour 1/4 cup boiling water over gelatin; stir to combine. Chill until it begins to set, about 30 minutes.
3. Combine trout, 2 tablespoons chives, onion, lemon juice, Worcestershire sauce, salt and hot pepper sauce in a bowl; mix well. Stir in gelatin mixture.
4. Beat cream with an electric mixer at high speed until stiff peaks form. Gently fold trout mixture into cream; chill until slightly set, about 20 minutes. Gently stir.
5. Spoon out the middle of each cucumber round, leaving a 1/8-inch border around edges and bottom. Spoon about 2 teaspoons mousse into each round.

6. Garnish with bacon and remaining tablespoon chives.

Smokey Horseradish Spread

Servings: 8 | Prep: 10 m | Style: American

Ingredients

- 2 cups shredded Cheddar Cheese
- 1/3 cup Real Mayonnaise
- 2 tsps Cream Style Horseradish
- 1/2 tsp Mustard
- 1/2 tsp smoked Paprika
- 1/2 tsp Worcestershire Sauce

Directions

1. Blend all ingredients together in a bowl. Refrigerate for 30 minutes before serving. Keep in an air-tight container for up to 1 week in the refrigerator.

Spiced Coconut Bark

Servings: 12 | Prep: 15 m | Style: American

Ingredients

- 7 oz Sugar Free Chocolate Chips
- 1 tsp Cinnamon
- 1/8 tsp Chili Powder
- 1/4 tsp Coarse Kosher Salt
- 5 tbsps Dried Coconut

Directions

1. Melt chocolate in the microwave at 30 second intervals (about 3 times) until it begins to melt. Stir in between and do not over heat.
2. Stir in ground cinnamon and chipotle pepper (as deisred for taste, amounts given are delicious but feel free to play with different levels to your taste). Stir in 2 tablespoons shredded coconut. Pour onto parchment paper, spread out evenly into a 6x8-inch rectangle and sprinkle remaining 3 tablespoons shredded coconut on top. Sprinkle coarse Kosher salt on top as well (optional).
3. Place in the refrigerator for 10-15 minutes to firm up then divide into 12 equal portions (squares of 2x2 inches are best for portioning).

Spiced Garlic Spread

Servings: 4 | Prep: 5 m | Style: American | Cook: 12 m

Ingredients

- 6 tsps Garlic
- 4 tbsps Light Olive Oil
- 1/2 tsp Curry Powder
- 1/4 tsp Cumin
- 1 tbsp Fresh Lemon Juice
- 1/4 tsp Salt

Directions

1. In a small saucepan, bring garlic and oil to a simmer, cook at a low simmer 9 to 11 minutes, until garlic is soft.
2. Stir in spices and remove from heat; let cool. Transfer to a mini-food processor and purée until smooth.
3. Add lemon juice and salt; purée again briefly to combine.

Spicy Chorizo Pumpkin Dip

Servings: 8 | Prep: 15 m | Style: American | Cook: 10 m

Ingredients

- 6 oz Pork and Beef Chorizo
- 8 oz Cream Cheese
- 1/2 cup Pumpkin (Without Salt, Canned)
- 3/4 cup chopped Red Sweet Pepper
- 1 oz, raw, yield Red Onions
- 1 Jalapeno Pepper
- 2 tsps Chili Powder
- 1/2 tsp Cinnamon
- 1/2 tsp Cumin
- 1/4 tsp Coriander Seed
- 1/8 tsp Salt

Directions

1. Break-up the chorizo into small pieces then cook over medium-high heat until cooked through; about 5 minutes. Drain on a paper towel and set aside.
2. Beat the softened cream cheese until smooth. Add the pumpkin and beat until incorporated. Add the chili powder, ground cinnamon, ground cumin, ground coridander, and salt; blend to combine.
3. Remove the seeds and gills of the red bell pepper and jalapeno. Chop the red pepper into 1/4 - inch pieces (measure out 3/4 cup; reserve the remaining as garnish if desired) and finely dice the jalapeno. Finely mince the red onion and add all to the cream cheese mixture along with the reserved chorizo.
4. Heat in the microwave for 2-3 minutes until hot; stirring in between and serve immediately with cut up vegetables. This dip keeps well in a small crockpot over low heat.

Spicy Crab Dip

Servings: 4 | Prep: 60 m | Style: Other

Ingredients

- 1 can (6.5 oz), drained Blue Crab (Canned)
- 2 medium (4-1/8" long) Scallions or Spring Onions

- 1/4 cup Real Mayonnaise
- 1/4 cup Sour Cream (Cultured)
- 1 Chipotle Peppers in Adobo Sauce
- 1 tsp Fresh Lemon Juice

Directions

1. Mix crab, onion, mayonnaise, sour cream, chipotle en adobo, and lemon juice in a sealable bowl.
2. Chill 1 hour for flavors to blend.

Spicy Shrimp Deviled Eggs

Servings: 2 | Prep: 10 m | Style: American

Ingredients

- 4 large Boiled Eggs
- 2 tbsps Real Mayonnaise
- 1/2 oz Pickles
- 1/2 tsp Dijon Mustard
- 1/2 tsp Horseradish
- 1/8 tsp Original Pepper Sauce
- 8 large Shrimps

Directions

1. Cut eggs in half and put yolks into small mixing bowl. Set whites aside.
2. Add mayonnaise to yolks and mash until smooth. Fold in pickle,mustard, horseradish and hot pepper sauce.
3. Fill egg white halves with mixture and top each with one shrimp. Garnish with fresh dill if desired.

Spinach and Shrimp Dip

Servings: 8 | Style: American

Ingredients

- 1 package (10 oz) Spinach (Chopped or Leaf, Frozen)
- 1 medium (4-1/8" long) Scallions or Spring Onions
- 1 clove Garlic
- 2 Jalapeno Peppers
- 1/2 cup Real Mayonnaise
- 6 tbsps Cream Cheese
- 1/2 oz Lemon Juice
- 1/4 tsp Old Bay Seasoning
- 12 oz Small Cooked Shrimp

Directions

1. Thaw spinach in the microwave for 1-2 minutes. Squeeze out excess water and place it into the bowl of a food processor. Coarsely chop the scallions, jalapeno and garlic and add to the food processor bowl. Process mixture until finely chopped.
2. Add the mayonnaise, softened cream cheese, lemon juice and Old Bay seasoning. Pulse until fully combined.
3. Add the shrimp and pulse just until the shrimp are finely chopped - about 10 seconds. Taste and adjust seasonings. Keep refrigerated until ready to serve. This recipe makes 2 cups. Serve with Cauliflower Fritters (see Atkins recipe) or with baked parmesan crisps or other low carb cracker.

Spinach Phyllo Triangles

*Servings: 8 | **Prep:** 45 m | **Style:** Other | **Cook:** 15 m*

Ingredients

- 1/2 cup Unsalted Butter Stick
- 1 tbsp Light Olive Oil
- 2 tsps Garlic
- 1 10 oz package Frozen Chopped Spinach
- 1/2 cup crumbled Feta Cheese
- 1/3 cup Ricotta Cheese (Whole Milk)
- 10 sheets Phyllo Dough
- 1 large Egg (Whole)

- 2 tbsps Parsley
- 1 1/2 tsps Paprika

Directions

1. Preheat oven to 375°F. Brush a jelly-roll pan or baking sheet lightly with butter.
2. In a large pan over medium heat, sauté garlic in oil until aroma is releases, about 3 seconds. Turn off heat and add spinach. Toss with garlic oil well and transfer to a large bowl. Mix in feta, ricotta and salt and pepper to taste.
3. Stir in egg and mix until ingredients are well combined. Arrange phyllo sheets atop one another and cut crosswise into thirds. Cover 2 stacks with plastic wrap and a kitchen towel to keep them from drying out.
4. Separate one strip from the exposed stack and brush it lightly with melted butter; fold in half lengthwise to form a narrow strip.
5. Place a scant tablespoon of filling at one end and fold up flag-style to form a triangular pastry. Place on prepared sheet. Repeat process to make 28 triangles (you will have 2 phyllo strips left over).
6. Brush tops and sides of triangles with butter every time you finish a row, and sprinkle with parsley and paprika. (If frozen, cover with plastic wrap, then heavy-duty foil, crimping edges tightly. Remove both coverings before baking, but do not defrost.)
7. Bake triangles until golden and slightly puffed in centers, about 12 to 15 minutes (or 20 to 25 minutes if frozen).

Spinach-Artichoke Dip

Servings: 8 | **Style:** Mediterranean / Greek

Ingredients

- 1 10 oz package Frozen Chopped Spinach
- 1 can (14 oz), drained Cooked Artichoke (Canned)
- 1 tsp Garlic
- 8 oz Cream Cheese
- 1 cup Parmesan Cheese (Grated)
- 1/4 tsp Black Pepper

Directions

1. Pre-heat oven to 350°F.
2. Grease a 1-quart ovenproof pan.
3. In a food processor, process spinach, artichokes, garlic, cream cheese, Parmesan and pepper until well combined, scraping down sides of processor, as needed.
4. Spread mixture in prepared pan. Bake until warmed through, about 30 minutes. Serve hot with sliced vegetables.

Star Spangled Berry Trifle

Servings: *12* | **Prep:** *180 m* | **Style:** *American*

Ingredients

- 1 fl oz Fresh Lemon Juice
- 1 fl oz Tap Water
- 2 1/2 tsps Vanilla Extract
- 1 tsp Pure Almond Extract
- 9 tbsps Xylitol
- 2 pinches Stevia
- 1/2 cup Organic High Fiber Coconut Flour
- 1/2 tsp Salt
- 2 large Eggs (Whole)
- 2 cups Heavy Cream
- 1 cup Coconut Milk Unsweetened
- 12 large Egg Whites
- 1 tsp Thick-It-Up
- 3 cup sliceds Strawberries
- 3 cups Blackberries

Directions

1. Preheat oven to 350°F. Prepare a large sheet pan with with parchment paper. Set aside.
2. Beat egg whites until frothy. Add the lemon juice and water. Continue to beat and slowly add in 4 tablespoons xylitol, a pinch of stevia, and 1 teaspoon each of vanilla and almond extracts. Fold in the coconut flour and salt until just incorporated. Place mixture on top of the parchment and smooth out with a spatula, making sure it stays on the parchment..

Bake for 15-20 minutes, remove and allow to cool 5 minutes on the pan. Quickly turn the cake over and gently lift the parchment off of the cake, set the cake aside to cool.

3. While the cake is baking make pastry cream. Place 1 cup heavy cream and 1 cup coconut milk into a 1 quart pan. Add 2 tablespoons xylitol and a pinch of stevia along with a pinch of salt. Heat over medium high heat until bubbles just start to appear around the edges of the pan.

4. In a small bowl combine the eggs, Thick-It-Up and 2 tablespoons xylitol. Whisk to combine. Continue whisking and slowly add about half of the hot cream mixture to the eggs. Return egg mixture to the rest of the cream in the pan. Cook for 5-10 minutes until the mixture has boiled for about 1-2 minutes and thickened; stir continuously. Strain through a mesh strainer into a bowl , place plastic wrap on the surface and set aside. Allow to cool to room temperature (speed this up by placing over an ice water bath); about 30 minutes, add in 1 teaspoon vanilla extract, and place into the refrigerator to cool for at least 2 hours.

5. Whip the cream with 1 tablespoon xylitol and 1/2 teaspoon vanilla until fully whipped. Fold whipped cream into cold pastry cream. Additional stevia may be added to taste.

6. Assemble Trifle. Cut out stars or other designs from the cake; set aside. Cut up the remaining pieces and gently mix into the pastry cream. Start by layering the strawberries on the bottom. Add 1/2 of the pastry cream mixture then place the blackberries on top of the pastry cream. Top it off with a final layer of pastry cream and decorate top with the reserved cake stars. If desired, place a few reserved stars along the inside of the bowl as you layer the ingredients up. The serving size is about 1 cup.

Strawberries and Walnuts

Servings: 1 | Prep: 5 m | Style: American

Ingredients

- 1/3 cup sliced Strawberries
- 1 oz (14 halves) English Walnuts

Directions

1. Combine strawberries with walnut halves. Or eat separately. Enjoy!

Sun-Dried Tomato Deviled Eggs

*Servings: 6 | **Prep:** 20 m | **Style:** American | **Cook:** 20 m*

Ingredients

- 12 large Eggs (Whole)
- 2 1/2 tbsps Real Mayonnaise
- 1 1/2 tbsps Sour Cream (Cultured)
- 1 oz Sun-Dried Tomato
- 2/3 tbsp chopped Shallots
- 1 tsp Dijon Mustard
- 1/4 tsp Tabasco Sauce

Directions

1. Place eggs in a large saucepan in a single layer covered with 1-inch of water. Bring to a boil; cover, remove from heat and let stand 20 minutes.
2. Run unpeeled eggs under cold water until cool to make them easy to peel.
3. Peel and halve eggs lengthwise. Set aside white halves on a plate.
4. Transfer yolks to a medium mixing bowl and mash with mayonnaise, sour cream, sun-dried tomatoes, shallots, mustard, hot sauce, salt and freshly ground black pepper to taste.
5. Spoon filling into egg halves evenly, mounding slightly. Serve immediately or refrigerate in an airtight container.

Sun-Dried Tomato Pesto

*Servings: 8 | **Prep:** 15 m | **Style:** Italian | **Cook:** 10 m*

Ingredients

- 3/4 cup Sun-Dried Tomatoes
- 1/4 cup Tap Water
- 3/4 cup Extra Virgin Olive Oil
- 16 tbsps Basil
- 1/4 cup Dried Pine Nuts
- 3/4 oz Romano Cheese

- 1 clove Garlic

Directions

A tasty twist on the classic Bail Pesto, this sauce can be mixed with sour cream or cream cheese for a tasty dip. Found near the produce section of the supermarket, dry-packed sun-dried tomatoes are much less expensive and fresher tasting than oil-packed ones. Each serving is 3 Tbsp.

1. Combine sun-dried tomatoes and 2 cups boiling water in a bowl; let stand until tomatoes are pliable, about 10 minutes. Drain; squeeze out excess liquid.
2. Combine tomatoes, 1/4 cup water, oil, 1/2 cup packed basil leaves, pine nuts, Romano cheese and garlic in a blender, pulse until fairly smooth. Serve immediately or refrigerate in an airtight container for up to 2 days or freeze for up to 1 week.

Sweet and Salty Almonds

Servings: 16 | Prep: 5 m | Style: Italian | Cook: 15 m

Ingredients

- 1 large Egg White
- 1/3 cup Sucralose Based Sweetener (Sugar Substitute)
- 3/4 dash Salt
- 2 tsps Cinnamon
- 2 cups whole Almonds

Directions

1. Heat oven to 350°F.
2. Combine the egg white, sugar substitute, salt, and cinnamon in a medium bowl. Beat with a fork until frothy. Add almonds and toss to coat. Spread out in a single layer on a nonstick baking sheet or a baking sheet lined with aluminum foil.
3. Bake for 12-15 minutes, turning once, until toasted and crisp. Remove from oven and place baking sheet on a baking rack. When the nuts are cool, remove from pan and store in an airtight container at room temperature up to one week.

Sweet and Spicy Nuts

*Servings: 8 | **Prep:** 10 m | **Style:** Other | **Cook:** 50 m*

Ingredients

- 1 large Egg White
- 1/2 cup half Pecan Nuts
- 1 fl oz Tap Water
- 2 tbsps Sucralose Based Sweetener (Sugar Substitute)
- 1/4 tsp Salt
- 1/4 tsp Black Pepper
- 1/4 tsp Cumin
- 1/4 tsp Cinnamon
- 1/8 tsp Red or Cayenne Pepper
- 1/2 cup whole Almonds
- 1/2 cup shelled (50 halves) English Walnuts
- 1/2 cup whole or halved Macadamia Nuts

Directions

1. Heat oven to 275°F. Line a baking sheet with aluminum foil; spray with nonstick cooking spray.
2. In a large bowl, mix egg white, water, sugar substitute, salt, pepper, cumin, cinnamon and 1/8 tsp cayenne (or to taste). Add nuts; mix until evenly coated.
3. Spread nuts in a single layer on prepared baking sheet. Bake 50 minutes to 1 hour until golden brown.

Swiss Cheese, Turkey and Asparagus Roll-Ups with Aioli

*Servings: 1 | **Style:** American*

Ingredients

- 3 oz Turkey Breast Meat (Fryer-Roasters, Cooked, Roasted)

- 1 3/4 slice (1 oz) Swiss Cheese
- 3 spear medium (5-1/4" to 7" long) Asparagus
- 1 serving Aioli

Directions

Use the Atkins recipe for Aioli.

1. Layer turkey and cheese together.
2. Carefully roll-up the asparagus in the turkey and cheese.
3. Serve with Aioli or spread Aioli between the layers of turkey and cheese before rolling up with asparagus.

Swiss Cheese, Turkey and Asparagus Roll-Ups

*Servings: 1 | **Prep**: 5 m | **Style**: American*

Ingredients

- 1 3/4 oz Swiss Cheese
- 3 oz Turkey Light Meat (Cooked, Roasted)
- 3 spear medium (5-1/4" to 7" long) Asparagus

Directions

1. Layer one slices of Swiss cheese over two slices of turkey.
2. Place both pieces of an asparagus spear at one end and roll up. Secure with a toothpick if desired.
3. Repeat twice for 3 roll-ups.

Tofu "Ricotta"

*Servings: 6 | **Prep**: 10 m | **Style**: American*

Ingredients

- 14 oz Firm Silken Tofu
- 1 fl oz Fresh Lemon Juice
- 1/2 packet Stevia
- 1/3 tsp Salt
- 1/3 tbsp Basil
- 1/4 tsp Garlic Powder
- 2 oz Mozzarella Soy Cheese

Directions

1. This is a great-tasting nondairy substitute for ricotta cheese to enjoy as a snack or use as an ingredient in recipes such as lasagna. Substitute it one for one in recipes.
2. Mash together tofu, lemon juice, chopped basil, Stevia, salt, garlic powder and "mozzarella" substitute.
3. Refrigerate for up to 5 days.

Tomatillo Salsa

*Servings: 10 | **Prep:** 15 m | **Style:** Mexican*

Ingredients

- 1 lb Tomatillos
- 1/2 small Red Onion
- 3/4 cup Cilantro (Coriander)
- 2 tbsps Fresh Lime Juice
- 2 tbsps Extra Virgin Olive Oil
- 1 Jalapeno Pepper
- 1/2 tsp Salt
- 1/8 tsp Black Pepper

Directions

1. Break out of your red salsa rut! This green salsa is tangy and slightly spicy and has a bit of crunch too. If you haven't experimented with tomatillo, a member of the tomato family that's particularly low in carbs, this is a good first recipe to try. Be sure to wear gloves and don't touch your eyes as (or

after) you chop up and de-seed the jalapeno pepper. Each serving is 1/4 cup.
2. Remove the husk from the tomatillo then chop it. Finely chop the onion and the jalapeno. Chop the cilantro.
3. Mix tomatillos, onion, cilantro, lime juice, oil, jalapeno, salt and pepper in a medium bowl. Let stand for 30 minutes to allow flavors to blend.
4. Serve chilled or at room temperature. Refrigerate leftovers in an airtight container for up to 3 days.

Tomato-Mozzarella Melt

Servings: 1 | Prep: 5 m | Style: American

Ingredients

1. 1 medium whole (2-3/5" dia) Red Tomato
2. 1/4 cup shredded Whole Milk Mozzarella Cheese

Directions

1. This is an easy recipe. Add some extra flavor by dusting the top of the tomato with salt, freshly ground black pepper and add other seasonings such as herbs (basil, oregano or thyme) or other spices (try a pinch of cayenne, powdered garlic).
2. Cut tomato in half. Cut off top and bottom so it will sit flat.
3. Place 1/2 of cheese on each tomato half.
4. Place in microwave for 30-60 seconds until cheese melts or place under broiler for 1 minute until cheese melts.

Vanilla Coffee Frappé

Servings: 1 | Prep: 5 m | Style: American

Ingredients

- 2 cup ice cubes Tap Water
- 11 fl ozs French Vanilla Shake

- 3 tsp, dries Instant Coffee (Dry Powder)
- 3 tbsps Heavy Cream

Directions

1. Combine 2 cups of ice in a blender with Atkins Advantage Vanilla Shake, heavy cream and instant coffee.
2. Blend until thoroughly combined and all the ice is crushed. Serve with a dollop of whipped cream if desired. Also terrific with 1/2 tsp ground cinnamon.

Vanilla-Spinach Shake

*Servings: 1 | **Prep:** 5 m | **Style:** American*

Ingredients

- 1 1/2 cups Almond Breeze Unsweetened Vanilla Milk
- 1 cup Spinach
- 1 tsp Vanilla Extract
- 3 tsps No Calorie Sweetener
- 1 oz or 1 scoop Vanilla Whey Protein

Directions

1. Place all ingredients in a blender with 2 cups of ice and blend until smooth.

Vegetarian "Ham," Cream Cheese and Dill Pickle Roll-Ups

*Servings: 1 | **Prep:** 5 m | **Style:** American*

Ingredients

- 6 slices Smart Deli Baked Ham Style
- 2 tbsps Cream Cheese

- 2 medium Pickles

Directions

1. Layer 3 slices of ham, spread 1 tablespoon cream cheese over the layers.
2. Place 1 pickle spear at one end and roll-up. Pin with a toothpick if desired.
3. Repeat for remaining ham, cream cheese and pickle spear.

Vegetarian "Ham," Monterey Jack and Jicama Roll-Ups

*Servings: 1 | **Prep:** 5 m | **Style:** American*

Ingredients

- 1 slice (1 oz) Monterey Jack Cheese
- 6 slices Smart Deli Baked Ham Style
- 4 slices Yambean (Jicama)

Directions

1. Place each slice of cheese over a slice of ham. Place a jicama spear on one end and roll up.
2. Secure each with a toothpick, if desired.

Vegetarian "Ham," Muenster and Asparagus Roll-Ups

*Servings: 1 | **Prep:** 5 m | **Style:** American*

Ingredients

- 6 slices Smart Deli Baked Ham Style
- 2 slice (1 oz) Muenster Cheese
- 3 spear medium (5-1/4" to 7" long) Asparagus

Directions

1. Layer 2 slices of "ham" with 1 slice of cheese. Place 2 halves of an asparagus spear on one end and roll up. Secure with a toothpick, if desired.
2. Repeat with remaining "ham," cheese and pickle.

Vegetarian "Turkey" and Provolone Cheese Roll-Ups

Servings: 1 | Prep: 5 m | Style: American

Ingredients

- 6 slices Smart Deli Roast Turkey Style
- 1 tsp Dijon Mustard
- 1/2 fruit without skin and seed California Avocados
- 6 oz Provolone Cheese

Directions

1. Spread each slice of "turkey" with mustard.
2. Layer with cheese and roll up.

Vegetarian "Turkey," Provolone and Pickle Roll-ups

Servings: 1 | Prep: 5 m | Style: American

Ingredients

- 6 slices Smart Deli Roast Turkey Style
- 2 oz Provolone Cheese
- 1 medium Pickle

Directions

1. Layer 3 slices provolone over 3 slices of "turkey." Place half pickle spear in center and roll up. Secure with a toothpick if desired.

2. Repeat with remaining 3 slices provolone, "turkey" and half pickle spear.

Vegetarian "Turkey," Swiss Cheese and Asparagus Roll-Ups

Servings: 1 | Prep: 5 m | Style: American

Ingredients

- 6 slices Smart Deli Roast Turkey Style
- 1 slice (1 oz) Swiss Cheese
- 3 spear medium (5-1/4" to 7" long) Asparagus

Directions

1. Lay down 2 slices of "turkey" then one slice of Swiss cheese.
2. Place 1 asparagus spear at one end and roll-up. Pin with a toothpick if desired.
3. Repeat with remaining ingredients.

Walnut and Jicama

Servings: 1 | Prep: 5 m | Style: American

Ingredients

- 1/4 cup slice Yambean (Jicama)
- 1 oz (14 halves) English Walnuts

Directions

1. Slice jicama and pair with walnuts.

Zucchini Bread Muffins

Servings: 6 | Prep: 10 m | Style: American | Cook: 25 m

Ingredients

- 2 large Eggs (Whole)
- 2 tbsps Canola Vegetable Oil
- 1 tsp Vanilla Extract
- 4 1/2 oz Zucchini
- 1 cup Organic 100% Whole Ground Golden Flaxseed Meal
- 1 oz Vanilla Whey Protein
- 1/3 cup Sucralose Based Sweetener (Sugar Substitute)
- 1 1/2 tsps Cinnamon
- 3/4 tsp Baking Powder (Straight Phosphate, Double Acting)
- 1/4 tsp Salt
- 1/8 tsp Allspice Ground
- 1/8 tsp Nutmeg (Ground)

Directions

1. Preheat an oven to 350°F. Grease 6 wells of a standard non-stick muffin tin.
2. Combine the eggs, oil and vanilla in a small bowl. Using a whisk beat until frothy about 1 minute. Shred the zucchini, add it to the bowl mixing to combine.
3. Add the flax meal, protein powder, granular sugar substitute, baking powder, salt, and spices. Mix with a spoon to combine.
4. Bake for 25 minutes until slightly puffed, golden and cooked through. Enjoy with cream cheese if desired.

Zucchini Crisps

Servings: 4 | Prep: 10 m | Style: American | Cook: 10 m

Ingredients

- 2 medium Zucchinis
- 2 tbsps Extra Virgin Olive Oil
- 1/4 tsp Salt
- 1/4 tsp Black Pepper

- 2 tbsps Parmesan Cheese (Grated)

Directions

1. Cut zucchini into 1/4-inch slices (on a diagonal if they're small). Brush both sides with extra-virgin olive oil and season with salt, pepper and Parmesan (add whatever else strikes your fancy - garlic powder, Italian seasoning, rosemary or dill). The nutritionals include 2 tablespoons of Parmesan.
2. Set on a baking sheet in a single layer and bake in a preheated 400°F oven for 10 minutes, turning once. Cool on a wire rack.

Zucchini Nut Bread

Servings: 18 | Prep: 25 m | Style: American | Cook: 45 m

Ingredients

- 1 cup dry Whole Grain Soy Flour
- 1 cup ground Almonds
- 1 cup Sucralose Based Sweetener (Sugar Substitute)
- 1 1/2 tsps Cinnamon
- 1/2 tsp Nutmeg (Ground)
- 1/2 tsp Salt
- 1/2 tsp Baking Soda
- 1/2 tsp Baking Powder (Straight Phosphate, Double Acting)
- 1/2 cup Canola Vegetable Oil
- 4 large Eggs (Whole)
- 1 medium Zucchini
- 1 tsp Vanilla Extract

Directions

1. Preheat oven to 350°F. Grease an 8x4-inch loaf pan generously with oil spray; set aside. In a large bowl whisk together soy flour , ground almonds, sugar substitute, cinnamon, nutmeg, salt, baking soda and baking powder.
2. In a medium bowl, whish together oil, eggs, grated zucchini and vanilla extract. Mix zucchini mixture into dry ingredients until just combined. Pour batter into prepared pan.

3. Bake 45 minutes until golden brown and a cake tester inserted in center comes out clean. Cool in pan for 10 minutes before removing loaf from pan. With a serrated knife, cut into 18 slices for serving.

Conclusion

Thank you again for downloading this book!

I hope you enjoyed reading about my book!

Finally, if you enjoyed this book, please take the time to share your thoughts and post a review on Amazon. It'd be greatly appreciated!

Write me an honest review about the book – I truly value your opinion and thoughts and I will incorporate them into my next book, which is already underway.

Leave your review of my book here:

http://www.amazon.com/author/anniekate

Thank you!

If you have any questions, feel free to contact at contact@smallpassion.com

An Awesome Free Gift for You

Download Gift

http://www.smallpassion.com/awesome-gift

I want to say "**Thank You**" for buying my book so I've put together a few, awesome free gift for you **Tips and Techniques for Cooking like a Chef & Delicious Desserts!**
This gift is the perfect add-on this book and I know you'll love it.
So click the link to go grab it.

Read more my book here:

http://www.amazon.com/author/anniekate
http://www.smallpassion.com/my-cookbooks

Annie Kate

Founder of www.SmallPassion.com

* * *

www.ingramcontent.com/pod-product-compliance
Lightning Source LLC
Chambersburg PA
CBHW072031280526
45788CB00006B/2091